Feedback Form
Acute Care of at-Risk Newborns (ACoRN)
First Edition, 2005

We value your feedback on the first edition of this book. Please complete and return this evaluation form by fax to **(604) 875-3106** or by mail to:

The ACoRN Editorial Board, c/o Dr. Alfonso Solimano,
Newborn Care Program, Children's and Women's Health Centre of BC,
4480 Oak Street, Vancouver, B.C., Canada V6H 3V4

What is your type of practice and professional affiliation? (Please check boxes and circle as appropriate)

Practice   ☐ Rural   ☐ Urban: Level I / Level II / Level III

Profession   ☐ MD: family doctor / pediatrician / neonatologist/ fellow/ resident   ☐ Nurse: general duty/ neonatal/ perinatal

☐ Neonatal nurse practitioner   ☐ Midwife

☐ Respiratory therapist   ☐ Other (Please specify)

On a scale of 4, how do you rate the following:

	Strongly disagree	Disagree	Agree	Strongly agree
The book is clearly and logically organized.	1	2	3	4
The objectives are relevant to my learning needs.	1	2	3	4
The content matches the objectives	1	2	3	4
The primary survey and sequences are clinically useful.	1	2	3	4
The sequences are easy to follow.	1	2	3	4
The case studies are helpful to illustrate step by step management.	1	2	3	4
Overall, this book is useful for the acute care of newborns	1	2	3	4

What was good about the book?

How could the book be improved?

How might you use the information in this book in your practice?

Did you attend an ACoRN workshop?   ☐ Yes   ☐ No

If no, would you be interested in attending one?   ☐ Yes   ☐ No

Please turn page!

Additional suggestions / comments

Optional:

Your name   ....

Your contact information   ....

                                 ....

                                 ....

We thank all professionals who attended the Preview presentation of ACoRN in June of 2003 and provided us with feedback and encouragement.

The ACoRN Editorial Board

The Canadian Paediatric Society has reviewed the ACoRN manual and has found the content to be relevant to the continuing professional development of health professionals who care for newborns.

The Canadian Paediatric Society
November 2004

As always in life,
when one teaches one learns,
and when one gives, one receives.
And one learns when one teaches because
the student asks questions
which the teacher no longer considers,
because they have become part
of the nearly automatic thought process
which each of us develop.

Suddenly,
it is the question about something
what forces us to rethink the origin,
the essence of the problem.

...

That is why,
when he and I played
those few minutes
of a Schubert Rondo...
I felt musically enriched
in a way that was completely unexpected.

Daniel Baremboim
La Nacion, Argentina, 17 October 2004
Translated from Spanish

ACoRN
Acute Care of at-Risk Newborns

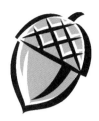

Acknowledgments

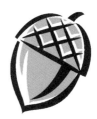

We gratefully acknowledge our major reviewers

Adele Harrison (Clinical Associate, Neonatology, Vancouver)
Daniel Husband (Family Physician, Three Hills, Alberta)
Krista Jangaard (Neonatologist, Halifax, Nova Scotia)
Roxanne Laforge (Perinatal Nurse Consultant, Saskatoon, Saskatchewan)
Al McDougal (Pharmacist, Vancouver, BC)
Douglas D. McMillan (Neonatologist, Halifax, Nova Scotia)
Michael Patterson (Cardiologist, Vancouver, BC)
Shubhayan Sanatani (Cardiologist, Vancouver, BC)
Diane Sawchuk (Perinatal Nurse Consultant, Vancouver, BC)
Avash Singh (Neonatologist, Vancouver, BC)
John Smyth (Neonatologist, Vancouver, BC)
Elene Vanderpas (Clinical Nurse Leader, Vancouver, BC)
Dan Waisman (Neonatologist, Haifa, Israel)
Hilary Whyte (Neonatologist, Toronto, Ontario)

We received a grant from

Health Canada

We acknowledge the support and encouragement received from the following organizations

British Columbia Reproductive Care Program
Calgary Health Region
Canadian Paediatric Society, Foetus and Newborn Committee
Canadian Paediatric Society, Section of Neonatal Perinatal Medicine
Children's and Women's Health Centre of British Columbia, Newborn Care Program
Memorial University of Newfoundland, Discipline of Pediatrics, Faculty of Medicine
Perinatal Partnership Program of Eastern and Southeastern Ontario
Regional Perinatal Outreach Program of Southwestern Ontario
Sunnybrook and Women's College Health Science Centre - Women's College Campus,
    Department of Newborn and Developmental Paediatrics
University of Calgary

We also thank

The American Academy of Pediatrics for giving us permission to reproduce diagrams from the
    AAP/AHA Neonatal Resuscitation Program in this textbook
Gerald J. Gill, MD, FRCPC, Associate Professor of Radiology, McMaster University, for
    providing many radiographic images
Lark Susak RN, BScN (Burnaby, British Columbia) for her technical assistance

Disclaimer

The ACoRN program is an educational tool. Its content is based on current knowledge and consensus of practice at the time of publication, is general in nature and does not constitute health care. It is the responsibility of each health care provider to evaluate the appropriateness of any recommendations in the context of actual situations and to determine the best treatment for each individual patient. As new research and clinical experience become available, changes in treatment and drug therapy may become necessary or appropriate. Readers are advised to check the most current information in the ever-changing field of neonatology, and to verify the drug dosage, schedule, administration with the most current product information provided by the manufacturer.

The statements and opinions expressed in this publication should not be construed as official policy of the ACoRN Editorial Board or its related organizations. Neither the publisher nor the editors/authors assume any liability or responsibility for any injury and/or damage to persons or property arising from this publication and the ACoRN program.

No endorsement of any product or service should be inferred or is intended.

First Edition, 2005

Library and Archives Canada Cataloguing in Publication

ACoRN : acute care of at-risk newborns / the ACoRN Editorial Board ; editorial direction and project leadership: Alfonso Solimano, Judith Littleford ; managing editors: Alfonso Solimano, Emily Ling, Debra O'Flaherty ; medical illustrator: Jim Fee ; cover design: Angela Desveaux-Patterson.

Includes bibliographical references and index.

ISBN 0-9736755-0-0

1. Neonatal intensive care. 2. Infants (Newborn) - Diseases. 3. Infants (Newborn) - Care. I. Solimano, Alfonso, 1950- II. Littleford, Judith III. Ling, Emily IV. O'Flaherty, Debra V. ACoRN Editorial Board VI. Title: Acute care of at-risk newborns.

RJ253.5.A28 2005   618.92'01   C2004-907246-3

Table of Contents

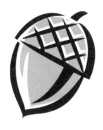

Table of Contents

Table of Contents

Tables

Sample Forms

Radiographs

Preface

For most health professionals, few events are more challenging or stressful than caring for a sick or preterm baby. It is therefore not surprising that the management and stabilization of these babies is repeatedly identified as a priority for new educational programs. The Acute Care of at-Risk Newborns (ACoRN) program was developed in response to this need. It is designed for any practitioner who may be called upon to care for at-risk babies and their families, regardless of experience or training in neonatal emergencies.

ACoRN provides a systematic approach to the identification and management of babies requiring stabilization. It serves as the foundation for an educational program that aims to teach the concepts and basic skills of neonatal stabilization and where necessary, preparation for transport to a referral facility. The ACoRN process applies to babies who need assistance in the transition from fetal life, and babies who become unwell or are at risk of becoming unwell in the first few hours or days after birth.

Through the creative efforts of individuals with diverse educational backgrounds and clinical practices, an innovative textbook has evolved that is designed to help the practitioner gather and organize information, establish priorities, and initiate interventions aimed at delivering a level of care that results in the best possible outcome.

ACoRN is based on established neonatal practice, commencing with principles from the International Liaison Committee on Resuscitation (ILCOR) guidelines for neonatal resuscitation (*Circulation* and *Pediatrics, 1999*). ACoRN also combines evidence- and consensus-based guidelines and acknowledges the clinical wisdom of those who have taught this material to health care professionals for many years. As new practices evolve, there will undoubtedly be changes and improvements in newborn care. We invite your comments and encourage constructive feedback for incorporation into future editions.

The ACoRN Editorial Board

ACoRN

Overview

What is ACoRN?

The Acute Care of at-Risk Newborns (ACoRN) is a priority-based, clinically oriented framework that sequentially integrates assessment, monitoring, diagnostic evaluation, intervention, and on-going management for at-risk and unwell newborns. ACoRN is also appropriate for further stabilization of babies who have been resuscitated at birth.

As the baby's condition changes and more information is collected during the process of stabilization, all components of the framework are systematically revisited.

What are the objectives of the ACoRN program?

The objectives of the ACoRN program are to:
1. Identify the at-risk or unwell baby who will benefit from the ACoRN process.
2. Determine whether the baby needs to be resuscitated immediately.
3. Conduct a systematic evaluation of the baby.
4. Develop working diagnoses and institute specific treatments for acute neonatal conditions.
5. Describe the types of support that may be required by the baby, the family, and the health care team.
6. Identify resources available for newborn care in local and referral facilities.
7. Identify and prepare babies who require transport to a referral facility.

What is the ACoRN textbook?

The textbook illustrates the ACoRN process and adds knowledge sequentially, chapter by chapter, and case by case.

In order to derive the greatest benefit, the textbook should be read from start to finish, within the context of the professional roles, responsibilities and level of training of the learner.

How are the chapters designed?

Each chapter is designed to illustrate the ACoRN process around one area of interest. All chapters contain:
- Learning Objectives, Key Concepts and a list of Skills required for the chapter
- Introduction
- The ACoRN Sequence specific to the area of interest being covered
- Core content specific to the ACoRN Sequence
- Illustrative case studies to advance the reader, step by step, through the ACoRN Process and to provide additional content
- Questions to reinforce previously presented content, or to introduce new knowledge
- Bibliography

This ACoRN symbol appears at various places throughout the text to introduce a particular skill that may require review.

The ACoRN symbol directs you to the Skills section in the Appendix where practical and technical information about that skill is provided.

©AAP/AHA

In this textbook, the NRP logo indicates resuscitation skills[1] that are taught by the AAP/AHA Neonatal Resuscitation Program. These skills are included with an ACoRN perspective for the purpose of providing a review for professionals with current training in NRP. Review or completion of this Appendix does not constitute an NRP activity.

What is in the Appendix?

The Appendix section of the ACoRN textbook contains the following additional information:
- Neonatal Assessment Tool: A sample assessment tool is provided for easy reference and documentation of clinical findings.
- Skills: The skills are grouped according to the following categories:
  o resuscitation
  o procedures
  o investigations
  o medications.

What is the ACoRN workshop?

The ACoRN workshop is an interactive session that utilizes case-based learning and practice stations to apply the concepts and skills presented in the textbook.

Learners are encouraged to participate in an ACoRN workshop in addition to reading this textbook.

The workshops should be designed to best meet the specific needs of the learners by the prior identification of the content and specific skills that will need to be emphasized and reviewed. Administration of a prior-learning assessment tool and identification of institutional objectives assist the ACoRN Education Team to tailor the design of each workshop.

Like neonatal resuscitation, stabilization is most effective when performed by a coordinated team. Teamwork and an interdisciplinary approach are emphasized along with sharing of clinical scenarios.

---

[1] All NRP diagrams reproduced in ACoRN have been kindly provided by the American Academy of Pediatrics (AAP) / American Heart Association (AHA).

Are there pre-requisites to participate in an ACoRN workshop?

ACoRN assumes familiarity with the American Academy of Pediatrics/American Heart Association's Neonatal Resuscitation Program (NRP) at the provider level. A brief review of core knowledge and skills in neonatal resuscitation is integrated into the ACoRN textbook and workshop.

In preparation for an ACoRN workshop, participants are asked to read the complete ACoRN textbook, or the sections pertaining to the workshop being offered. This preparation should always include a thorough understanding of Chapter 1, and a review of the eight Sequences as they apply to the professional roles, responsibilities and level of training of the learners.

The Skills section of the Appendix contains information on equipment, procedures and medications. These should be reviewed as applicable to the workshop being offered and the roles and responsibilities of the learners.

Does workshop completion imply clinical competence?

Participation in an ACoRN workshop does not imply the participant has achieved clinical competence. The responsibility to determine the readiness of an individual for their clinical responsibilities belongs to the institution and professional organization with which the learner is associated.

An ACoRN workshop is a learning experience. At the conclusion of a workshop, participants are asked to complete a case-based evaluation of key ACoRN concepts (for example, how to apply the Primary Survey). The evaluation may also include demonstration of knowledge and skills using simulations or models.

Do I get CME credit for completing an ACoRN program?

ACoRN workshops can be designed to comply with the requirements set by professional organizations to provide their members with educational credits. Regional networks and/or professional organizations are encouraged to apply for continuing professional education credits for participants in an ACoRN workshop.

Standard Precautions   Health care providers are advised to use standard precautions against disease transmission. These precautions are used for contact with blood; all body fluids, secretions, and excretions except sweat (regardless of whether these fluids, secretions, or excretions contain visible blood); non-intact skin; and mucous membranes. Barrier techniques are designed to decrease exposure of health care personnel to body fluids containing human immunodeficiency virus or other blood-borne pathogens. Precautions are used at all times because medical history and examination cannot reliably identify all patients infected with these agents. Standard precautions decrease transmission of microorganisms from patients who are not recognized as harbouring potential pathogens, such as antimicrobial-resistant bacteria. Standard precautions include the following techniques:

- hand hygiene
- gloves
- masks, eye protection, and face shields
- non-sterile gowns
- proper handling of patient care equipment, used linen, mouthpieces, resuscitation bags, and other ventilation devices
- proper cleaning and disposition of needles, scalpels, and other sharp instruments and devices.[i]

---

[i] From: American Academy of Pediatrics. Infection control for hospitalized children. In: Pickering LK, ed. Red Book: 2003 Report of the Committee on Infectious Diseases. 26th ed. Elk Grove Village, IL: American Academy of Pediatrics; 2003

Chapter 1
The ACoRN Process

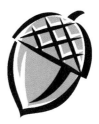

Objectives

Upon completion of this chapter, you should be able to:
1. Describe the ACoRN Framework and its components.
2. Identify the baby who will benefit from the ACoRN Process.
3. Describe how to apply the ACoRN Process to assess and manage unwell or at-risk babies.

Key Concepts

1. Babies who are unwell or at-risk require anticipatory care, close observation, and early detection and management.

2. The ACoRN Process uses an 8-step clinical framework, which integrates assessment, monitoring, diagnostic evaluations, interventions and on-going care.

3. Alerting Signs are used to identify babies who will benefit from the ACoRN Process.

4. The need for immediate resuscitation to establish adequate cardiorespiratory function takes precedence over all other newborn needs.

5. A prioritized Problem List is generated using the ACoRN Primary survey, which can be completed with minimal disturbance to the baby.

6. For each area of concern in the Problem List, an ACoRN Sequence is applied. It allows for the systematic acquisition of information, organization of care, implementation of interventions, diagnostic evaluation leading to a specific diagnosis or diagnostic category, and institution of appropriate specific management.

7. As the baby's condition changes and more information is collected during the process of stabilization, all components of the Framework are systematically revisited.

Consider the following scenario:

> A baby boy was born at 36 weeks gestation, weighing 2950 grams. The Apgar score was 9 at 1 minute and 9 at 5 minutes. The baby is now 10 minutes of age. He is lying on the radiant warmer in a flexed position. He is breathing regularly with a respiratory rate of 56/minute, but is grunting and indrawing. Heart rate is 140 beats per minute (bpm). Free-flow oxygen is required to maintain a pink colour. You are unable to wean him from supplemental oxygen.

How will you care for this baby?

The ACoRN Framework

ACoRN provides a logical and systematic approach to gathering and organizing information, establishing priorities, and intervening appropriately for those babies who become unwell or are at risk of becoming unwell in the first few hours or days after birth. The approach is designed to be useful regardless of the complexity of the condition or the frequency with which the practitioner is called upon to manage it.

The ACoRN process is based on an 8-step framework to:

1. Identify the Baby at-Risk who will benefit from the ACoRN Process. The Baby at-Risk is the one who is unwell, at risk of becoming unwell, or has been resuscitated and requires stabilization.
2. Determine if immediate Resuscitation is required.
3. Conduct an ACoRN Primary Survey of the six main areas of potential concern:
   - Respiratory
   - Cardiovascular
   - Neurology
   - Surgical Conditions
   - Fluid & Glucose Management
   - Thermoregulation
4. Consider the presence of Infection.
5. Generate a prioritized Problem List.
6. Complete the Sequences that address the Problem List in order of priority.
7. Consider the need for early consultation and/or transport.
8. Overarching the framework is support for the baby, family, and health care team.

The schematic version of the 8-step ACoRN framework described above is illustrated on the next page.

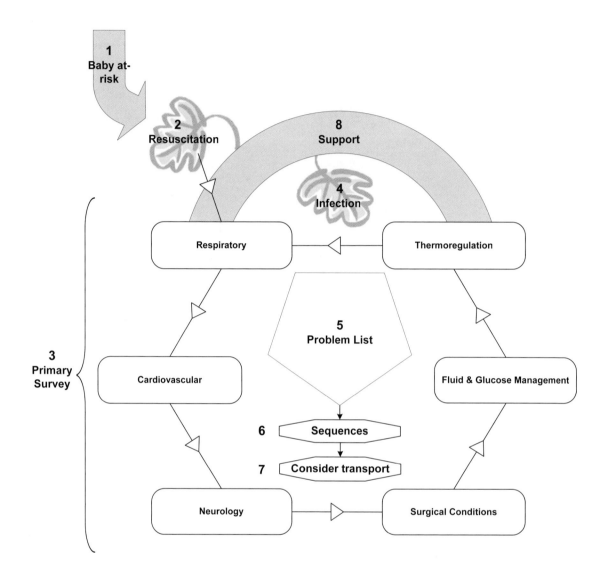

Steps 1 to 4 of the ACoRN framework contain components or elements called Alerting Signs. These Alerting Signs identify babies

1. at-Risk
2. who need immediate Resuscitation
3. who have areas of potential or actual concern
4. in whom Infection needs to be considered.

Step 5, the Problem List, is generated after completion of the Primary Survey. The Problem List, shown in the center of the ACoRN framework, ensures that all the appropriate Sequences are addressed in a prioritized order.

The ACoRN Process

The ACoRN Process is illustrated below, and explained in more detail in subsequent pages of this chapter.

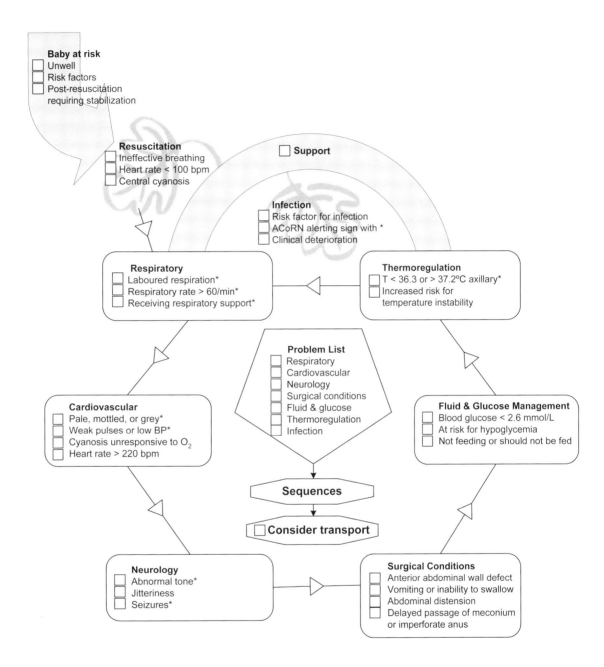

**Step 1:
Identification of the
Baby at-Risk**

The process begins with distinguishing the baby who seems well from the baby who does not. The well baby has normal vital signs, color, activity, feeding pattern, and has passed meconium and urine within the first 24 hours following birth.

Indications that a baby is unwell may be as subtle as a weak sucking reflex or as obvious as cyanosis unresponsive to oxygen. Rely on the power of observation, findings on physical examination, and the maternal and birth history. An intuitive sense that something is just not right with a baby is as valid as more overt signs. Both should trigger the ACoRN Process.

Of the babies who initially appear well, some are at greater risk of becoming unwell than the general newborn population. These "at-risk" babies are broadly identified on the basis of their gestational age, size, and the presence of risk factors in the antepartum, intrapartum, and/or neonatal history. Examples include
- babies who are preterm (< 37 weeks) or small for gestational age (SGA)
- infants of diabetic or substance-using mothers
- babies born following prolonged rupture of membranes
- babies who have been subjected to an abnormally warm or cold environment.

Managing at-risk babies using the ACoRN Process provides a means of close observation and early detection, intervention, treatment, and possible prevention of problems. Specific neonatal risk factors are discussed in the relevant chapters of this textbook.

The ACoRN Process is also appropriate for further stabilization of babies who have been resuscitated at birth.

**Step 2:
Immediate
resuscitation if
required**

The need for immediate resuscitation to establish adequate cardiorespiratory function takes precedence over all other newborn needs. Three signs distinguish the baby who requires resuscitation:

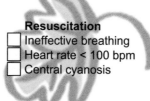

Resuscitation
- [ ] Ineffective breathing
- [ ] Heart rate < 100 bpm
- [ ] Central cyanosis

Any baby who demonstrates one or more of these Resuscitation Signs will first proceed through the Resuscitation Sequence (see page 1-15). This Sequence is adapted from the International Liaison Committee on

Resuscitation (ILCOR) advisory statement (1999)[1] so that it can be applied to babies who require resuscitation at or after birth.

It may be necessary to return to the Resuscitation Sequence at any time should the baby's condition deteriorate.

Step 3:
Conduction of an
ACoRN Primary
Survey

The ACoRN Primary Survey is a rapid, thorough, systematic and sequential assessment of the baby in six areas of potential concern: Respiratory, Cardiovascular, Neurology, Surgical Conditions, Fluid & Glucose Management, and Thermoregulation. The Primary Survey is completed with minimal disturbance to the baby.

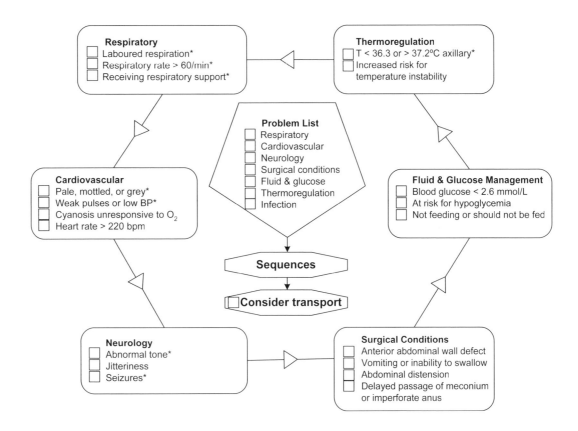

[1] Kattwinkel J, Niermeyer S, Nadkarni V, Tibballs J, Philllips B, Zideman D, Van Reempts P, Osmond, M. ILCOR advisory statement: Resuscitation of the newly born infant. An advisory statement from the pediatric working group of the International Liaison Committee on Resuscitation. Circulation 1999; 99(14):1927-38.

Each area of potential concern is distinguished by its own Alerting Signs, for example:

> **Respiratory**
> ☐ Laboured respiration*
> ☐ Respiratory rate > 60/min*
> ☐ Receiving assisted ventilation*

As each Alerting Sign is examined, it is marked as:

☑ check mark if present

☐ box left blank if absent

☐? question mark if pending evaluation (for example, awaiting results of blood pressure or blood glucose).

Interventions already initiated are continued while the survey is being conducted.

Any Alerting Sign with an asterisk (*) also constitutes an Alerting Sign for Infection, and a corresponding mark should be inserted in the Infection box.

Step 4: Consideration of Infection

The presence of Alerting Signs for Infection should be identified as soon as the Primary Survey is completed.

Infection is suspected in a baby who has a risk factor for infection, an ACoRN alerting sign with *, or clinical deterioration.

> **Infection**
> ☐ Risk factor for infection
> ☐ ACoRN alerting sign with *
> ☐ Clinical deterioration

Early diagnosis and prompt treatment with antibiotics will improve the outcome in babies with bacterial infections.

Step 5: Generation of a prioritized Problem List

Inserting a mark in areas of concern will generate a Problem List which automatically prioritizes the order in which these concerns need to be addressed.

ACoRN

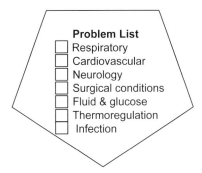

If a baby demonstrates one or more of the Alerting Signs in an area of potential concern, for example Cardiovascular, a corresponding check mark is placed in the Problem List.

When an Alerting Sign is pending evaluation (for example, the blood glucose result is not yet available), the corresponding box in the Problem List (Fluid & Glucose in this case) should be marked with a question mark as a reminder to obtain the missing data as soon as possible while other aspects of the ACoRN Process are occurring simultaneously.

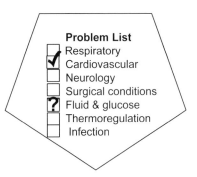

Step 6:
Completion of
Sequences that
address the
Problem List

For each area of concern, there is a sequence of steps that culminates in a working diagnosis and specific treatment.

The evaluation-decision-action cycle is repeated throughout the ACoRN Sequence.

In the Sequence design, the process of evaluation is represented by ovals, decisions are depicted by arrows, and actions (including monitoring, interventions, and diagnostic tests) are indicated by rectangles.

The schematic structure of the sequences is shown on the next page.

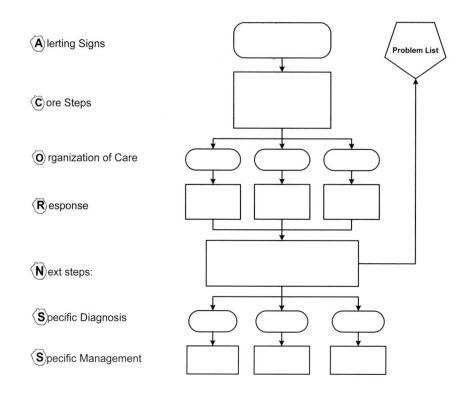

A lerting Signs	Confirm the presence of the Alerting Signs identified in the Primary Survey.
C ore Steps	Perform Core Steps applicable to all babies entering a given Sequence.
O rganization of Care	Organize your planned course of action according to predominant physical findings.
R esponse	Respond with immediate interventions.
N ext Steps	Perform Next Steps – take a focused history, conduct a physical examination, order diagnostic tests relevant to the specific area of concern, establish a working diagnosis, and consider consultation. Concurrently, plan specific management and return to the Problem List to address the next area of concern.
S pecific Diagnosis	Establish a working diagnosis or diagnostic category.
S pecific Management	Provide ongoing management specific to the working diagnosis while addressing any other areas of concern.

As one progresses through a Sequence, information is acquired, beginning with the Alerting Signs, proceeding through Core Steps, Organization of Care, Response, and Next Steps. Evaluations and actions guide decision-making at each stage. The ACoRN Process culminates in a Specific Diagnosis or Diagnostic Category and the appropriate Specific Management.

A check mark is placed in each applicable box in the sequence, starting with the Core Steps. These check marks indicate that an observation and/or action has been completed.

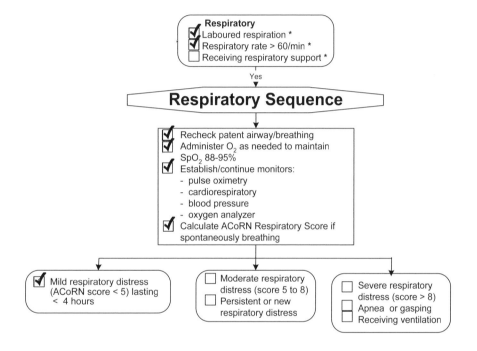

Each Sequence has a point in time when it is appropriate to address the next problem in the Problem List. This is shown by an arrow that returns to the Problem List.

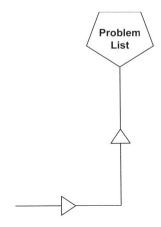

All the ACoRN Sequences are shown at the end of this chapter, and are described in detail in their own specific chapters.

Step 7:
Consideration of the need for Transport

The need for transport depends on many things, such as the baby's condition, expertise and resources available at the local and receiving facilities, and travel conditions. Arrangements for transport to another centre should begin as soon as the need becomes apparent.

Each of the ACoRN Sequences indicates when to consider obtaining consultation for management and possible transport.

Step 8:
Providing Support for the baby, the family and health care team

Care that minimizes physiological stress for babies is intrinsic to all phases of stabilization.

The baby is the focus of everyone's attention, but the needs of the family and health care team are important and should not be overlooked.

Illustrative Case Study

Recall the story of the baby from the beginning of this chapter:

> A baby boy was born at 36 weeks gestation, weighing 2950 grams. The Apgar score was 9 at 1 minute and 9 at 5 minutes of age. The baby is now 10 minutes of age. He is lying on the radiant warmer in a flexed position. He is breathing regularly with a respiratory rate of 56/minute, but is grunting and indrawing. His heart rate is 140 bpm. Free-flow oxygen is required to maintain a pink color. You are unable to wean him from supplemental oxygen. How will you care for this baby?

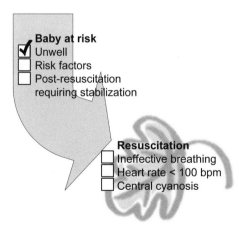

Baby at risk
- ☑ Unwell
- ☐ Risk factors
- ☐ Post-resuscitation requiring stabilization

Resuscitation
- ☐ Ineffective breathing
- ☐ Heart rate < 100 bpm
- ☐ Central cyanosis

This baby is unwell. He exhibits no Alerting signs for immediate resuscitation. You proceed through the Primary Survey and generate a Problem List.

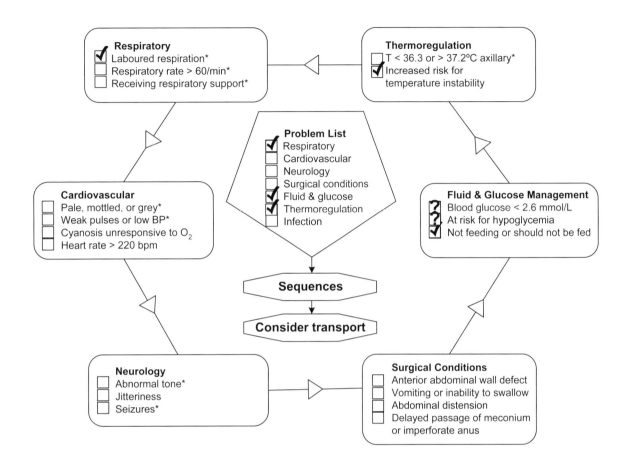

Respiratory
☑ Laboured respiration*
☐ Respiratory rate > 60/min*
☐ Receiving respiratory support*

Thermoregulation
☐ T < 36.3 or > 37.2°C axillary*
☑ Increased risk for temperature instability

Problem List
☑ Respiratory
☐ Cardiovascular
☐ Neurology
☐ Surgical conditions
☑ Fluid & glucose
☑ Thermoregulation
☐ Infection

Cardiovascular
☐ Pale, mottled, or grey*
☐ Weak pulses or low BP*
☐ Cyanosis unresponsive to O_2
☐ Heart rate > 220 bpm

Fluid & Glucose Management
☑? Blood glucose < 2.6 mmol/L
☑? At risk for hypoglycemia
☑ Not feeding or should not be fed

Sequences

Consider transport

Neurology
☐ Abnormal tone*
☐ Jitteriness
☐ Seizures*

Surgical Conditions
☐ Anterior abdominal wall defect
☐ Vomiting or inability to swallow
☐ Abdominal distension
☐ Delayed passage of meconium or imperforate anus

Having completed the Primary Survey, you note there is one ACoRN alerting sign with an asterisk (*) in Respiratory. This constitutes an alerting sign for Infection.

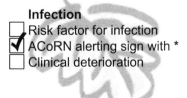

Infection
☐ Risk factor for infection
☑ ACoRN alerting sign with *
☐ Clinical deterioration

You modify your Problem List, adding Infection as a fourth area of concern. Your updated List now contains all the problems that need to be addressed in order of priority:
- Respiratory
- Fluid & Glucose Management
- Thermoregulation
- Infection.

You work through the Respiratory Sequence, carrying out the Core Steps, Organization of Care and Next Steps to develop a working diagnosis. As specific treatment is instituted, you work through the other three Sequences in order of priority, bearing in mind that thermal management is integral to all aspects of neonatal care.

Once the Infection Sequence is completed, the last steps of stabilization are to ensure that Support is being provided to the Family and Team, and to assess whether the baby will need Transport to a facility that can provide a higher level of care.

The Primary Survey will be repeated at regular intervals, and at any stage if the baby's condition changes.

Summary

The ACoRN Process provides a systematic approach to the identification, assessment and management of unwell and at-risk babies, babies who require further support following resuscitation at birth, or babies who require preparation for transport to a facility that can provide a higher level of care. It serves as the foundation for an educational program that aims to teach the concepts and basic skills of neonatal stabilization.

The Resuscitation Sequence

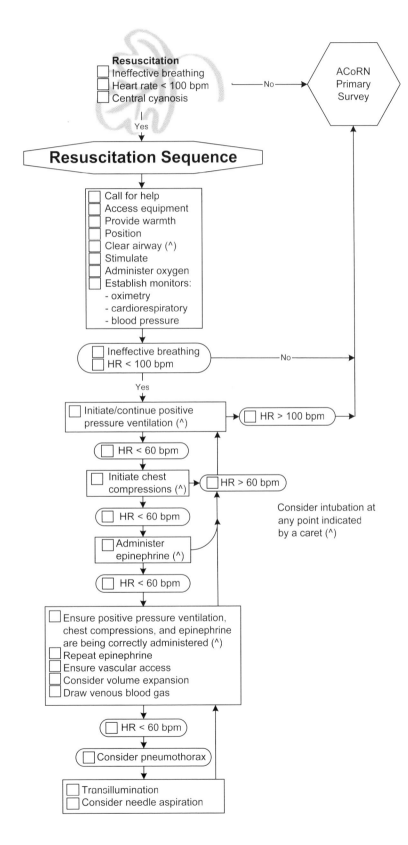

The Respiratory Sequence

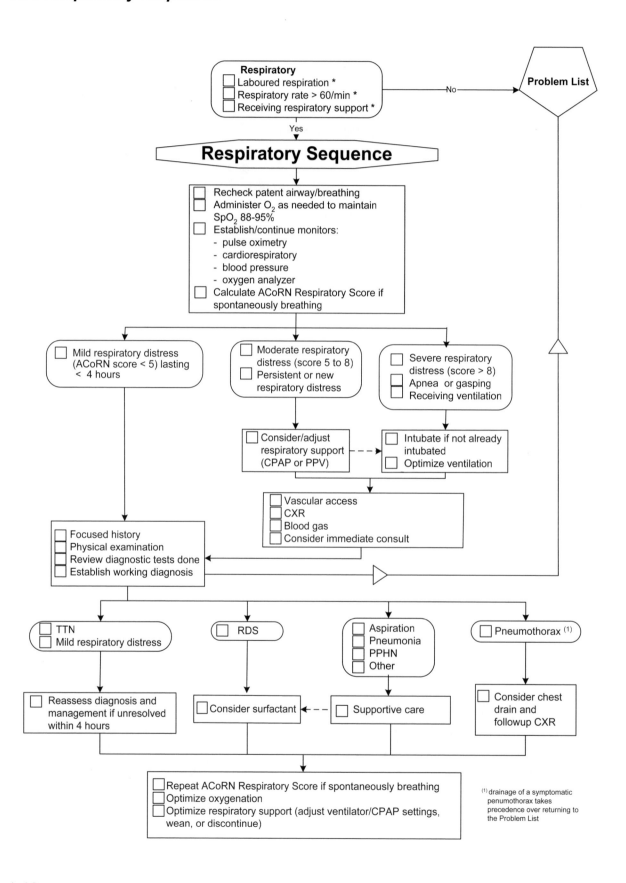

The Cardiovascular Sequence

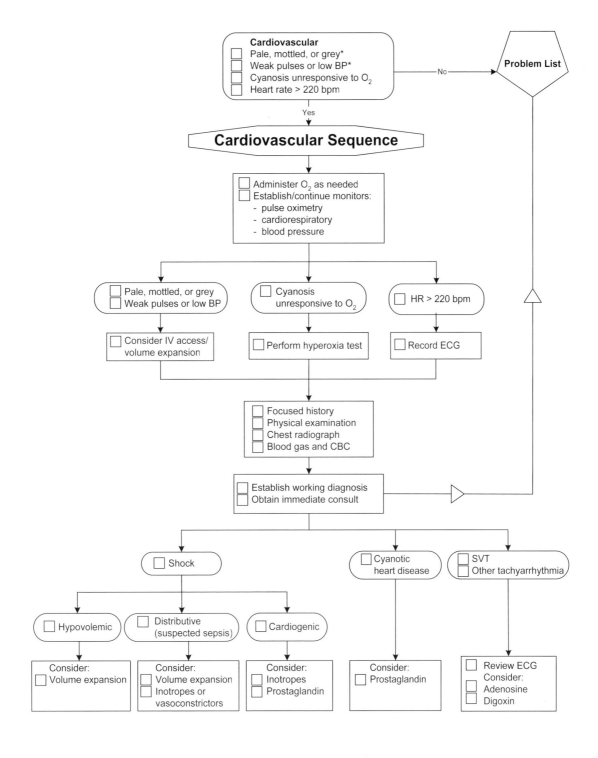

Chapter 1

The Neurology Sequence

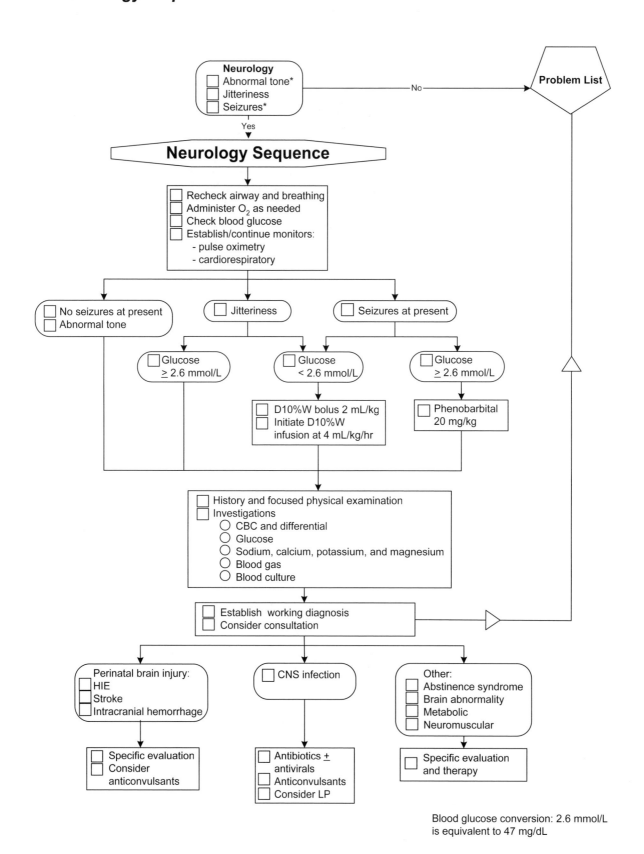

Blood glucose conversion: 2.6 mmol/L
is equivalent to 47 mg/dL

The Surgical Conditions Sequence

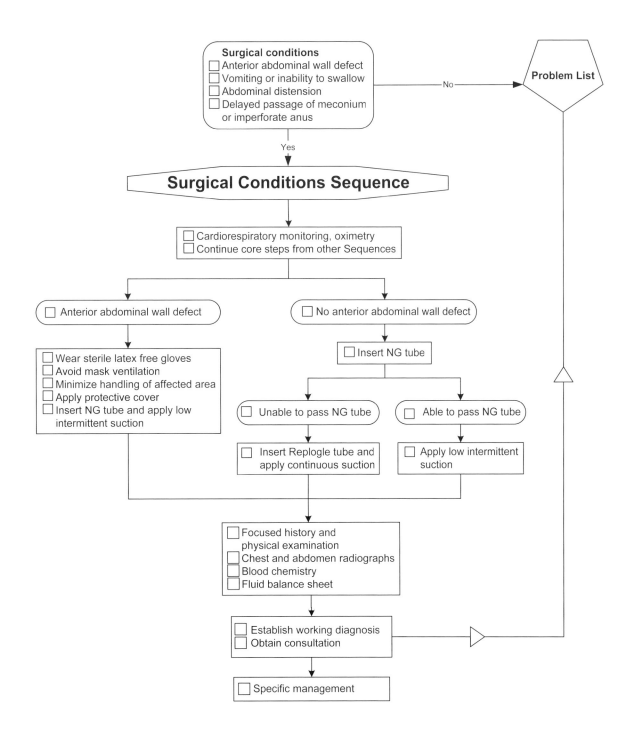

Chapter 1

The Fluid & Glucose Management Sequence

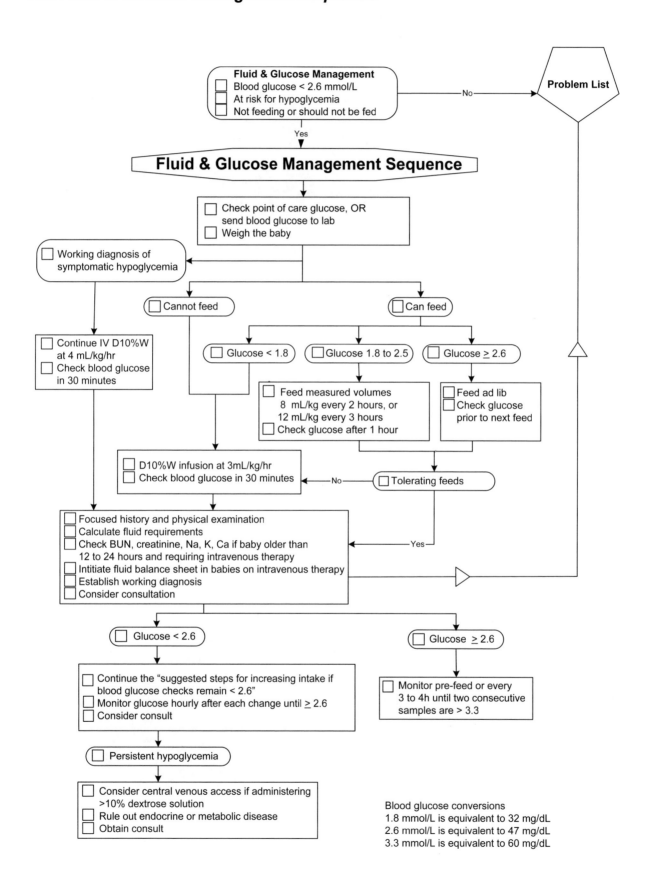

The Thermoregulation Sequence

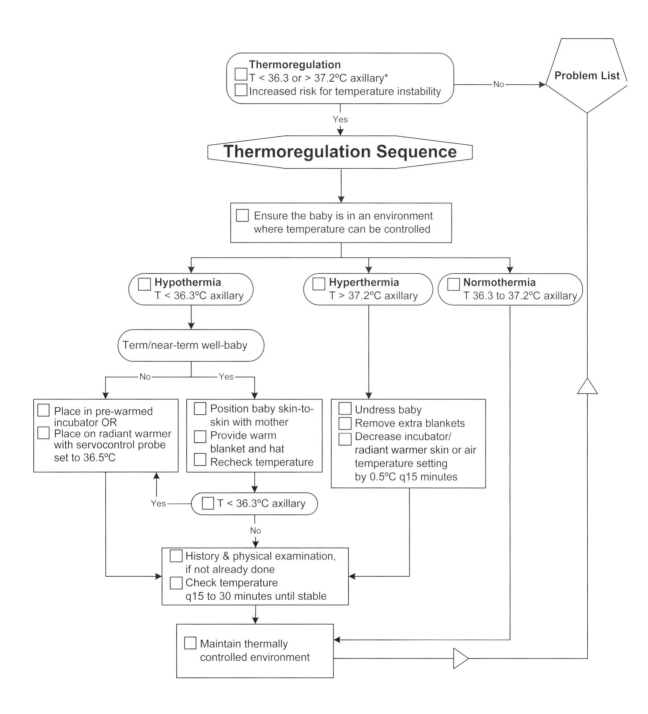

The Infection Sequence

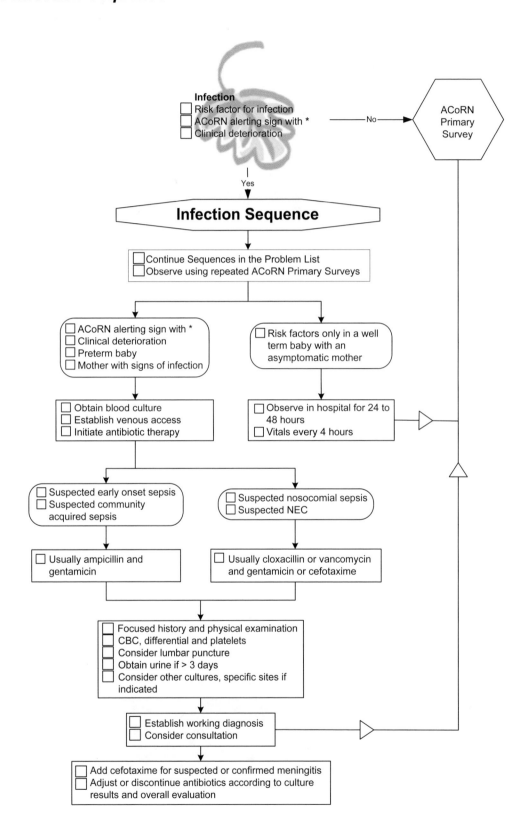

Chapter 2
Resuscitation

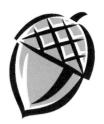

Objectives:

Upon completion of this chapter, you should be able to:
1. Identify babies who require immediate resuscitation.
2. Describe techniques required for neonatal resuscitation.
3. Apply the Resuscitation Sequence.
4. Recognize when to exit into the ACoRN Sequences.

Key Concepts

1. The time frame for resuscitative interventions is short and their importance is high.
2. The most common cause of cardiorespiratory instability in the newborn is hypoxemia as a result of respiratory problems.
3. Resuscitation equipment and trained personnel must be readily available in any facility where babies receive care (planned or unplanned) because the need to resuscitate a baby can occur at any time.
4. It may be necessary to return to the Resuscitation Sequence if the baby's condition deteriorates.
5. Thermal management is integral to all aspects of neonatal care and begins when the baby is first encountered.

Skills

- Resuscitation skills
- End-tidal CO_2 detector

Introduction	The first priority in caring for an at-risk or unwell baby is to determine whether immediate resuscitation is needed to establish adequate cardiorespiratory function. The most common cause of cardiorespiratory instability in the newborn is hypoxemia, and the most common cause of poor response to resuscitation is failure to correct the hypoxemia. Thus, the interventions in the Resuscitation Sequence are aimed at establishing effective ventilation, which in turn should improve oxygenation and cardiac output.

The Resuscitation Sequence is adapted from the International Liaison Committee on Resuscitation (ILCOR) advisory statement to make it applicable to unwell and at-risk newborns after birth.

The skills required for neonatal resuscitation after birth are the same as those needed at birth. These skills are best taught by the American Academy of Pediatrics (AAP)/American Heart Association (AHA) Neonatal Resuscitation Program (NRP).

Resuscitation Signs

A baby who demonstrates one or more of the following Resuscitation Signs enters the Resuscitation Sequence.

Resuscitation
- ☐ Ineffective breathing
- ☐ Heart rate < 100 bpm
- ☐ Central cyanosis

Ineffective breathing

Ineffective breathing includes:
- decreased respiratory drive – apnea or gasping respiration
- airway obstruction resulting from poor positioning, secretions, aspiration, or anatomic abnormality.

Babies who are breathing ineffectively cannot generate sufficient air movement to ventilate their lungs effectively or consistently.

Heart rate < 100 bpm (bradycardia)

A heart rate < 100 bpm in an unwell baby usually reflects ineffective breathing and hypoxemia, and signals the need for entry into the Resuscitation Sequence.

Some healthy term babies have a slow resting heart rate, in the range of 80 to 100 bpm. These babies look otherwise well, and their cardiac rhythm is sinus. Babies with a slow heart rate caused by congenital heart block are rare and usually present with a fixed heart rate < 80 bpm. The persistent bradycardia is usually identified during the antepartum/intrapartum periods. These babies do not enter the Resuscitation Sequence.

Central cyanosis Central cyanosis is clinically observed as a bluish discoloration (duskiness) of the body, lips, and mucous membranes. However, cyanosis is not always clinically appreciated as a bluish discoloration and thus should always be suspected if a baby's color is not obviously pink.

The presence of central cyanosis is abnormal and indicates hypoxemia (decreased oxygen content in the blood).

The most common causes of central cyanosis are ineffective ventilation and lung disease with respiratory distress.

Central cyanosis may also occur in conditions where venous and arterial blood mix, such as persistent pulmonary hypertension of the newborn (previously called persistent fetal circulation) and congenital cardiac anomalies. Mixing of venous blood with arterial blood results in reduced oxygen content in the arterial blood.

A bluish discoloration of the hands and feet with a pink body and mucous membranes is called peripheral cyanosis or acrocyanosis. It is normally seen in the first hours after birth, and can also occur in cold stress. This finding is a result of peripheral vasoconstriction, not hypoxemia, and does not require oxygen therapy.

Core Steps

The interventions and monitoring activities that occur simultaneously or in rapid sequence and are applicable to all babies who enter the Resuscitation Sequence, include:

Call for help Neonatal resuscitation requires a minimum of two people, both of whom should be able to initiate resuscitative interventions independently. One of the individuals should have the knowledge and skills to carry out all aspects of the Resuscitation Sequence.

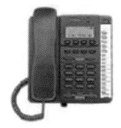

In complicated resuscitations, more personnel may be needed to help set up equipment, perform procedures, run errands, and/or make chart entries.

Every health care facility needs a procedure for summoning personnel to manage clinical emergencies and clear guidelines for when and how to call for additional assistance. Contact information for both internal and external resources (facilities and consultants) should be kept readily available and regularly updated.

The Resuscitation Sequence

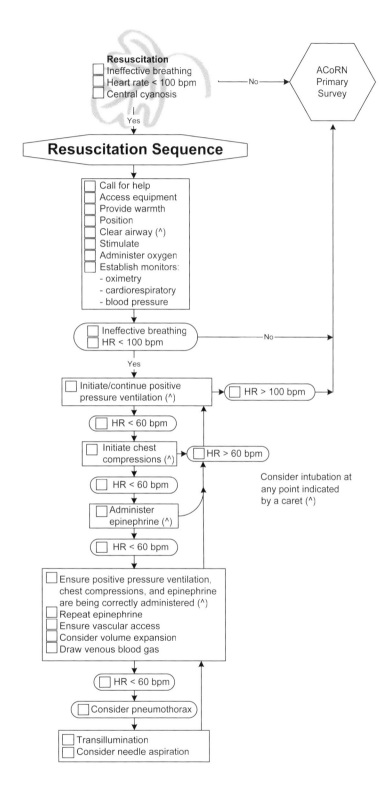

Adapted from: Kattwinkel J, Niermeyer S, Nadkarni V, Tibballs J, Philllips B, Zideman D, Van Reempts P, Osmond, M. ILCOR advisory statement: Resuscitation of the newly born infant. An advisory statement from the pediatric working group of the International Liaison Committee on Resuscitation. Circulation 1999; 99(14):1927-38.

Access equipment

Airway and ventilation equipment:

1. laryngoscope with blade size 1
2. laryngoscope blade size 0; spare bulbs and batteries
3. endotracheal tubes (2.5, 3.0, 3.5, 4.0 mm ID)
4. stylette
5. end-tidal CO_2 detector
6. suction catheters (# 6, 8, 10, 12 Fr)
7. tape
8. scissors
9. oral airway
10. meconium aspirator
11. stethoscope
12. flow inflating or self inflating bagging system with face masks for term and premature babies

© AAP/AHA

Other equipment:

- syringes (10, 20 mL)
- orogastric tube (8 Fr)
- blankets
- intravenous fluid (0.9% NaCl, D10%W)

- umbilical catheter (3.5, 5 Fr)
- vascular access supplies
- infusion pump
- chest needling supplies

Provide warmth

Providing warmth to a baby is essential.

The baby must be dry and in a warm environment (on a radiant warmer or in an incubator).

A radiant warmer is the optimal surface for resuscitation as it allows an unobstructed view and ready access to the naked baby from three sides. The heat output must be servocontrolled using a skin probe in order to avoid both hypothermia and hyperthermia

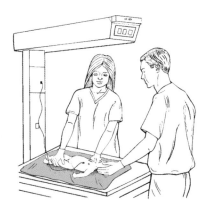

Adapted from © AAP/AHA

Position the baby and clear the airway

Position the baby's head and body to align the pharynx, larynx, and trachea, creating a continuous passage from mouth to trachea.

Clear the airway by suctioning if necessary.

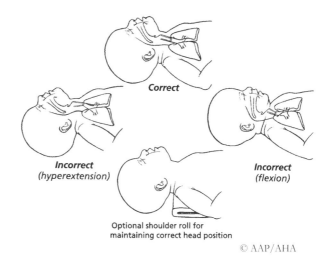

Correct

Incorrect (hyperextension)

Incorrect (flexion)

Optional shoulder roll for maintaining correct head position

© AAP/AHA

Stimulate

Stimulation may induce respiration in the apneic baby.

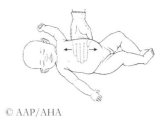

© AAP/AHA

Administer oxygen

Oxygen should be administered to babies who are spontaneously breathing or receiving mechanical ventilation to correct hypoxia. The objective is to

- relieve cyanosis
- attain pulse oximetry values in the 88 to 95% range

Avoidance of hyperoxia is an important consideration when administering oxygen to a baby, especially a premature baby, during and after resuscitation.

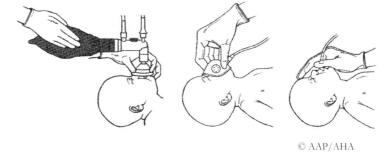

© AAP/AHA

Oxygen administration during resuscitation:

Flow inflating bag   Oxygen mask   Oxygen tubing

Establish monitors Pulse oximetry, cardiorespiratory and blood pressure monitors allow ongoing assessment of vital signs.

Organization of Care

After completing the Core Steps, the decision whether to continue through the Resuscitation Sequence or go directly to the ACoRN Primary Survey is based on whether the baby is breathing effectively and has a heart rate > 100 bpm.

Babies who have ineffective respirations or a heart rate < 100 bpm require resuscitation until their heart rate is ≥ 100 bpm, at which point an ACoRN Primary Survey is initiated.

Babies who remain cyanotic after the Core Steps, but who have effective respirations and a heart rate ≥ 100 bpm do not require resuscitation, and move directly to the ACoRN Primary Survey.

Response

The Response in resuscitation is urgent and involves a progression of sequential interventions, assessments and exit points. The Resuscitation Sequence shows the sequential interventions and assessment in the vertical axis. Exit points are shown in the horizontal axis, next to an assessment with satisfactory results.

The essential intervention in neonatal resuscitation is the initiation or continuation of positive pressure ventilation as almost all babies requiring resuscitation do so because of inadequate ventilation/oxygenation.

Bag mask ventilation should be avoided in babies with a known or suspected congenital diaphragmatic hernia or anterior abdominal wall defect. These babies should be intubated immediately and an orogastric tube inserted to reduce problems related to gastric distention and aspiration of gastric contents.

© AAP/AHA

NRP is a prerequisite to ACoRN.

The NRP symbol appears at various points in the Resuscitation Case Studies as a reminder of the skills presented in The Textbook of Neonatal Resuscitation. For a quick review of neonatal resuscitation skills, you may refer to Appendix section of this textbook.

Other skills (such as cardiorespiratory monitoring, pulse oximetry, blood pressure measurement, chest transillumination, and needle aspiration of the chest) that appear in the Resuscitation Sequence will be discussed in the Cardiovascular and Respiratory Chapters and also presented in the Appendix section of this textbook.

Next Steps

An ACoRN Primary Survey is initiated once ineffective breathing has been addressed and the heart rate is ≥ 100 bpm, whether or not ongoing support is being administered. This process generates a Problem List, which identifies the relevant Sequences to be completed.

Resuscitation Case # 1 – Apnea during feeding

A mother calls for help as you are making rounds on the mother/baby unit. You respond quickly. She tells you that her baby suddenly turned blue and stopped breathing just as she finished feeding him. The baby is apneic.

This baby demonstrates two Resuscitation Signs for immediate resuscitation.

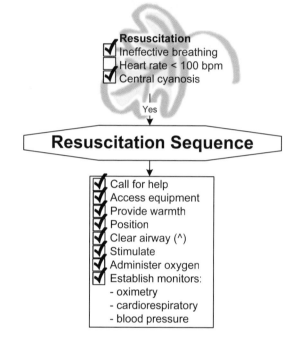

You quickly take the baby to your resuscitation area. You call for help, place the baby on a radiant warmer, and initiate resuscitation.

Who and how do you call for help when resuscitation is required in your facility?

Who? _____

How? _____

Fill out the sample contact form provided on the next page.

Contact Form for Newborn Resuscitation and Stabilization

Internal contacts

	Telephone #	Pager #	Emergency code #	Crash cart location
Emergency response team				
Labour and delivery area				
Nursery • Observation • Level 2 • Level 3				
Mother/baby unit				
Emergency dept.				

External contacts

	Contact	Telephone	Fax	Website or postal address
Regional perinatal centre				
Transport access				

You continue through the Resuscitation Sequence.

You position the baby to open the airway, recalling that the mother mentioned she had just finished feeding him. You turn on the suction apparatus and initiate oropharyngeal suctioning as help arrives.

II.   **List areas were you can find resuscitation equipment in your facility.**

_____   _____

_____   _____

Equipment appropriate for neonatal resuscitation must be available at or near all locations where it may be needed.

© AAP/AHA

You suction the oropharynx with a #10 Fr suction catheter for a moderate amount of milk, and the baby gasps.

Your colleague indicates that the heart rate is < 100 bpm.

Bag-and-mask ventilation with 100% oxygen is initiated.

Twenty seconds later, the baby begins to breathe spontaneously and the heart rate is 120 bpm. The skin begins to turn pink. You cease bag-and-mask ventilation and give free-flow oxygen.

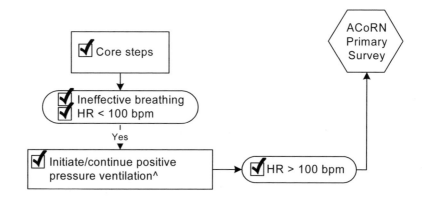

This baby meets no criteria for further resuscitation and you proceed to the ACoRN Primary Survey.

Resuscitation Case #2 – Apneic episodes in a preterm baby

© AAP/AHA

A 2100 gram baby, born by vaginal delivery at 34 weeks gestation, was admitted to the nursery for mild respiratory distress.

At four hours of age, the baby has a severe apneic episode.

This baby demonstrates one Resuscitation Sign for immediate resuscitation.

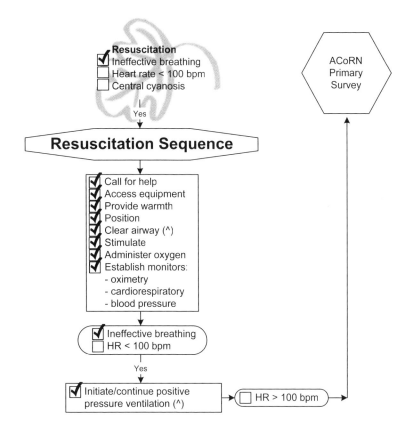

Resuscitation
- ☑ Ineffective breathing
- ☐ Heart rate < 100 bpm
- ☐ Central cyanosis

Yes

Resuscitation Sequence

ACoRN Primary Survey

- ☑ Call for help
- ☑ Access equipment
- ☑ Provide warmth
- ☑ Position
- ☑ Clear airway (^)
- ☑ Stimulate
- ☑ Administer oxygen
- ☑ Establish monitors:
  - oximetry
  - cardiorespiratory
  - blood pressure

- ☑ Ineffective breathing
- ☐ HR < 100 bpm

Yes

- ☑ Initiate/continue positive pressure ventilation (^)

→ ☐ HR > 100 bpm →

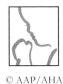

© AAP/AHA

You perform the Core Steps of the Resuscitation Sequence. You call for help. You position the baby, suction to ensure the airway is clear, and provide stimulation.

The baby continues to have apneic episodes.

You decide to initiate positive pressure ventilation.

As you begin bag-and-mask ventilation, a respiratory therapist arrives and begins auscultating the chest to determine the adequacy of ventilation and heart rate. The heart rate is 140 bpm. Bag-and-mask ventilation results in good chest expansion and equal air entry. As soon as this support is withdrawn, the baby becomes apneic again.

You and the respiratory therapist agree the baby's condition warrants intubation.

I.   **What factor in this case helps you decide to intubate at this point (remember NRP)?**

© AAP/AHA

> The baby's heart rate drops to 80 bpm as you attempt to visualize the vocal cords. The intubation attempt is aborted. You resume bag-and-mask ventilation.
>
> After 30 seconds, the heart rate is 140 bpm and the chest expansion is poor despite repositioning and suctioning. A second intubation attempt is successful. There is good chest expansion, and breath sounds can be heard on both sides symmetrically.

Neonatal intubation is a difficult skill in the best of hands. The placement of the tracheal tube has to be confirmed immediately after insertion.

Endotracheal tube placement is usually confirmed clinically by visualizing the passage of the tube through the vocal cords, auscultation over the lung fields and stomach, and observing good chest movement and improvement of heart rate and oxygen saturations.

Proper tube placement can also be confirmed with an end-tidal carbon dioxide (CO_2) detector. These devices change color with exhaled carbon dioxide, and are reliable after three to six breaths in babies that have good perfusion through their lungs. End-tidal CO_2 detectors

- have been shown to shorten the time of confirmation that a tube has been in an endotracheal position, and
- decrease clinical error in making this assessment.

 End-tidal CO_2 detector

> This baby meets no criteria for further resuscitation. You continue ventilation via the endotracheal tube, exit the Resuscitation Sequence, and begin the ACoRN Primary Survey.

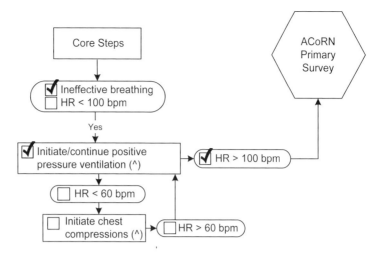

Answers to the questions in Chapter 2

Case # 1:

I.   Who and how do you call for help when resuscitation is required in your facility?

Who?   Fill out and refer to your contact list

How?   Fill out and refer to your contact list

II.   Examples of areas were you should have resuscitation equipment in your facility.

Delivery room area   Operating room

Nursery area   Post-partum area

Case # 2:

I.   What factor in this case helps you decide to intubate at this point?

Recurrent apnea (prolonged bag and mask ventilation).

Bibliography

Kattwinkel J, Niermeyer S, Nadkarni V, Tibballs J, Philllips B, Zideman D, Van Reempts P, Osmond M. ILCOR advisory statement: Resuscitation of the newly born infant. An advisory statement from the pediatric working group of the International Liaison Committee on Resuscitation. Circulation 1999; 99(14):1927-38.

Kattwinkel J, ed. Textbook of Neonatal Resuscitation. Dallas: American Academy of Pediatrics and American Heart Association, 2000.

Chapter 3
Respiratory

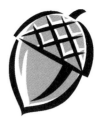

Objectives

Upon completion of this chapter, you should be able to:
1. Identify babies who require respiratory support or interventions.
2. Apply the Respiratory Sequence.
3. Determine oxygen requirements and select an appropriate oxygen delivery method.
4. Use the Respiratory Score to organize care on the basis of the severity of respiratory distress.
5. Recognize the need for and how to initiate respiratory support.
6. Perform basic interpretation of chest radiographs and blood gas results.
7. Recognize and manage the common causes of respiratory distress.
8. Recognize when to exit to the other ACoRN Sequences.

Key Concepts

1. Establishment of ventilation and prevention of hypoxia are required for successful transition from fetal to neonatal circulation.
2. Oxygenation is critical for cellular, tissue, and organ function.
3. The most common cause of cardiorespiratory failure in the newborn is hypoxemia; this is corrected by adequate ventilation and oxygenation.
4. Processes that interfere with the inflation and subsequent ventilation of the newborn lungs cause respiratory distress.
5. The goal of early detection and intervention for respiratory distress is to optimize ventilation and oxygenation.
6. Severe respiratory distress is a precursor of respiratory failure.
7. Babies with severe respiratory distress, or frequent or intermittent apnea or gasping respirations require immediate attention including intubation and ventilation.
8. Respiratory distress may be a sign of infection requiring immediate treatment.
9. Preterm babies have poor respiratory reserve and may require earlier intervention.
10. The ACoRN Respiratory Score provides guidance for intervention.
11. Babies with increasing oxygen requirements require close observation.

Skills

- Blood gas interpretation
- Chest radiograph interpretation
- Continuous positive airway pressure (CPAP)
- Emergency vascular access - Umbilical vein catheterization
- End-tidal CO_2 detector
- Free flow oxygen administration
- Mechanical ventilation
- Pneumothorax - Chest transillumination
- Pneumothorax - Chest tube insertion
- Pneumothorax - Needle aspiration
- Premedication for intubation
- Pulse oximetry
- Surfactant

Introduction

The Respiratory Sequence is the first area of concern in the ACoRN Primary Survey, reflecting the critical importance of establishing and maintaining adequate ventilation and oxygenation in the management of the unwell and at-risk newborn.

Transient or ongoing respiratory disorders are among the most common conditions encountered in neonatal care, particularly in preterm babies. Attention to the early signs and symptoms of respiratory insufficiency will often prevent later deterioration or instability.

Successful cardiopulmonary transition from intrauterine to extrauterine life involves a series of changes. It starts with the aeration, and ventilation of the lungs immediately after birth.

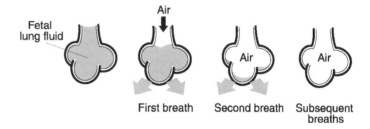

During this process, fluid in the alveoli is replaced by air, and blood flow to the lung increases as the pulmonary blood vessels dilate.

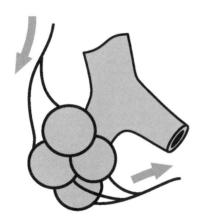
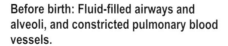

Before birth: Fluid-filled airways and alveoli, and constricted pulmonary blood vessels.

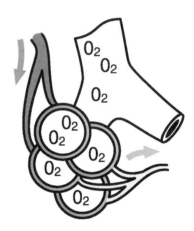

After birth: air-filled airways and alveoli, and dilated pulmonary blood vessels.

At the same time, with the clamping of the umbilical cord, the systemic vascular resistance rises and exceeds the pulmonary vascular resistance, resulting in the closure of the foramen ovale. Gas exchange at the alveolar level increases oxygen levels in the blood, further decreasing the pulmonary vascular resistance, and eliminates carbon dioxide. The ductus arteriosus constricts, and the normal newborn ventilation and circulation are established.

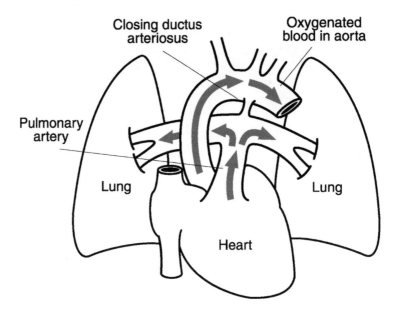

A delay or inability to complete the normal transition to extrauterine life results in neonatal respiratory problems, such as when,

- reabsorption of alveolar fluid is delayed: transient tachypnea of the newborn
- alveoli do not stay inflated after the alveolar fluid is reabsorbed due to surfactant deficiency: respiratory distress syndrome
- small airways and alveoli become obstructed: aspiration syndromes
- lungs become infected: pneumonia
- pulmonary pressure remains high: persistent pulmonary hypertension of the newborn
- lungs suffer external compression: pneumothorax
- lungs are hypoplastic: congenital diaphragmatic hernia or prolonged severe oligohydramnios starting in the second trimester.

The Respiratory Sequence

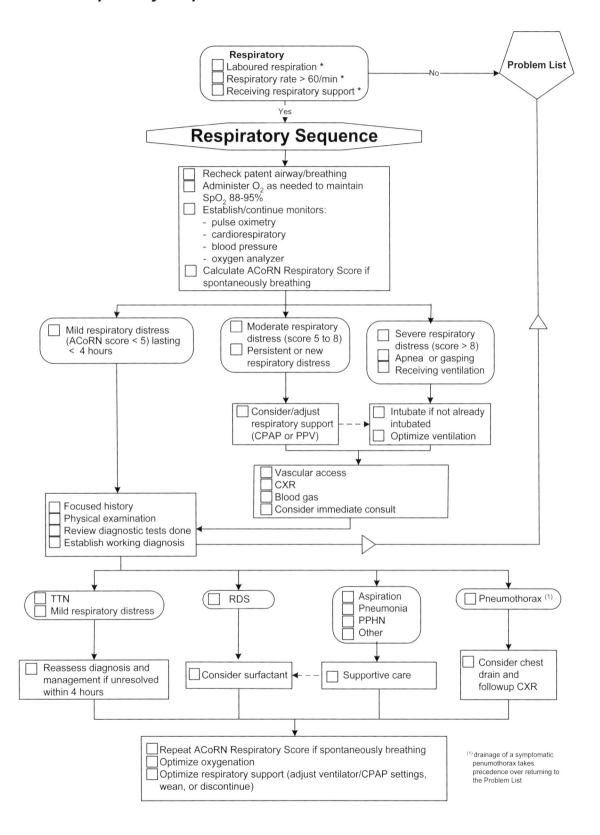

Alerting Signs   A baby who demonstrates one or more of the following Alerting Signs enters the Respiratory Sequence:

> **Respiratory**
> ☐ Laboured respiration *
> ☐ Respiratory rate > 60/min *
> ☐ Receiving respiratory support *

Laboured respiration   A baby with laboured respiration is also described as having respiratory distress, difficulty breathing, or increased work of breathing. The signs of laboured respiration are:
- nasal flaring – outward flaring movements of the nostrils on inspiration in an attempt to move more air into the lungs.
- grunting – audible sounds produced as the baby exhales against a partially closed glottis in an effort to maintain end-expiratory pressure.
- intercostal indrawing – retractions of the intercostal spaces due to increased negative pressure within the chest.
- sternal retractions – paradoxical backward movements of the sternum on inspiration due to increased negative pressure within the chest.
- gasping – an ominous sign of cerebral hypoxia characterized by deep, single or stacked, slow and irregular, terminal breaths.

Respiratory rate 60/minute   The normal newborn respiratory rate is 40 to 60/minute. A respiratory rate > 60/minute (tachypnea) usually indicates respiratory difficulty or distress.

Receiving respiratory support   This Alerting Sign identifies babies who are receiving ongoing respiratory support, with continuous positive pressure ventilation (CPAP) or positive pressure ventilation (manual or mechanical). Their respiratory insufficiency is ongoing and they require further evaluation and management.

Core Steps   Core steps are the interventions and monitoring activities applicable to all babies entering the Respiratory Sequence. These include,
- recheck patent airway/breathing
- administer O_2 as needed to maintain SpO_2 88 to 95%
- establish/continue monitors
  - pulse oximetry
  - cardiorespiratory
  - blood pressure
  - oxygen analyzer
- calculate the Respiratory Score in spontaneously breathing babies.

Respiratory Score Judging the severity of respiratory distress is a skill acquired with experience. The Respiratory Score assists the clinician to recognize the components that need assessment. The Score is utilized in babies who are breathing spontaneously, including those being treated with CPAP. It is not utilized in babies who are receiving ventilation assistance.

The Table lists the 6 components of respiratory assessment and their descriptors. The first 5 components help quantify the degree of respiratory distress. The degree of prematurity has been included in the score as it is the main modifier of the baby's ability to cope with a given degree of respiratory distress.

Each component is scored from 0 to 2.

The Respiratory Score

Score	0	1	2
Respiratory rate	40 to 60/minute	60 to 80/minute	> 80/minute
Oxygen requirement[1]	None	≤ 50%	> 50%
Retractions	None	Mild to moderate	Severe
Grunting	None	With stimulation	Continuous at rest
Breath sounds on auscultation	Easily heard throughout	Decreased	Barely heard
Prematurity	> 34 weeks	30 to 34 weeks	< 30 weeks

[1] A baby receiving oxygen prior to the setup of an oxygen analyzer should be assigned a score of "1"

Adapted from Downes JJ, Vidyasagar D, Boggs TR Jr, Morrow GM 3rd. Respiratory distress syndrome of newborn infants. I. New clinical scoring system (RDS score) with acid-base and blood-gas correlations. Clin Pediatr 1970; 9(6):325-31.

The Respiratory Score is the sum of the 6 individual scores.

The Respiratory Score is also useful for tracking the severity of respiratory distress over time in a baby who is breathing spontaneously.

The interpretation of the Respiratory Score and its use by itself or in conjunction with other findings is described under Organization of Care.

Organization of Care

The objectives in the care of babies with respiratory problems are to ensure that ventilation and oxygenation are adequate, and to provide early intervention and support as required.

The organization of care is based primarily on the severity of respiratory distress as identified using the Respiratory Score, and secondarily on additional clinical information.

Mild respiratory distress
- Respiratory Score < 5, starting at birth and lasting < 4 hours.

Moderate respiratory distress
- Respiratory Score of 5 to 8
- mild respiratory distress (Respiratory Score < 5), but persisting over 4 hours
- babies who were previously well but develop new respiratory distress. These babies are at risk of progressing to respiratory failure. Babies with persistent or new respiratory distress may be symptomatic due to other causes such as infection.

Severe respiratory distress
- Respiratory Score > 8
- babies with severe apnea or gasping
- babies who are already receiving ventilation due to respiratory failure diagnosed during the Resuscitation Sequence or a previous passage through the Respiratory Sequence.

Other factors that increase the risk a baby will be unable to sustain breathing (respiratory failure) include,
- the degree of prematurity
  - babies whose gestational age is < 27 weeks usually require respiratory support
  - babies whose gestational age is < 30 weeks and/or birth weight < 1500 grams are at increased risk of requiring respiratory support
- oxygen requirements > 50%, which indicate that the baby has little reserve.

Response

Babies with **mild respiratory distress** lasting less than four hours require,
- ongoing observation
- oxygen supplementation to maintain blood oxygen levels in the desired range (such as, SpO_2 between 88 to 95%)
- further work-up if they meet criteria for entry into the Infection Sequence.

Babies with **moderate respiratory distress** may need some degree of respiratory support, such as CPAP or, sometimes, mechanical ventilation to prevent progression to severe respiratory distress and respiratory failure.

Babies with **severe respiratory distress,** including severe apnea or gasping, require immediate attention including intubation and ventilation, as these are ominous signs of respiratory failure.

Once initiated, ventilation needs to be optimized to,
- decrease the work of breathing
- maintain the Sp_{O_2} in the desired range, such as between 88 to 95%
- restore acid base balance (pH between 7.25 and 7.40)
- maintain P_{CO_2} between 45 and 55.

Babies receiving respiratory support (CPAP or ventilation) require,
- vascular access to initiate D10%W solution
- chest radiograph
- blood gases
- consideration for immediate consult, depending on expertise and resources.

 ### Continuous positive airway pressure (CPAP)

 ### Mechanical ventilation

Next Steps The Next Steps are to obtain a focused history, conduct a physical examination, order diagnostic tests and establish a working diagnosis.

Focused respiratory history Important information to gather during the focused respiratory history includes:

Antepartum
- gestation and accuracy of dates
- antenatal ultrasound findings
- maternal diabetes
- maternal Group B streptococcus (GBS) status (positive, negative, unknown)
- administration of antenatal steroids
- maternal substance use
- family history of neonatal respiratory disorders

Intrapartum
- presence of non-reassuring fetal health surveillance during labour and delivery
- presence of meconium stained liquor
- duration of rupture of membranes
- evidence of chorioamnionitis (maternal fever and/or fetal tachycardia)
- nature of labour and route of delivery
- medications
- administration of intrapartum antibiotics for GBS prophylaxis

Neonatal
- results of umbilical cord blood gas (arterial and venous) determination, if done
- condition at birth, including Apgar score
- resuscitation efforts required and response
- time of onset of symptoms, i.e., present from birth or developed after a period of normal respiratory function
- gestational age and birth weight

Physical examination   The essential components of the physical examination include:

Observation
- work of breathing and symmetry of chest movement
- indicators of laboured respiration (nasal flaring, intercostal indrawing, sternal retraction, and gasping)
- skin colour and mucous membranes for evidence of central cyanosis
- respiratory support (for example, size and position of endotracheal tube, ventilator settings, and inspired oxygen)

Measurement of vital signs: respiratory rate, heart rate, temperature, blood pressure, and oxygen saturation.

Examination
- auscultate both lung fields laterally for equality and nature of breath sounds. Diminished breath sounds unilaterally may signal intubation of the right bronchus, pneumonia, an area of atelectasis, or presence of a pneumothorax or other space-occupying lesion (for example, a diaphragmatic hernia).
- presence of grunting, inspiratory stridor, audible expiratory wheeze, crackles)
- presence of cleft palate or micrognathia (small jaw)

Diagnostic tests Diagnostic tests are performed on all babies entering the Respiratory Sequence. The exceptions are term babies with mild respiratory distress lasting less than four hours.

Two diagnostic tests that can assist in quickly reaching a working diagnosis for respiratory conditions are:

1. **Chest radiograph**
   - To determine the cause of respiratory distress and guide intervention.

 Chest radiograph interpretation

2. **Blood gases**
   - Arterial, capillary and venous blood gases are used to assess the adequacy of ventilation (P_{CO_2}) and the presence of acidosis (pH and base deficit)
   - Arterial blood gases are used to assess the adequacy of oxygenation (P_{O_2}).

Blood gases should be used in conjunction with pulse oximetry which provides a continuous assessment of oxygenation.

 Blood gas interpretation

Establish a Working Diagnosis

Formulation of a working diagnosis relies heavily on knowledge of the more common conditions that present as respiratory distress in the newborn, and their radiographic findings. These include,
1. transient tachypnea of the newborn
2. respiratory distress syndrome
3. meconium aspiration syndrome
4. pneumothorax and other air leaks
5. pneumonia

1. Transient Tachypnea of the Newborn (TTN)
- Lung fluid production does not cease prior to birth and there is a delay in clearance of residual lung fluid after birth.
- Occurs as a primary cause of respiratory distress in term or near-term babies, and is more common in newborns born by cesarean section, especially when there has been no labor.
- Babies present with mild to moderate respiratory distress, with oxygen requirements usually < 40%.
- Respiratory distress due to transient tachypnea of the newborn will often resolve over the first few minutes to hours after birth as residual lung fluid is reabsorbed.

Mild TTN:

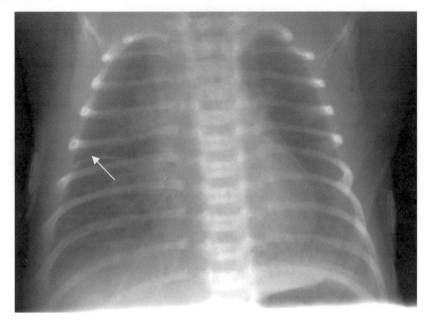

- o normal or increased lung inflation (increased in the example)
- o fairly clear lung fields
- o diaphragm and heart borders are easy to see throughout
- o increased vascular markings near the heart shadow give lungs a streaky appearance
- o fluid in the major fissure (arrow); may have small amount of pleural fluid

Severe TTN:

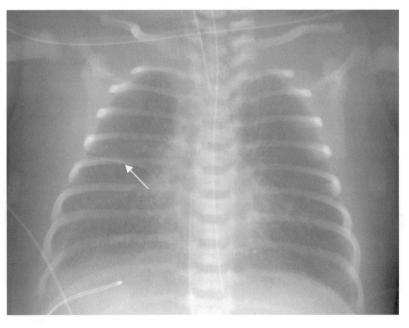

- o same as above but with increased haziness of lung fields

2. Respiratory Distress Syndrome (RDS)

- Lack of surfactant production/release in the lungs, resulting in progressive collapse of the terminal bronchioles/alveoli.
- Primarily a disease of preterm babies; its incidence increases with decreasing gestational age.
- Babies present with any degree of respiratory distress and oxygen requirements.
- Respiratory distress will worsen if respiratory effort or support is unable to prevent progressive lung collapse. When RDS is not treated with exogenous surfactant it will generally improve after 72 hours as endogenous surfactant production and release are established.

Mild RDS:

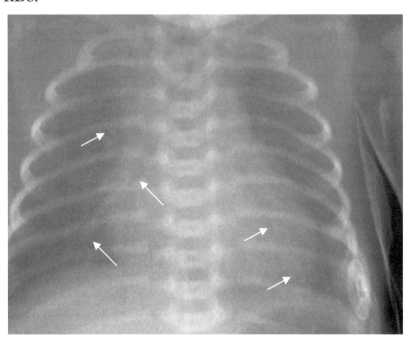

- o normal or slightly decreased lung inflation
- o fairly clear lung fields with slight diffuse haziness
- o diaphragm and heart borders mildly obscured
- o few air bronchograms (airways containing air become visible against collapsed lung), longitudinally (arrows) and in cross section (cross section of airway appears as a donut with a black centre and white circumference)

Moderate RDS:

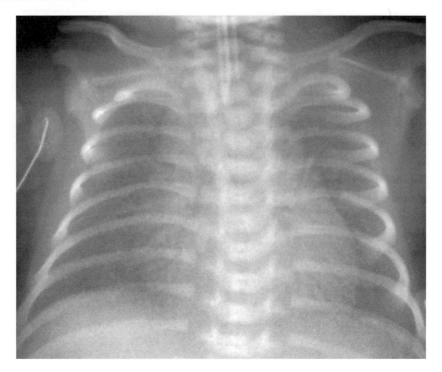

- moderately decreased lung inflation
- lung fields diffusely hazy, with "ground glass" appearance
- heart borders and diaphragm approximately 50% obscured.
- air bronchograms more widely seen in upper and lower lobes

In the above radiograph:

1) Mark with a T the tip of the endotracheal tube.

2) Mark with an X all the air bronchograms you can see.

Severe RDS:

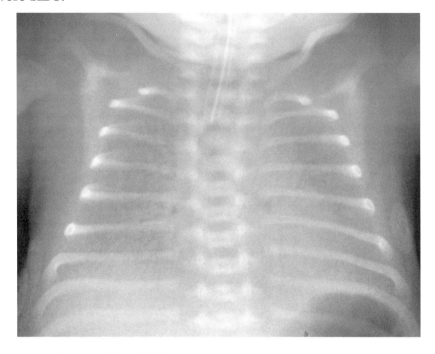

- ○ decreased lung inflation
- ○ lung fields diffusely hazy, total or near total "white out" appearance
- ○ heart borders and diaphragm > 50% obscured
- ○ air bronchograms in upper and lower lobes

In the above radiograph:

1) Mark with a **T** the tip of the endotracheal tube.

2) Mark with a **C** the carina

3) Draw a line along any area of heart border or diaphragm that can be <u>clearly</u> seen.

3. Meconium Aspiration Syndrome (MAS)

- Perinatal aspiration of meconium resulting in a combination of large and small airway obstruction, pneumonitis, surfactant inactivation, and ventilation:perfusion mismatch.
- A disease of post-term, term and, sometimes, near-term babies (with a functionally mature gastrointestinal tract) who are born in the presence of meconium. More common if the baby is depressed at birth or if meconium is thick or particulate.
- Babies may present with any degree of respiratory distress and oxygen requirements.
- May be accompanied by persistent pulmonary hypertension of the newborn.
- Severe MAS is life threatening and requires prompt specialized care.

Moderate to severe MAS:

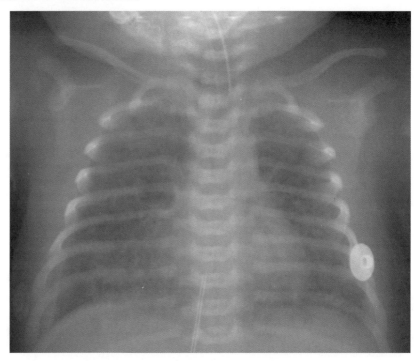

- o normal or increased lung inflation
- o lung fields show fluffy, patchy and coarse infiltrates, and asymmetric areas of hyperinflation interposed with areas of atelectasis
- o heart borders and diaphragm are usually significantly obscured by areas of atelectatic lung

4. Pneumothorax
- Air leak within the pleural space.
- Primarily occurs in babies with lung disease (aspiration syndromes and RDS) receiving respiratory support (CPAP or ventilation). May also occur with spontaneous respirations and in the absence of lung disease (during initial spontaneous breaths).
- Babies present with an acute increase in respiratory distress and oxygen requirements.
- Tension pneumothorax may present with sudden onset of cardiovascular collapse.
- A small pneumothorax is often minimally symptomatic.
- A moderate or large pneumothorax requires drainage via chest tube.
- A smaller pneumothorax with minimal respiratory distress (tachypnea only) and no cardiovascular deterioration can be observed until it resolves spontaneously.

Small pneumothorax:

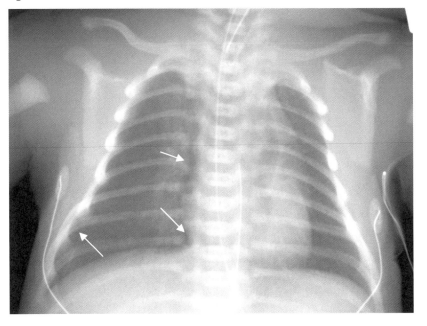

- ○ hemithorax volume is similar in the affected and unaffected side
- ○ the affected side is more lucent and a black rim of air (arrows) may be noted between the chest wall and the lung tissue which contains no lung markings
- ○ the cardiac silhouette is not shifted towards the unaffected side

Medium sized pneumothorax:

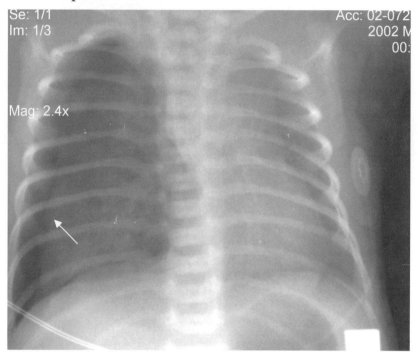

- o hemithorax volume is slightly larger in the affected side than in the unaffected side
- o the affected side is more lucent and a black rim of air is noted between the chest wall and the lung tissue (arrow) which contains no lung markings
- o the cardiac silhouette is slightly shifted towards the unaffected side

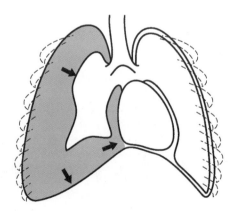

Large (tension) pneumothorax – antero-posterior (AP) view:

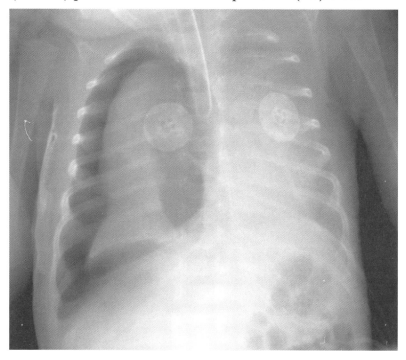

- o hemithorax volume is markedly larger in the affected side than in the unaffected side, and the diaphragm may be flattened
- o the affected side is more lucent and a black rim of air is noted between the chest wall and the lung tissue which contains no lung markings
- o the cardiac silhouette is markedly shifted towards the unaffected side

Large (tension) pneumothorax – lateral view:

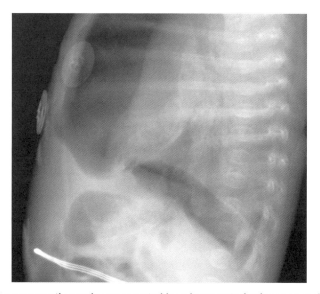

- o the pneumothorax is represented by a large anterior lucency and lucency at the level of the diaphragm
- o the diaphragm is flattened

Other radiographic signs found in air leaks:

- In **pneumomediastinum**, the thymus is outlined and may appear lifted from the cardiac surface giving the impression of a "butterfly" or "sail".
- In **pneumopericardium**, a halo is seen around the heart.

Pneumomediastinum and left sided pneumothorax:

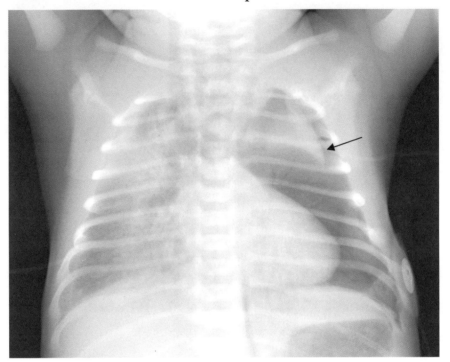

Signs of pneumomediastinum:
- ○ the arrow shows a lifted thymus, radiologically referred to as the "sail sign"
- ○ air is seen on the right side of the heart, tracking up the neck

Signs of pneumothorax:
- ○ the entire left hemithorax is hyperlucent
- ○ most of the air is anterior to the lung (the lung "rim" cannot be seen)
- ○ the size is moderate (no mediastinal shift or depression of the diaphragm)

5. Pneumonia
- Infectious infiltrate of the lungs, usually interstitial and diffuse rather than lobar in appearance.
- It is more likely to occur in the presence of risk factors for sepsis (for example, prolonged rupture of membranes, maternal colonization with GBS, or chorioamnionitis).
- Babies may or may not be systemically ill at onset, but the clinical course may be fulminant.
- The inability to rule out pneumonia by clinical or radiographic appearance gives rise to the recommendation to treat all respiratory disease in the newborn with intravenous antibiotics.

Radiographic findings:

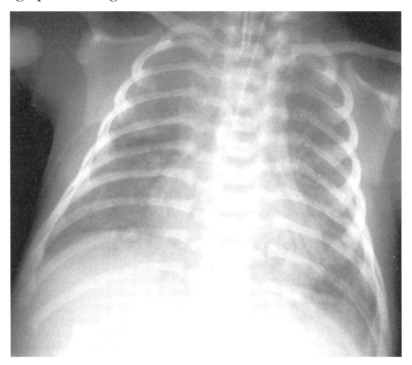

- radiographic diagnosis is always tentative as the chest radiograph may mimic RDS, TTN and, occasionally, MAS
- there may be moderately to markedly increased lung inflation
- lung fields may show patchy densities and various degrees of "white out" and air bronchograms
- diaphragm and heart borders may be obscured
- discrete segmental or lobar involvement may be present but is not common

Other causes of newborn respiratory insufficiency

1. Persistent Pulmonary Hypertension of the Newborn (PPHN)

- Failure of the normal drop in pulmonary vascular resistance after birth, resulting in decreased pulmonary blood flow and in bi-directional or right-to-left shunting of blood through the ductus arteriosus or foramen ovale, and tricuspid regurgitation.
- Usually has an underlying vascular component of prenatal origin, which includes increased vascular muscularization and reactivity, decreased pulmonary vascularization, and/or abnormal vascular distribution.
- PPHN is usually triggered by respiratory conditions such as RDS, MAS, pneumonia, or congenital diaphragmatic hernia, but may also occur as a primary disturbance of transition in the absence of parenchymal lung disease
- Presents with hypoxic respiratory failure (high oxygen requirements), labile oxygenation, and may be able to demonstrate higher preductal than post ductal oxygenation by blood gas analysis or pulse oximetry. The diagnosis should always be confirmed by cardiology consultation and echocardiography to rule out abnormal cardiovascular anatomy.
- PPHN is life threatening and requires prompt specialized care.

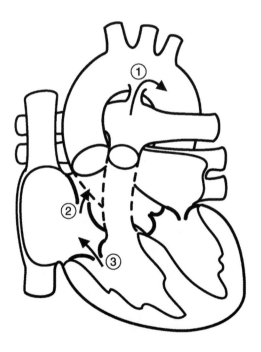

Persistent Pulmonary Hypertension

1. **Right to left shunt via the PDA**
2. **Right to left shunt via patent foramen ovale**
3. **Functional tricuspid insufficiency and regurgitation due to right ventricular dysfunction**

2. Lung hypoplasia
- Overall decrease in the number of airways and gas-exchange spaces (alveolar sacs, or alveoli).
- Occurs in babies who experienced insufficient lung inflation in-utero due to:
  - severe oligohydramnios as a result of
    - rupture of the membranes in the second trimester
    - renal agenesis
    - urinary outflow obstruction.
  - congenital diaphragmatic hernia (CDH)
  - neuromuscular disease with decreased fetal respiration
- Presents at birth as profound respiratory distress.
- There is increased risk of PPHN and pneumothorax.
- Lung hypoplasia is life threatening and requires prompt specialized care.

Radiographic findings:
- Small lung fields, often with clear lung fields.
- In congenital diaphragmatic hernia, a space-occupying lesion is seen which is more commonly found on the left side.

Left sided congenital diaphragmatic hernia

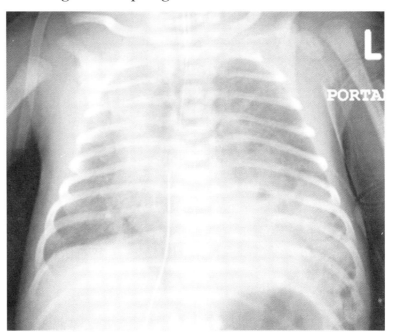

- stomach bubble is in the abdomen
- there is some mediastinal shift to the right
- air is present in the bowel located within the left chest

Severe left sided congenital diaphragmatic hernia

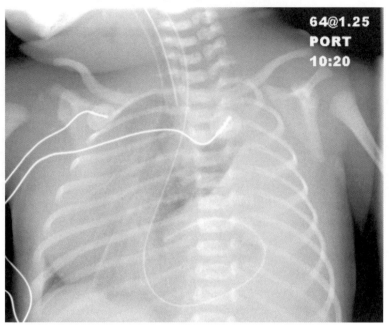

○ stomach is in the chest (see NG tube coiled in the chest)
○ there is marked mediastinal shift to the right, with the heart
    border "touching" the chest wall, due to the left CDH

Note: air is not present in the bowel because the baby was
intubated immediately after birth (no bag and mask
ventilation), and given neuromuscular blockade (unable to
swallow air).

**Specific
Management**

Specific Management depends on the working diagnoses, and is discussed in
the illustrative cases that follow.

Respiratory Case # 1 - Mild respiratory distress in a term newborn

> A baby girl is born by Cesarean section at 38 weeks gestation. This was a planned elective section in view of a breech presentation. She was vigorous at birth. You are called to assess her in the recovery room at 30 minutes of age because the baby is grunting.
>
> You find her to be dusky in room air, with regular respirations, mild nasal flaring, and audible grunting with stimulation. She has intercostal indrawing and mild sternal retractions. Her heart rate is 120 bpm.

What is duskiness?

Duskiness is a common term often used to describe central cyanosis.

> Although her breathing is laboured, it is effective as the heart rate is > 100 bpm and respiration is regular, however, cyanosis is one of the Alerting Signs for immediate resuscitation.
>
> You take the baby across the hall to the radiant warmer in the newborn resuscitation area.

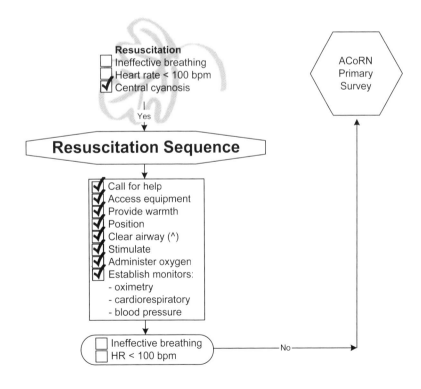

You perform the Core Steps of the Resuscitation Sequence, and provide free flow oxygen by mask.

The baby's breathing remains laboured but regular, respiratory rate is 70/minute, and heart rate 140 bpm. You note the baby's color has improved in response to oxygen administration.

You exit the Resuscitation Sequence and complete the ACoRN Primary Survey.

Additional observations made in order to complete the ACoRN Primary Survey indicate that the baby is at risk for hypoglycemia because she is exhibiting respiratory distress and has not been fed, and the blood glucose is not known. The baby's temperature is also unknown and she is at risk for temperature instability.

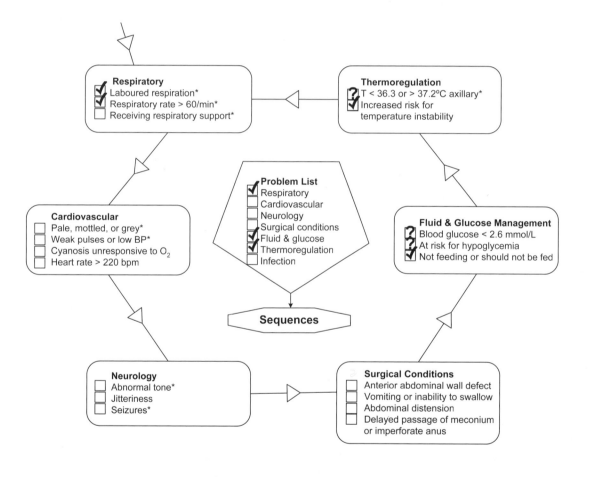

The baby exhibits two of the Alerting Signs for the Respiratory Sequence.

You enter the Respiratory Sequence and perform the Core Steps.

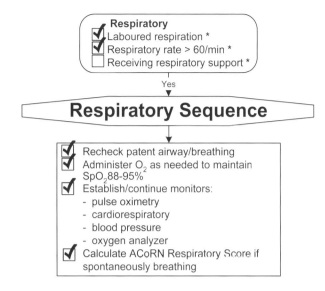

Respiratory
- ☑ Laboured respiration *
- ☑ Respiratory rate > 60/min *
- ☐ Receiving respiratory support *

Yes
↓

Respiratory Sequence

- ☑ Recheck patent airway/breathing
- ☑ Administer O_2 as needed to maintain SpO_2 88-95%
- ☑ Establish/continue monitors:
  - pulse oximetry
  - cardiorespiratory
  - blood pressure
  - oxygen analyzer
- ☑ Calculate ACoRN Respiratory Score if spontaneously breathing

---

You ensure that the airway is patent and that she has been positioned and suctioned. Breath sounds are easily heard throughout the lungs on auscultation.

Free-flow oxygen is being administered by facemask.

How can supplemental oxygen be administered to a spontaneously breathing baby?

During resuscitation
- administered using a flow inflating bag, oxygen mask or oxygen tubing placed close to the baby's face
- equipment is easy to use and immediately available
- administer oxygen or blended gas at a flow rate of 5 L/minute
- flow inflating bags allow delivery of desired oxygen concentration, according to the setting on the blender
- oxygen masks and oxygen tubing do not allow delivery of desired oxygen concentration, according to the setting on the blender
  - o oxygen masks administer up to 50% oxygen
  - o oxygen tubing administers up to 30% oxygen.

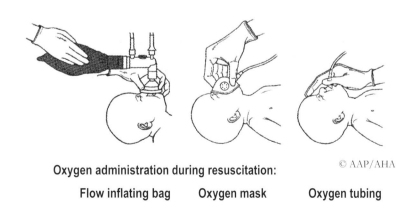

© AAP/AHA

Oxygen administration during resuscitation:

Flow inflating bag   **Oxygen mask**   **Oxygen tubing**

Free-flow oxygen administration during resuscitation

Oxygen hood
- blended, humidified oxygen is administered at 5 to 10 L/minute into a hood placed over the baby's head to,
  - ensure desired oxygen concentration
  - prevent CO_2 accumulation
- able to administer desired oxygen concentration, according to the setting on the blender
- the exact amount of oxygen delivered can be determined using an oxygen analyzer placed close to the baby's mouth
- oxygen concentration is adjusted by changing the setting on the blender to achieve the desired SpO_2, such as between 88 to 95%
- the initial temperature of the gas entering the hood should be 32 to 34° C.

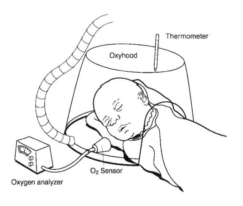

Incubator
- incubators manufactured after 1990 are able to consistently administer high oxygen concentration, humidity and warmth, and have built-in oxygen analyzers that continuously adjust the oxygen flow to maintain a preset concentration
- older incubators may provide as little as 30% oxygen despite being flooded with 100% oxygen and are not able to maintain the oxygen concentration when the port-hole or door is opened
  - reliable oxygen administration requires simultaneous use of an oxygen hood when using older incubators.

Nasal prongs (newborn size)
- 100% oxygen is administered at a flow < 2 L/minute. Higher flows,
  - can cause inadvertent positive end expiratory pressure (PEEP)
  - irritate and dry the nasal mucosa
- oxygen flow is adjusted up or down to achieve the desired SpO_2, such as between 88 to 95%

- not a preferred method of oxygen delivery during initial management because,
  - of the inability to determine the precise amount of oxygen the baby is receiving,
  - oxygen administered in this way is easily diluted by entrained air during crying, mouth breathing, or increased respiratory rate and depth of respiration.

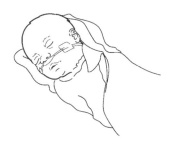

Why should the oxygen concentration delivered be determined using an oxygen analyzer?

- it is important to know if the baby's oxygen requirements are increasing or decreasing over time.
- oxygen requirements > 40 to 50% indicate a higher risk that the baby will not be able to sustain breathing.

What do we measure to determine the amount of oxygen in the baby's circulation?

- hemoglobin oxygen saturation (S_{O_2})
  - pulse oximetry (Sp_{O_2})
  - arterial sample (Sa_{O_2})
- partial pressure of oxygen (P_{O_2})
  - arterial sample (Pa_{O_2})
  - capillary sample

It is important to understand the difference between hemoglobin oxygen saturation (S_{O_2}) and the partial pressure of oxygen (P_{O_2})

Oxygen is carried by the blood either bound to hemoglobin molecules, or dissolved in plasma in an approximate ratio of 40 to 1.

- S_{O_2}, measured in %, represents hemoglobin saturation, the percentage of hemoglobin molecules that are bound to oxygen.

- P_{O_2}, measured in mmHg, is the partial pressure exerted by the oxygen molecules dissolved in the plasma; P_{O_2} determines how much oxygen binds to hemoglobin.
  - as P_{O_2} drops in the capillary circulation, oxygen is released to the tissues
  - when P_{O_2} increases in the alveolar capillaries oxygen binds to hemoglobin.

For practical purposes it is correct to assume that,
- S_{O_2} determines how much oxygen is carried in the blood
- the maximum oxygen carrying capacity of the blood is reached once S_{O_2} reaches 100%.

The relationship between P_{O_2} and S_{O_2} is figuratively expressed as the oxyhemoglobin dissociation curve.

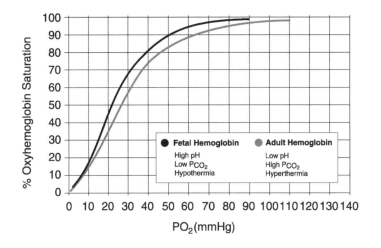

- On the steep portion of the oxyhemoglobin dissociation curve, S_{O_2} increases rapidly with P_{O_2} until S_{O_2} reaches approximately 75% and P_{O_2} approximately 35 to 40 mmHg.
- On the flat portion of the curve, once S_{O_2} exceeds 95%, large changes in P_{O_2} result in small changes in S_{O_2}.
  - S_{O_2} of 98 to 100% may reflect any value of $P_{O_2} \geq 90$ mmHg.

SaO_2   Indicates how much oxygen is bound to hemoglobin in arterial blood. The amount of oxygen carried by the blood is proportional to the Sa_{O_2} and hemoglobin concentration, and not to the Pa_{O_2}.
- the target range of Sa_{O_2} in newborns receiving oxygen is 88 to 95%
- Sa_{O_2} is a sensitive indicator of hypoxemia
- Sa_{O_2} is a poor indicator of hyperoxemia
  - once the P_{O_2} is > 80 to 90 mmHg, S_{O_2} will be 100% regardless of the P_{O_2} value
- minimal additional oxygen is carried by blood with Sa_{O_2} > 95%.

PaO$_2$ Indicates how well the lung is transferring inspired oxygen to the blood. The magnitude of impairment in lung function is proportional to the difference between inspired oxygen (%) and arterial oxygen (PaO$_2$).

- the target range of PaO$_2$ in a newborn is 50 to 70 mmHg
- hypoxemia (PaO$_2$ < 50 mmHg) decreases blood flow to the lungs by increasing pulmonary vascular resistance
- hyperoxemia (PaO$_2$ > 70 to 90 mmHg) increases the risk of oxygen associated retinal injury in preterm infants (retinopathy of prematurity).

The ideal oxygen saturation range for babies is controversial, but values between 88 to 95% are generally recommended. Oxygen saturation values > 95% may be associated with high levels of blood oxygen which are potentially damaging to immature tissues, such as the retina of premature babies.

In the presence of good cardiac function, oxygen saturation in the normal range indirectly indicates adequate oxygen delivery to the tissues, and prevents the development of acidosis and pulmonary vasoconstriction.

Oxygen saturation monitoring provides a good indication of the effectiveness of respiratory interventions in oxygenating the blood, but is not an indicator of effective breathing or ventilation.

Pulse oximetry (SpO$_2$) Pulse oximetry is used frequently to monitor a baby's oxygenation because it is non-invasive, easy to use, and provides immediate readings in a continuous display. SpO$_2$ closely reflects SaO$_2$.

 Pulse oximetry

You change the mode of oxygen administration to an oxygen hood, and determine the oxygen % required to maintain the SpO$_2$ in the 88 to 95% range.

You calculate the Respiratory Score, assigning 1 point for each component: respiratory rate (60 to 80/minute), baby is receiving oxygen, mild retractions, and grunting only when disturbed. The baby's gestational age is 38 weeks so you assign 0 points for prematurity.

Score	0	1	2
Respiratory rate	40 to 60/minute	60 to 80/minute	> 80/minute
Oxygen requirement[1]	None	≤ 50%	> 50%
Retractions	None	Mild to moderate	Severe
Grunting	None	With stimulation	Continuous at rest
Breath sounds on auscultation	Easily heard throughout	Decreased	Barely heard
Prematurity	> 34 weeks	30 to 34 weeks	< 30 weeks

[1] A baby receiving oxygen prior to the setup of an oxygen analyzer should be assigned a score of "1"

You organize care on the basis of the Respiratory Score.

The baby has mild respiratory distress, with a respiratory score of 4 and no apnea.

She requires observation and continued monitoring.

The Focused history reveals that the mother's pregnancy and cesarean section delivery were uneventful, and that there are no risk factors for infection: there was no maternal fever, membranes were ruptured at birth, and group B streptococcus screening was negative.

On Physical examination you note that she is pink on 30% oxygen and that SpO_2 is 92%. The baby looks well despite her respiratory symptoms.

The clinical evaluation of a baby's response to administration of oxygen includes the assessment of color and oxygenation, and effect on breathing.

You make a tentative diagnosis of transient tachypnea of the newborn and return to the ACoRN Problem List in order to address the Fluid & Glucose Management and Thermoregulation Sequences.

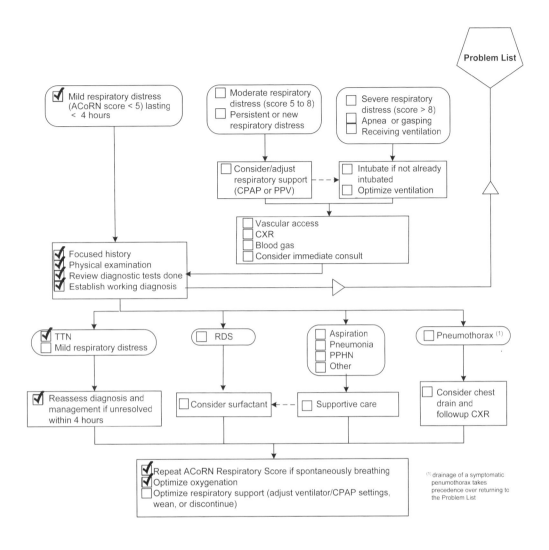

I. Why is the diagnosis of TTN likely?

_____   _____

_____   _____

Mild respiratory distress due to transient tachypnea of the newborn will often resolve over the first few minutes to hours after birth as residual lung fluid is reabsorbed. Babies will require further assessment to confirm the diagnosis and guide further management if the,
- respiratory distress persists for ≥ 4 hours or worsens
- oxygen requirements increase over this time.

This re-evaluation involves,
- reassessment of the diagnosis and management
- repeat of the Respiratory Score if spontaneously breathing
- optimization of oxygenation
- optimization of respiratory support
- re-entry into the ACoRN Process

As a reminder that Infection often presents with respiratory symptoms in the newborn, all three Respiratory Alerting Signs are ACoRN alerting signs with *.

- Term babies with mild respiratory distress should enter the Infection Sequence only if they exhibit one or more of,
  - respiratory distress $\geq$ 4 hours after birth
  - risk factors for infection
  - clinical deterioration (for example, an increase in oxygen requirements)
  - requirement for ventilatory support
- All preterm babies with any degree or duration of respiratory distress should enter the Infection Sequence and receive antibiotics.

You enter a question mark in the second box of the Alerting Signs for Infection, to remind you to reassess the diagnosis within 4 hours.

Infection
- [ ] Risk factor for infection
- [?] ACoRN alerting sign with *
- [ ] Clinical deterioration

Over the next hour, the nurse reports that the baby is no longer grunting, has a respiratory rate of 50/minute, and is alert and active. She has a saturation of 93% in room air.

Respiratory Case # 2 - Respiratory distress in a preterm newborn – Initiating CPAP

> A 2240 gram baby boy is born at 34 weeks gestation by spontaneous vaginal vertex delivery following a pregnancy complicated by rupture of the membranes and preterm labor. The baby cried at birth and required minimal resuscitation. The Apgar score was 7 at 1 minute and 8 at 5 minutes.
>
> After initial resuscitation, he develops regular but labored respiration, audible grunting at rest, and sternal retractions. The respiratory rate is 72/minute, and the heart rate 160 bpm. He requires oxygen to remain pink.

Cyanosis or oxygen requirement is an Alerting Sign for immediate resuscitation.

Resuscitation
- ☐ Ineffective breathing
- ☐ Heart rate < 100 bpm
- ☑ Central cyanosis

I.   **What is the definition of ineffective breathing? Does the description of this baby meet the definition?**

_____

_____

> You work through the Core Steps of the Resuscitation Sequence. The respiratory rate remains regular and the heart rate 156 bpm. You then exit the Resuscitation Sequence and complete the ACoRN Primary Survey.

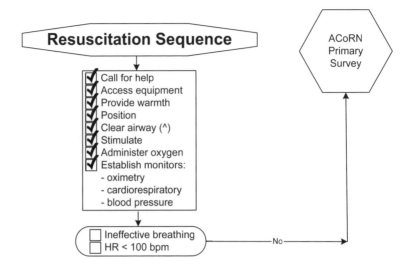

The baby is in the special care nursery area of your community hospital. He is under a radiant warmer with servo control receiving 35% oxygen by oxygen hood. The pulse oximeter reading is 92%. The respiratory rate is 72/minute and heart rate 160 bpm. The blood pressure by cuff is 48/30, mean of 36 mmHg, which is normal for a baby of 34 weeks gestation.

You observe the baby and notice he is pink, and is lying in a semi-flexed posture characteristic of a baby of his gestational age. He continues to grunt at rest, and has moderate sternal retractions and intercostal indrawing. You auscultate his chest and find that breath sounds are decreased bilaterally.

II. Complete the Primary Survey below to generate your problem list.

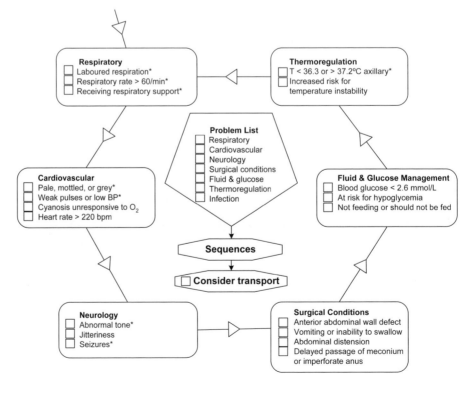

Your Primary Survey generates a Problem List that indicates that there are three areas of concern

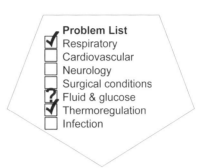

Problem List
- ☑ Respiratory
- ☐ Cardiovascular
- ☐ Neurology
- ☐ Surgical conditions
- ？ Fluid & glucose
- ☑ Thermoregulation
- ☐ Infection

You enter the Respiratory Sequence and carry out the Core Steps and calculate the ACoRN Respiratory Score:

Score	0	1	2
Respiratory rate	40 to 60/minute	60 to 80/minute	> 80/minute
Oxygen requirement[1]	None	≤ 50%	> 50%
Retractions	None	Mild to moderate	Severe
Grunting	None	With stimulation	Continuous at rest
Breath sounds on auscultation	Easily heard throughout	Decreased	Barely heard
Prematurity	> 34 weeks	30 to 34 weeks	< 30 weeks

[1] A baby receiving oxygen prior to the setup of an oxygen analyzer should be assigned a score of "1"

The ACoRN Respiratory Score adds up to 7, indicating moderate respiratory distress and that respiratory support may be needed.

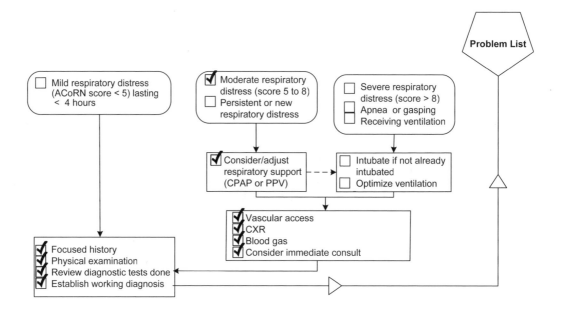

III.   **Name two types of respiratory support that may assist babies in moderate respiratory distress.**

_____

_____

Continuous positive airway pressure (CPAP)   The administration of continuous positive airway pressure (CPAP) during spontaneous breathing stabilizes the small airways and chest wall, and prevents atelectasis at end expiration. CPAP decreases the need for endotracheal intubation and mechanical ventilation in babies with moderate respiratory distress and good respiratory effort.

CPAP must only be administered and monitored by on-site and trained personnel, in a setting with adequate resources for the care of a baby needing respiratory support.

The purpose of CPAP is,
- to improve arterial P_{O_2} in order to reduce inspired oxygen concentration in babies with respiratory distress who do not require mechanical ventilation
- to wean the baby from mechanical ventilation
- to treat apnea in some preterm babies
  - CPAP reduces mixed and obstructive apnea, but has no effect on central apnea.

CPAP is contraindicated in babies,
- in respiratory failure
- incapable of spontaneous breathing efforts (for example, central nervous system disorders)
- who are easily agitated or do not tolerate CPAP
- where excessive air swallowing is undesirable
  o gastrointestinal obstruction
  o necrotizing enterocolitis
  o congenital diaphragmatic hernia.

CPAP can be delivered using,
- nasal prongs
- nasal masks
- nasopharyngeal tube.

CPAP can be generated by,
- ventilators on CPAP mode
- circuits with free flow of gas exiting through an underwater seal ("bubble CPAP") or valve
- infant flow drivers
- a flow inflating bag and mask (transiently).

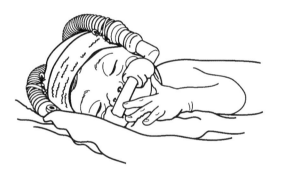

 Continuous positive airway pressure (CPAP)

You decide to initiate nasal CPAP because the baby has moderate respiratory distress. There is on-site personnel who are familiar with CPAP and the hospital has adequate resources to care for a baby needing respiratory support.

Vascular access is started via a peripheral vein and a chest radiograph is ordered. Venous blood is drawn for a blood gas, CBC, glucose and blood culture.

- Vascular access is needed to administer fluids and medications.
- A chest radiograph is requested to diagnose lung pathology, such as TTN or RDS, or complications, such as pneumothorax.
- Blood gases are drawn to assess the adequacy of ventilation and the presence of acidosis.
- The need for internal or external consultation is decided on the basis of the availability of resources needed to care for the baby on a continuous basis.

The mother is a 24-year-old primigravida with an unremarkable past medical history and family history. She had an uneventful pregnancy until the onset of labor at 34 weeks. On admission, her cervix was 7 cm dilated and contractions were occurring every 3 minutes. In discussion with the regional centre, it was decided that transfer would be unsafe as delivery was imminent. Intrapartum antibiotic prophylaxis was suggested, and one dose of Penicillin G was given shortly after admission, about four hours before birth. Membranes had ruptured 5 hours before birth.

Currently the baby is on CPAP of 5 cmH$_2$O, 40% oxygen, and the SpO$_2$ is stable around 92%. Respiration is less labored and the respiratory rate 60/minute. Heart rate, blood pressure, and temperature remain within normal limits. The chest radiograph is shown below

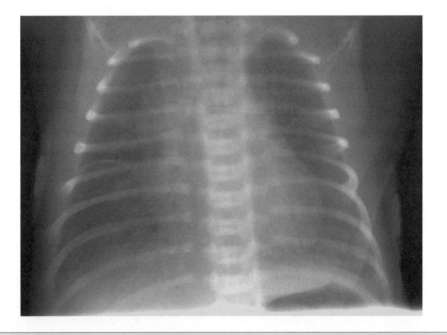

You interpret the chest radiograph as showing
- fluid in the right horizontal fissure
- the heart borders are easy to see, but the hemi-diaphragms are not
- although the lung fields look "grainy" or with "ground glass" appearance, you do not see any air bronchograms extending past the cardiac silhouette.

In view of the history, physical examination, and chest radiograph findings, a presumptive diagnosis of moderate to severe TTN is made. It is likely that there is some loss of lung volume in the bases, making the hemi-diaphrams difficult to see.

At this time you exit the Respiratory Sequence, returning to the ACoRN Problem List in order to address Fluid & Glucose Management and Thermoregulation.

You also note that there are several Alerting Signs with an *, indicating that you will also have to address the Infection Sequence.

Infection
- ☐ Risk factor for infection
- ☑ ACoRN alerting sign with *
- ☐ Clinical deterioration

IV. **Why do this baby's Alerting Signs indicate that he should enter the Infection Sequence?**

_____

_____

What is the Specific Management for moderate to severe TTN?

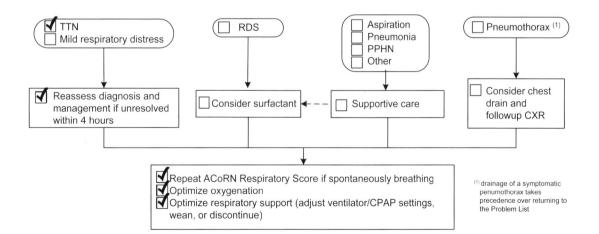

Once CPAP has been initiated, ongoing assessment is necessary to optimize oxygenation and the level of respiratory support. In a spontaneously breathing baby this is done through,

- reassessment of the Respiratory Score
- measurement of blood gases
- continuous assessment of oxygenation using pulse oximetry (SpO_2)

> The capillary blood gas result shows: pH 7.30, PCO_2 45, PO_2 30, BD 3.

Blood gases   **pH** estimates the blood total acid load, which mostly reflects dissolved CO_2 but may also include metabolic acids such as lactic acid.

PCO_2 indicates how well the lung is removing CO_2 from the blood (ventilation).

PaO_2 (arterial PO_2) indicates how well the lung is transferring oxygen to the blood (oxygenation) in relation to % inspired oxygen.

Base deficit, BD, estimates how much metabolic acid is present in the blood. Base excess (BE), the negative value of BD, and bicarbonate are also used to describe the acid-base status.

Arterial, capillary or venous samples are nearly equally useful for the determination of PCO_2, pH and base deficit.

SpO_2 can be used as a continuous estimate of oxygenation.

Blood gases are considered satisfactory in acute respiratory illness when the pH is 7.25 to 7.40 and PCO_2 45 to 55 mmHg.

The presence of an acidosis (pH ≤ 7.25) with PCO_2 ≥ 55 is an indication of poor ventilation (respiratory acidosis).

 Blood gas interpretation

> You decide that the blood gas result is satisfactory, the pH is between 7.25 and 7.40 and PCO_2 45 to 55 mmHg. You note the baby's grunting now occurs only with stimulation. You reassess the Respiratory Score.

Score	0	1	2
Respiratory rate	40 to 60/minute	60 to 80/minute	> 80/minute
Oxygen requirement[1]	None	≤ 50%	> 50%
Retractions	None	Mild to moderate	Severe
Grunting	None	With stimulation	Continuous at rest
Breath sounds on auscultation	Easily heard throughout	Decreased	Barely heard
Prematurity	> 34 weeks	30 to 34 weeks	< 30 weeks

[1] A baby receiving oxygen prior to the setup of an oxygen analyzer should be assigned a score of "1"

The Respiratory Score of 6 indicates the baby still has moderate respiratory distress.

You decide to continue providing CPAP, paying close attention to the baby's clinical course by repeating a formal assessment of the Respiratory Score and blood gases every 4 to 6 hours. Continuous pulse oximetry is used as your main guide to escalate or wean oxygen therapy.

Over the next 6 hours the baby's oxygen requirements decrease to 30% with SpO_2 around 92%, respiratory rate of 50/minute, and less audible grunting.

Two days later, CPAP is discontinued, and breast milk feeds are initiated.

The day after, the baby is in room air.

Respiratory Case # 3 – Respiratory distress in a preterm newborn – Initiating mechanical ventilation

> An 1800 gram baby boy is born at 32 weeks gestation by Cesarean section following antepartum bleeding because of a placenta previa. The baby developed respiratory distress at birth and was given oxygen and CPAP using a flow-inflating bag and mask in the delivery room and during transfer to the nursery for stabilization. The Apgar score was 7 at 1 minute and 8 at 5 minutes.
>
> On admission to the nursery, the baby has regular but laboured respiration, audible grunting at rest, and marked sternal retractions. The respiratory rate is 80/minute, and the heart rate 160 bpm.

Cyanosis or oxygen requirement is an Alerting Sign for immediate resuscitation. Breathing is laboured but effective. Heart rate is > 100 bpm.

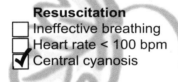

Resuscitation
- ☐ Ineffective breathing
- ☐ Heart rate < 100 bpm
- ☑ Central cyanosis

> You work through the Core Steps of the Resuscitation Sequence. The respiratory rate remains regular and the heart rate approximately 160 bpm. You exit the Resuscitation Sequence and complete the ACoRN Primary Survey.
>
> Your Primary Survey generates a Problem List that indicates that there are three areas of concern: Respiratory, Fluid & Glucose Management, and Thermoregulation.

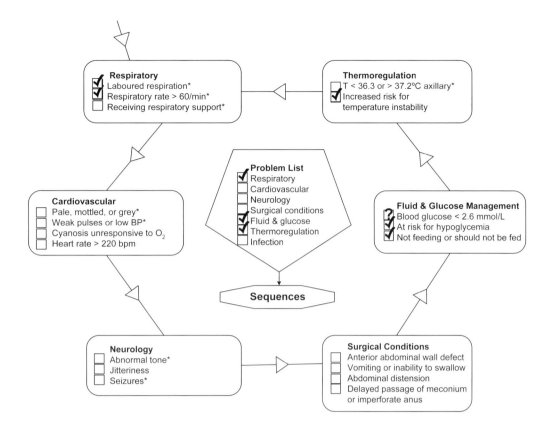

The baby is now in the special care nursery under a radiant warmer with servo control. He is receiving 55% oxygen according to the oxygen blender, and CPAP using a flow-inflating bag and mask system. The respiratory rate is 72/minute. The pulse oximeter reads 92%. He is pink, but continues to grunt at rest, has moderate sternal retractions and intercostal indrawing. You auscultate his chest and find that breath sounds are decreased bilaterally. Non-invasive blood pressure is 48/30 and the mean 36 mmHg (normal range). The heart rate is 160 bpm. The baby's axilla temperature is 36.5°C.

You enter the Respiratory Sequence and carry out the Core Steps and calculate the Respiratory Score.

Score	0	1	2
Respiratory rate	40 to 60/minute	60 to 80/minute	> 80/minute
Oxygen requirement[1]	None	≤ 50%	> 50%
Retractions	None	Mild to moderate	Severe
Grunting	None	With stimulation	Continuous at rest
Breath sounds on auscultation	Easily heard throughout	Decreased	Barely heard
Prematurity	> 34 weeks	30 to 34 weeks	< 30 weeks
[1] A baby receiving oxygen prior to the setup of an oxygen analyzer should be assigned a score of "1"			

The Respiratory Score total is 8, indicating moderate respiratory distress and that respiratory support may be needed.

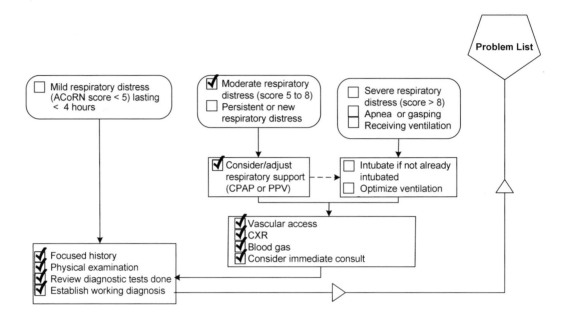

According to the Respiratory Sequence, you should consider or adjust respiratory support for babies with moderate respiratory distress. Administration of oxygen without respiratory support is also an option in moderate respiratory distress, however this increases the risk of gradual deterioration in pulmonary function due to progressive atelectasis.

Respiratory support can be provided as CPAP or mechanical ventilation.

The baby is already receiving CPAP by face mask. However, that is usually not a long term option. You must now decide how you will continue administering CPAP or whether you should initiate mechanical ventilation

I.   **What criteria must be met to consider a baby suitable for CPAP?**

_____

_____

_____

You have the resources needed to initiate CPAP or mechanical ventilation, however keeping a baby in house who is receiving respiratory support is beyond the capability of your hospital.

You request that the baby be transported to a facility where ongoing ventilation is available. In preparation for transport, you then intubate the baby with a 3.0 ETT and initiate mechanical ventilation. You remain in periodic telephone contact with the transport coordinator.

Premedication before elective intubation

Laryngoscopy and intubation are painful procedures that can provoke detrimental responses such as hypertension, increased intracranial pressure, bradycardia, and hypoxia. The goals of premedication are to provide analgesia and to blunt undesirable hemodynamic consequences. Ideally, a premedication regimen includes a combination of opiates (e.g. morphine or fentanyl), atropine, and a short acting paralyzing agent (e.g. succinylcholine). A paralyzing drug should only be administered by personnel familiar with its use and who are skilled in neonatal intubation.

In view of the discomfort and physiologic responses associated with intubation, newborns should be premedicated when possible. Intubation should not be delayed for IV access and premedication in babies requiring urgent or emergent intubation (e.g. during resuscitation).

 Premedication for intubation

Mechanical ventilation

The administration of mechanical ventilation (cycled positive pressure) with positive end expiratory pressure (PEEP) stabilizes the small airways and chest wall, prevents atelectasis at end expiration, and re-expands the lung during inspiration.

Mechanical ventilation is delivered via an endotracheal tube,
- manually (for example, with a flow inflating bag) or
- mechanically, using a ventilator.

The indications for ventilation include,
- ineffective respiration with decreased respiratory drive (irregular breathing or apnea)
- severe respiratory distress (Respiratory Score > 8)
- moderate respiratory distress (Respiratory Score 5 to 8) with unsatisfactory blood gases (pH ≤ 7.25 and $P_{CO_2} \geq 55$) or inability to oxygenate despite CPAP
- as an alternative to CPAP in babies requiring transport.

Mechanical ventilation must be administered and monitored by on-site and trained personnel in a setting with adequate resources for the care of a baby needing respiratory support, or until the baby can be transported out.

Mechanical ventilation

> The Transport Coordinator suggests you obtain vascular access using a
> - peripheral intravenous or
> - an umbilical venous catheter

Vascular access using an umbilical venous line inserted 2 to 3 cm under the skin level, and secured using a silk suture to the remaining umbilical stump allows for short-term blood sampling and infusion of fluids and medications.

© AAP/AHA

Emergency venous access: Umbilical vein catheterization

> You obtain a chest radiograph and venous blood for a blood gas.
>
> You proceed to obtain a focused history and physical examination and review the results of the diagnostic tests requested.
>
> The mother is a 28-year-old in her second pregnancy with an unremarkable past medical history and family history.
>
> She was admitted to hospital 2 days prior for vaginal bleeding. An ultrasound had shown a low placenta and no evidence of abruption. The amount of bleeding increased this morning. A Cesarean section was performed for this reason after discussion with the regional perinatal centre.
>
> Intrapartum antibiotic prophylaxis was initiated before the Cesarean section because of a positive Group B streptococcus screen in her previous pregnancy.
>
> The baby is now receiving mechanical ventilation using a time-cycled, pressure limited ventilator, with pressure of 20/5, rate of 40, and inspiratory time of 0.4 seconds. Oxygen concentration has been weaned to 40% based on pulse oximetry. The SpO_2 is stable around 92%.
>
> The baby appears comfortable. The heart rate, blood pressure, and temperature remain within normal limits. The chest radiograph is shown on the next page.

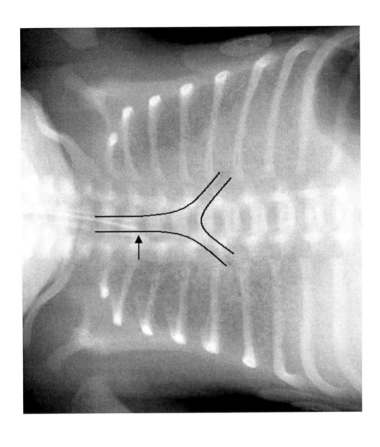

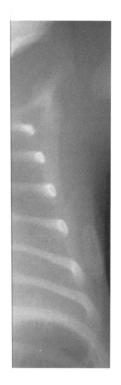

...educed lung volumes with a
...ou also note some air
...he cardiac silhouette, and that
...tured

...ow), appropriately above the

...chest radiograph findings, a
...drome is made.

...the ACoRN Problem List in
...d Thermoregulation.

...th an *, indicating that you will

...spiratory Sequence for RDS.

Errata:

Page 3-49:

The arrow pointing at
the tip of the
endotracheal is
displaced in the
textbook. The
intended position of
the arrow is shown in
the radiograph.

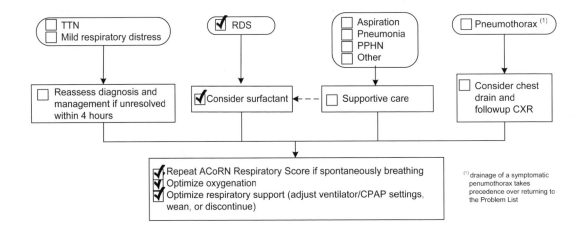

Respiratory distress syndrome (RDS)

RDS is a condition caused by lack of pulmonary surfactant, a soapy material that is normally present in mature lungs. Surfactant reduces the surface tension within the alveoli, preventing their collapse and allowing them to inflate more easily.

In the absence of surfactant, there is widespread atelectasis (alveolar collapse) resulting in decreased lung volume and increased work of breathing. The lung surface area for gas exchange is reduced, resulting in hypoxemia and hypercarbia.

Symptoms usually appear shortly after birth and become progressively more severe. RDS commonly affects preterm babies and is rare in full-term babies.

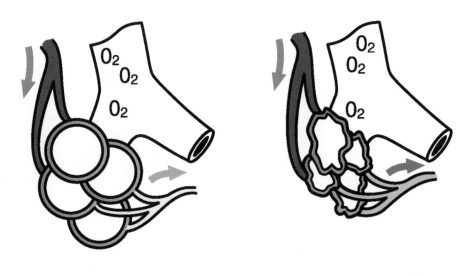

Healthy lung   **Respiratory distress syndrome**

The treatment of RDS is aided by the administration of exogenous surfactant.

Surfactant should be given as early as possible in babies with RDS.
- The early use of surfactant has been shown to reduce mortality, pneumothorax and other complications of RDS
- Surfactant also improves pulmonary function in babies with meconium aspiration syndrome, however,
  - the decision to administer surfactant in babies with MAS should be taken with great caution as these babies may deteriorate due to labile pulmonary hypertension.

How is surfactant administered?

Exogenous surfactant is given directly into the trachea and bronchial tree via the endotracheal tube as shown in the diagram below. The usual dose (depending on the type or brand) is 4 to 5 mL/kg.

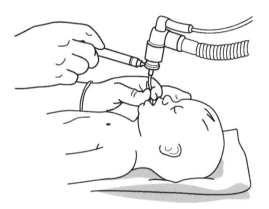

During surfactant administration, many babies desaturate and become transiently bradycardic due to brief obstruction of the airway.
- This usually resolves with positive pressure ventilation
- Sometimes the ventilator settings and the % inspired oxygen need to be increased temporarily
- If desaturation and bradycardia persist, it may be necessary to slow or halt the administration until the baby improves.

Following surfactant administration, as lung inflation improves, the pressures required to inflate the lungs (produce an easy rise of the chest) and % inspired oxygen required often drop dramatically. It is important to,
- closely monitor changes in oximetry readings and serial blood gases
- reduce the peak ventilator pressures as needed to avoid complications of over inflation, including pneumothorax
- reduce the % inspired oxygen to maintain SpO_2 in the desired range.

An improvement in respiratory status may be temporary and does not eliminate the need for transport to a center capable of a higher level of neonatal care.

Health care providers administering surfactant must be skilled in neonatal intubation and be prepared to deal with the rapid changes in lung compliance and oxygenation during and after surfactant is given. They must also be aware of the potential complications of this treatment.

 Surfactant

Post surfactant administration the baby is comfortable in 25% oxygen with SpO_2 of 93%.

The umbilical venous blood gas result is: pH 7.30, PCO_2 45, PO_2 30, BD 3.

You are satisfied that blood gases show a pH between 7.25 and 7.40, and that the PCO_2 is between 45 and 55 mmHg. You disregard the venous PO_2 as the SpO_2 offers a more accurate assessment of oxygenation.

You decide to continue providing mechanical ventilation, paying close attention to the baby's clinical status while awaiting the arrival of the transport team.

Continuous oximetry will be used as your main guide to escalate or wean oxygen therapy, and blood gases will be repeated every 4 to 6 hours if the baby remains stable. You decide that blood gases will be repeated sooner if there is deterioration in the baby's respiratory status such as increased oxygen requirements > 10 to 20%.

At 4 hours of age, the transport team arrives.

The baby's oxygen requirements have remained at 25% with SpO_2 92%. A new blood gas has shown that pH and PCO_2 remain within the desired range. Ventilation settings are: pressure of 20/5, rate of 40/minute, and inspiratory time of 0.4 seconds.

Two days later, you hear that the mother and baby are doing well. The baby is no longer on a ventilator, and feeds are advancing.

Respiratory Case # 4 - Sudden deterioration in a ventilated baby

You are waiting for the transport team to transfer a 1500 gram baby girl, born at 30 weeks gestation, who developed respiratory distress at birth and required intubation, mechanical ventilation and surfactant.

The baby was born 2 hours ago to a mother who presented in active labor, near full dilatation, after a short labor. Intrapartum and post-partum, her temperature was 38°C, and she has been treated with antibiotics for suspicion of chorioamnionitis possibly due to an amniotic fluid leak of 24 hours.

You have worked through all the areas of concern in the ACoRN Primary Survey and the Infection Sequence.

The baby is on a radiant warmer with servo control, and has an umbilical venous catheter for short-term infusions and blood sampling. Pulse oximetry reads 92% and an umbilical venous blood gas, obtained one-hour ago, showed pH 7.34, and P_{CO_2} 45 mmHg on 40% oxygen on ventilator settings of 20/5, rate of 50, and inspiratory time of 0.4 seconds.

As you return to complete your charting after talking to the parents, the nurse tells you that the oxygen requirements have rapidly increased from 40% to 100% in the last 5 minutes and that the baby is "fighting against the ventilator".

You ask the nurse for assistance and rapidly assess the baby using the Alerting Signs of the Resuscitation Sequence. The ventilator is cycling as preset, and air entry can be heard on auscultation of both lungs; the baby is on 100% oxygen, looks pink but mottled and her SpO_2 is 92%. The heart rate on the monitor and by auscultation is 180 bpm.

Resuscitation
- [ ] Ineffective breathing
- [ ] Heart rate < 100 bpm
- [ ] Central cyanosis

Your reassessment indicates the baby needs no resuscitation.

You proceed to the ACoRN Primary Survey.

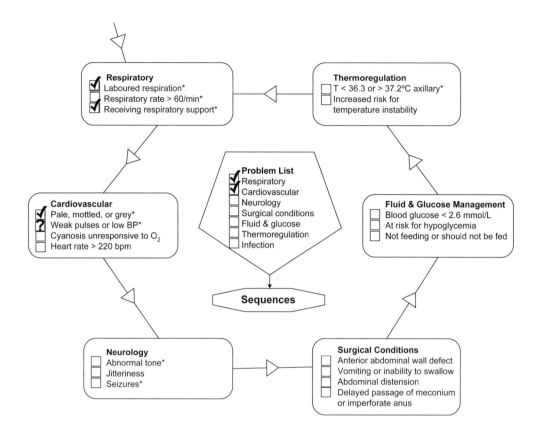

The Primary survey identifies two areas of concern: Respiratory and Cardiovascular. The blood pressure is 40/22 with a mean of 30, which is in the normal range for this baby. Fluid & Glucose Management and Thermoregulation have been monitored regularly and not been a problem.

You enter the Respiratory Sequence.

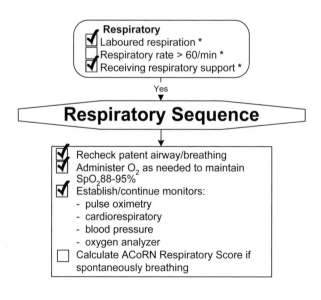

> You check if the airway is patent.

Airway patency Checking for airway patency in an intubated baby includes ensuring that the endotracheal tube (ETT) is not,
- kinked
- obstructed by secretions
- displaced from proper position (baby extubated or tube too far in).

Ensuring that the endotracheal tube is not displaced from its proper position involves,
- making certain that it is at the same cm mark as when inserted
- using an end-tidal CO_2 detector to determine if the tube is in the trachea
- auscultating for presence and symmetry of breath sounds in chest but not over the stomach area (may not be a reliable sign in small babies)
- inspecting the tube position using a laryngoscope.

End-tidal CO_2 detector

> You inspect the endotracheal tube ensuring it is not kinked, and suction for scant amount of loose white secretions. You ensure that the endotracheal tube is not displaced from its proper position.
>
> The baby is already receiving 100% oxygen.
>
> You quickly ensure all monitors are properly placed, but do not calculate the Respiratory Score as the baby is receiving mechanical ventilation.

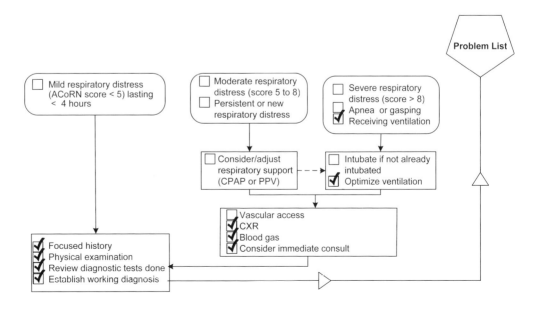

> You proceed to optimize ventilation.

Optimize ventilation Optimizing ventilation involves ensuring that,
- the baby is connected to the ventilator
- the ventilator is delivering the settings indicated and is not malfunctioning
  - check equipment while providing manual ventilation
- chest expansion can be observed and breath sounds are equal and symmetrical
- baby is breathing in synchrony with the ventilator
- pulse oximetry and blood gases are within the target range
  - SpO_2 88 to 95%
  - pH 7.25 to 7.40 and PCO_2 40 to 55 in a capillary, venous or arterial gas.

> You ensure that the ventilator is properly connected to the baby and is not malfunctioning, observe that there is chest expansion and hear bilateral breath sounds. The baby already has a peripheral intravenous line and an umbilical venous catheter in place.
>
> You prepare to obtain an umbilical venous blood gas and request a chest radiograph.
>
> The nurse tells you the baby deteriorated rapidly over the last 5 minutes, needing an increase in oxygen concentration from 40% to 100% in order to maintain a SpO_2 approximately 90% and that bilateral air entry could be heard.
>
> The baby remains mottled. The heart rate is 188 bpm, and the precordium is very active but does not appear to be displaced.

What can cause a sudden deterioration in a ventilated baby?

As you followed the Sequence you have been able to troubleshoot the causes for acute deterioration in a ventilated baby. However, the acronym D.O.P.E. is useful in remembering potential causes:

D…displaced endotracheal tube? Has the baby accidentally extubated or is the endotracheal tube too far in?

O…obstructed airway or endotracheal tube?

P…pneumothorax or other critical diagnosis? Other causes may include pulmonary interstitial emphysema or atelectasis.

E…equipment working and ventilation optimized?

> You decide the working diagnosis needing to be ruled out at this time is the presence of a pneumothorax.

Pneumothorax   A pneumothorax occurs when there is regional or global overdistension of the lung leading to rupture of alveoli or terminal bronchioles and release of intrapulmonary air into the pleural space.

A pneumothorax may occur when there is,
- rapid improvement in lung compliance after surfactant therapy
- excessive airway pressure
- plugging of small airways causing a ball-valve effect.

A "spontaneous pneumothorax" is one that occurs in spontaneously breathing babies, usually around the time of initial lung inflation.

Babies who are at high risk of pneumothorax include those,
- with RDS, MAS or hypoplastic lungs
- receiving respiratory support, especially mechanical ventilation.

The risk of pneumothorax is highest in the first 24 to 48 hours after birth.

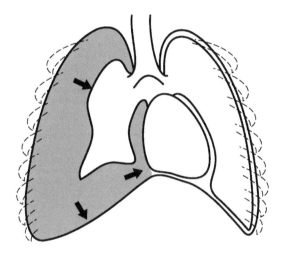

How is a pneumothorax diagnosed?

1. Chest radiograph   A chest radiograph is the definitive test to diagnose a pneumothorax.

2. Chest transillumination   Comparative transillumination of the chest may be useful when a baby is deteriorating rapidly and a chest radiograph cannot be obtained in a timely fashion. Transillumination is less sensitive when used in term and near term babies.

Transillumination **must** be done in a darkened environment using a fiberoptic device capable of delivering high illumination.
- The fiberoptic device must be in direct contact with the baby's chest.
- A unilateral pneumothorax is suspected when the halo around the point of contact is significantly larger on one side of the chest compared to the other.

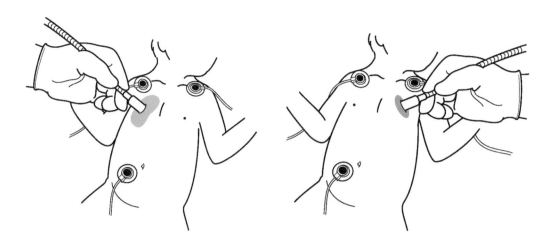

 Pneumothorax - Chest transillumination

You review the chest radiograph.

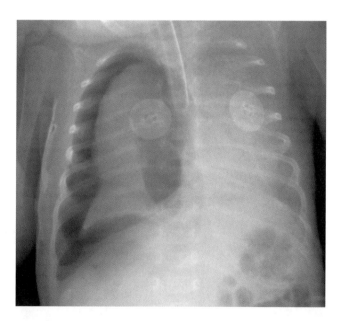

I.   What does the radiograph show?

_____

_____

II.   **List three characteristics of a pneumothorax that does not need drainage.**

_____

_____

_____

Management of a symptomatic pneumothorax

A symptomatic pneumothorax, especially one under tension, needs to be drained urgently and takes precedence over exiting the Respiratory Sequence to complete the Problem List.

There are two ways to drain a pneumothorax: chest tube insertion or needle aspiration.

1. Chest tube insertion

The insertion of a chest tube provides continuous drainage of a pneumothorax, allowing re-expansion of the ipsilateral collapsed lung and release of pressure on the heart and other mediastinal structures.

A chest tube should never be left open to the environment,
- this would allow air to be drawn back into the pleural space with spontaneous respiratory effort.

To prevent air re-entry, before unclamping the chest tube it should be connected to,
- a drainage system with an underwater seal, or
- a Heimlich flutter valve if preparing the baby for transport.

Initial indications that a chest tube is within the pleural space are,
- palpation of the tube between the ribs rather than up the chest wall, just after the tube insertion
- bubbling into the underwater seal at the time of unclamping
- appearance of condensation and serous drainage in the tube
- fluid meniscus moving along the tube
- improvement of the baby's oxygenation and perfusion.

Drainage of frank blood is unusual and may indicate that a blood vessel has been disrupted (e.g. intercostal artery).

Definitive confirmation that the chest tube placement is intrapleural and the pneumothorax is drained is by chest radiograph.

Pneumothorax - Chest tube insertion

2. Needle aspiration   This procedure should only be undertaken as an emergency in a baby with significant compromise and a positive transillumination or chest radiograph.

- In severely symptomatic babies it may be necessary to proceed with needle aspiration prior to a confirmatory chest radiograph after ensuring the endotracheal tube has not been displaced or obstructed.

Needle aspiration is usually an interim measure pending placement of a chest tube.

The needle can be held in place for ongoing removal of air or be connected to an underwater seal.

 Pneumothorax - Needle aspiration

You insert the needle through the second intercostal space, just above the third rib, over the midclavicular line, and remove 50 mL of air. The SpO_2 improves to 95% and she looks less mottled. Gradually, the oxygen is weaned to 60%. The heart rate is now 165 bpm and the blood pressure 42/28 mmHg (mean is 34 mmHg).

The nursery staff prepares equipment for the chest tube insertion. An assistant holds the needle in place and aspirates intermittently, using a stopcock, to withdraw any re-accumulation of air.

You exit the Respiratory Sequence and return to the Problem List. As you enter the Cardiovascular Sequence you note the baby's perfusion and blood pressure have normalized and the baby no longer meets the alerting signs.

Because antibiotics were initiated 2 hours ago you do not need to re-enter the Infection Sequence.

You proceed to insert a chest tube. After the chest tube is inserted you see condensation in the tube along with a small amount of serous fluid. The chest tube is sutured in place and attached to an underwater drainage system.

A chest radiograph is ordered to check the position of the chest tube and to ensure the pneumothorax has been drained.

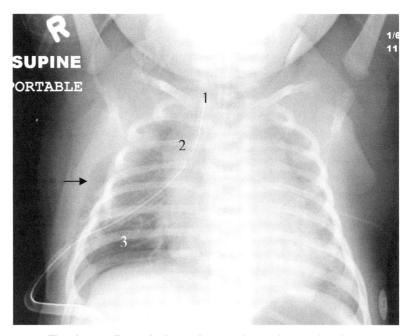

- The chest radiograph above shows a chest tube entering the chest through the 6th intercostal space.
- The tip of the chest tube is high (1); a more desirable position is shown with the number (2).
- The arrow shows that there is some air trapped under the skin (subcutaneous emphysema).
- There is a small residual pneumothorax identified by the increased lucency in the area between the chest tube and the right hemidiaphragm (3) and by the ease with which the dome of the right hemidiaphragm can be seen.

You can now assess and optimize oxygenation and ventilation by repeating the blood gases and adjusting the amount of oxygen being delivered and the ventilator settings.

When the transport team arrives the baby is stable on 50% oxygen and the ventilator settings have been weaned.

Several hours later, you hear from the admitting physician that the baby and mother have arrived in good condition.

Respiratory Case # 5 – Meconium aspiration

You are called to the Cesarean delivery of a baby at 41 weeks and 3 days gestation. There is copious meconium noted at birth and the baby is not vigorous. Following resuscitation guidelines, the baby is carried to the radiant warmer and is endotracheally suctioned twice for moderate amounts of thick green meconium.

The baby requires positive pressure ventilation and chest compressions before the heart rate rises above 100 bpm at 2 minutes of age. Recovery of heart rate is followed by respiratory effort and improvement in color by 4 minutes. Tone and reflex irritability are beginning to improve by 6 minutes of age. The assigned Apgar score is 1, 5 and 8 at one, five and ten minutes respectively.

Post resuscitation the baby is pink with free flow oxygen by face mask and has labored respiration with nasal flaring, retractions and grunting. Respiratory rate is 90/minute, heart rate 156 bpm, BP 64/41 mmHg, and axillary temperature 36.3°C.

You determine that the baby shows no resuscitation signs for immediate resuscitation now and proceed to complete the ACoRN primary survey to generate the problem list.

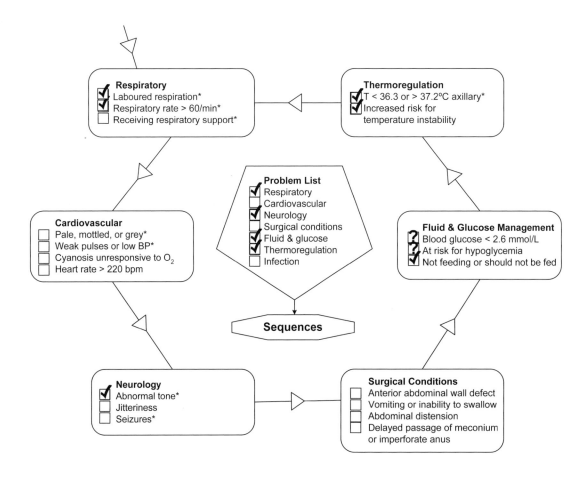

ACoRN

You enter the Respiratory Sequence and carry out the Core Steps.

The baby is already on a radiant warmer with servocontrol, in an oxygen hood with 45% oxygen, and monitors are attached. The SpO_2 reads 90%.

You calculate the Respiratory Score.

Score	0	1	2
Respiratory rate	40 to 60/minute	60 to 80/minute	> 80/minute
Oxygen requirement[1]	None	≤ 50%	> 50%
Retractions	None	Mild to moderate	Severe
Grunting	None	With stimulation	Continuous at rest
Breath sounds on auscultation	Easily heard throughout	Decreased	Barely heard
Prematurity	> 34 weeks	30 to 34 weeks	< 30 weeks

[1] A baby receiving oxygen prior to the setup of an oxygen analyzer should be assigned a score of "1"

The Respiratory Score adds up to 7, indicating moderate respiratory distress and that respiratory support may be needed.

You ask the Respiratory Therapist to start nasal CPAP of 5 cm H_2O, and request a chest radiograph.

You also prepare to insert an umbilical venous catheter in order to have intravenous access and obtain blood for a blood gas. A blood glucose determination is needed to complete the Primary Survey.

Based on the presenting history and signs of respiratory distress you are concerned that the baby may have aspirated meconium, and decide to obtain a consult alerting your regional transport coordinator.

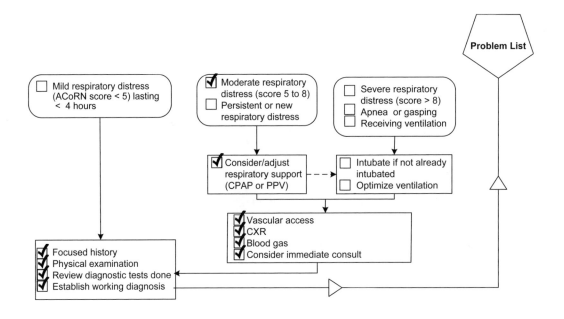

Your focused physical examination shows the baby is receiving CPAP 5 cm H_2O and 45% oxygen. The respiratory rate is 76/minute, heart rate 154 bpm, and blood pressure 58/32 mmHg (mean 46). The oxygen saturation is 92%.

You note he is a well grown, post dates male weighing 3890 grams. He is centrally pink with acrocyanosis. Meconium staining is noted in the skin creases and around his umbilical cord. There are no dysmorphic features or other abnormalities found on physical examination.

Satisfied that he is stable for the present, you go to the parents to obtain a focused history and inform them of their baby's current condition and the management plans.

Mother is a healthy 32-year-old whose pregnancy was uneventful. The maternal serum screen and screening ultrasounds were normal and GBS swab was negative at 36 weeks. Labor was induced due to post dates. Membranes were ruptured artificially 6 hours prior to birth at which time meconium was noted. Electronic fetal monitoring was non-reassuring during the second stage and a caesarean section was performed.

The admission chest radiograph is shown on the next page.

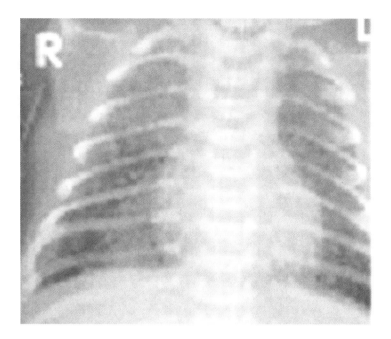

I. **What does the radiograph above show?**

_____

> Having established a working diagnosis, you move to address the rest of the ACoRN Problem List to address Neurology, Fluid & Glucose Management and Thermoregulation.
>
> You note that in the Primary Survey there are four Alerting Signs with * which necessitate entering the Infection Sequence. You would initiate antibiotic therapy as this baby is receiving respiratory support and respiratory distress is unlikely to resolve by 4 hours of age.

Babies with respiratory distress should be treated with antibiotics after obtaining blood cultures.
- Early sepsis and pneumonia are indistinguishable clinically and radiologically from other forms of respiratory distress.

II. **Can you manage this baby in your hospital? Why or why not?**

_____

_____

You enter the Specific Management section of the Respiratory Sequence.

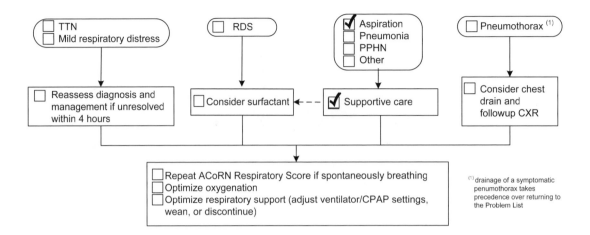

[¹] drainage of a symptomatic penumothorax takes precedence over returning to the Problem List

What is Meconium Aspiration Syndrome (MAS)

In MAS, respiratory distress is secondary to the aspiration of meconium.

Respiratory distress in MAS can be mild and transient, or severe leading to respiratory failure with hypoxemia, acidosis and persistent pulmonary hypertension (PPHN). MAS always warrants close observation as even babies who are initially stable can deteriorate quickly and develop refractory PPHN

Aspiration of meconium has three main effects on pulmonary function,
- airway obstruction
- surfactant inactivation
- chemical pneumonitis.

Because MAS is a disease that begins with fetal compromise in utero, it appears that most cases are not preventable with interventions at birth, such as endotracheal suctioning.

The main complications of MAS are,
- respiratory failure
- PPHN
- pulmonary air leaks, especially pneumothorax.

1. Avoiding respiratory failure The best strategy to avoid respiratory failure is to maintain optimal lung inflation and prevent atelectasis.
- In babies with moderate respiratory distress associated with MAS, this is best accomplished using CPAP.

2. Avoiding PPHN

PPHN is a pulmonary vascular disorder that may have its onset in utero. The mechanisms for its development are not fully understood.

The pulmonary arterioles may show,
- increased muscularization
- increased contraction and reactivity
- decreased responsiveness to endogenous vasodilating stimuli
- increased responsiveness to endogenous vasocontrictive stimuli

In addition, babies with CDH and lung hypoplasia have decreased airway and pulmonary arteriolar branching.

Interventions that help decrease the pulmonary arterial pressures during or following transition in babies prone to PPHN include,
- minimizing handling and disturbance
- maintaining oxygenation in the high end of the normal range
  - PO_2 70 to 90 mmHg, and SpO_2 approximately 95%
- minimizing atelectasis while avoiding overdistension in babies with moderate to severe respiratory distress
  - CPAP
  - surfactant therapy
  - mechanical ventilation
- avoiding and correcting respiratory and metabolic acidosis to maintain initially
  - pH 7.30 to 7.40
  - PCO_2 40 to 50 mmHg.

Once established, PPHN is very difficult to treat.

3. Avoiding pulmonary air leaks

The best strategy to avoid pulmonary air leaks is to prevent lung overdistension. For babies receiving mechanical ventilation, this is best accomplished by,
- avoiding overdistension by limiting levels of CPAP to 5 to 6 cmH_2O
- avoiding overventilation (PCO_2 < 35 mmHg)
- administering surfactant
- suctioning the ETT when needed.

Inspired oxygen concentration remains at 45%, and at SpO_2 95%. The umbilical venous blood gas results show pH 7.28, PCO_2 52, PO_2 30, BD 2.

The hemoglobin is 162 g/L, WBC 22.1 x 10^9 /L and platelets 216 x 10^9 /L.

Blood glucose is 2.9 mmol/L.

You reassess and optimize oxygenation and respiratory support, and repeat the Respiratory Score.

Baby remains tachypneic with moderate sternal and intercostal retractions and nasal flaring. His grunting is less prominent than prior to starting CPAP. Air entry is equal bilaterally but crackly and diminished at the bases. The ACoRN Respiratory Score is now 5.

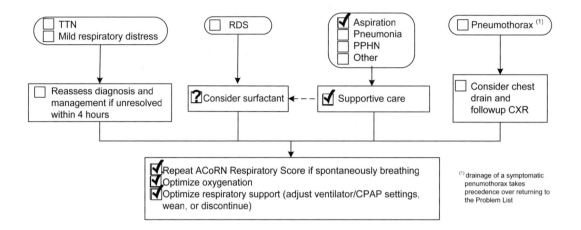

After reassessing the ACoRN Respiratory Score and blood gases, you decide the baby is managing well on CPAP, and it is not necessary to consider escalation of therapy with mechanical ventilation at this point.

Mechanical ventilation in MAS

Mechanical ventilation is usually reserved for babies with,
- oxygen requirement > 60% to maintain SpO_2 > 90%,
- PCO_2 > 55 or pH < 7.25.

However,
- the acts of intubation and initiation of mechanical ventilation can cause a baby with MAS to react adversely and PPHN to worsen
  - this complication may be decreased by use of premedication for intubation, and sedation during mechanical ventilation
- babies with MAS often have low lung compliance, and require high ventilation pressure (> 25 to 28/5 cmH_2O)
  - muscle paralysis may become necessary to achieve control of ventilation and oxygenation.

Surfactant therapy

Meconium aspiration causes secondary surfactant deficiency. Clinical trials have shown that surfactant replacement therapy is beneficial in MAS. However, surfactant must be administered cautiously, avoiding hypoxia and excessive stimulation with negative effects on the labile pulmonary circulation.

As you wait for the transport team to arrive, you discuss with the staff in the nursery other considerations that are important when stabilizing a baby with MAS.

Blood pressure and intravascular volume

Babies with MAS and PPHN may have a pulmonary arterial pressure that exceeds their systemic blood pressure. This leads to right to left shunting through the ductus arteriosus, and post-ductal hypoxemia.

When right ventricular pressure is supra-systemic, the amount of blood pumped by the heart may decrease (right ventricle failure). The right atrial pressure increases leading to right to left shunting through the foramen ovale.

These babies also third-space considerable amounts of intravascular volume.

Maintenance of systemic blood pressure at least level with the pulmonary arterial pressure is important in the management of MAS with PPHN. Volume expansion and inotropic therapy may be necessary to maintain blood pressure. Dopamine is the inotropic drug most commonly used for initial therapy.

Minimizing stimulation

Babies with MAS and others predisposed to PPHN have labile pulmonary circulation, and drop their oxygenation in response to stimuli such as excessive handling, painful procedures, bright lights or loud noises.

The following interventions are useful:
- shielding the baby's eyes from light
- speaking in a low voice, and away from the baby's bed
- minimizing handling
- nesting
- providing adequate pain relief
- considering the need for sedation (only in a ventilated baby).

You discuss the baby's condition with the neonatologist at the regional level III center. There are no additional management suggestions. A decision is made jointly that this baby should be transferred to the level III center as soon as possible.

You ask for that transport arrangements be also made for the mother, to minimize separation from her baby.

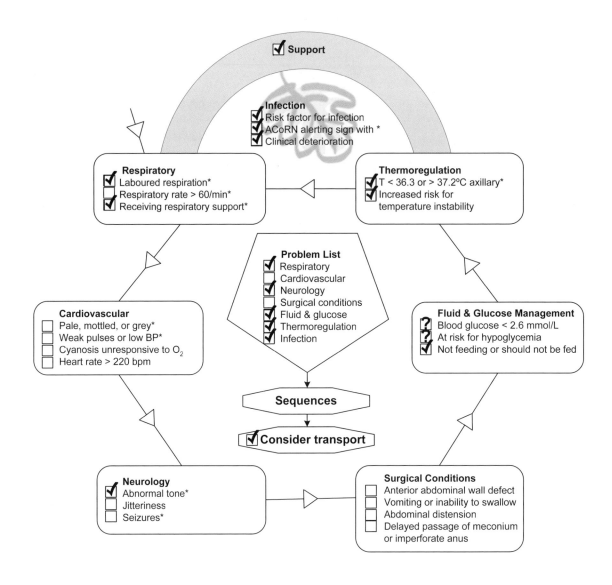

The transport team arrives two hours later. The baby remains in stable condition, and is now on 30% oxygen. After transferring the baby to the transport incubator and talking to the parents, the team departs indicating that they will call as soon as they arrive to at the referral hospital. They also indicate that arrangements have been made for admission of the mother to a ward in close proximity to the baby.

One week later, the mother calls to say that her baby is being discharged home in good condition.

Answers to the questions in Chapter 3

Case # 1:

I. **Why is the diagnosis of TTN likely?**

Born at term	Cesarean section
No labor	Mild respiratory distress (ACoRN Respiratory Score < 4)

Case # 2:

I. **What is the definition of ineffective breathing? Does the description of this baby meet the definition?**

Heart rate < 100 bpm or irregular respirations with apnea or airway obstruction

No, the baby does not meet the definition

II. **Complete the primary survey above to generate your problem list.**

Labored respirations	Respiratory rate > 60
? Blood glucose < 2.6 mmol/L	? at risk for hypoglycemia
? Not feeding or should not be fed	? T < 36.3 or > 37.2°C axillary
Increased risk for temperature instability	

III. **Name two types of respiratory support that may assist babies in moderate respiratory distress.**

CPAP

Ventilation

IV. **Why do this baby's Alerting Signs indicate that he should enter the Infection Sequence?**

Respiratory distress is a common presentation of infection in the newborn

Infection may mimic any persistent radiographic abnormality

Case # 3:

I.   **What criteria must be met to consider a baby suitable for CPAP?**

Moderate respiratory distress

Spontaneous breathing with adequate ventilation (pH 7.25 to 7.40 and P_{CO_2} 45 to 55)

Trained personnel on site

Case # 4:

I.   **What does the radiograph show?**

A large right sided tension pneumothorax. The diaphragm is depressed on the

right side and the mediastinum shifted to the left.

II.   **List three characteristics of a pneumothorax that does not need drainage.**

Small, with no signs of tension

Minimal respiratory (tachypnea only) signs

No cardiovascular effects

Case # 5:

I.   **What does the radiograph above show?**

Bilateral coarse infiltrates consistent with meconium aspiration syndrome

Bibliography

Goldsmith JP, Karotkin EH. Assisted Ventilation of the Neonate. 4th ed. Philadelphia, PA: Saunders; 2003.

Czervinske M. Perinatal and Pediatric Respiratory Care. WB Saunders Co. Aug 2002.

Management of neonatal respiratory distress syndrome. RCPCH Guidelines for good practice, Dec 2000. Accessed 5th Nov 2004
http://www.rcpch.ac.uk/publications/clinical_docs/GGPrespiratory.pdf

Dinwiddie R. Diagnosis and Management of Paediatric Respiratory Disease: Chapter 3, Neonatal Respiratory Disorders. Churchill Livingstone, 1997.

Chapter 4
Cardiovascular

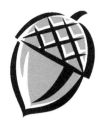

Objectives

Upon completion of this chapter, you should be able to:
1. Describe babies who require cardiovascular stabilization.
2. Apply the Cardiovascular Sequence.
3. Assess the adequacy of circulation.
4. Recognize and manage circulatory shock.
5. Recognize and manage cyanosis.
6. Recognize and manage tachycardia.
7. Recognize when to exit to the other ACoRN Sequences.

Key Concepts

1. Shock, cyanosis despite oxygen therapy, or tachycardia are indicators of cardiovascular instability.
2. Respiratory distress may be a presenting sign of cardiac instability.
3. Babies with serious congenital heart disease may appear well initially.
4. The underlying cause of shock is often difficult to ascertain at presentation, but all causes are characterized by under-perfusion of vital organs; therefore, volume expansion should be considered in advance of making a diagnosis.
5. Shock may also be the initial presentation of sepsis; these babies should be treated with antibiotics.
6. The classic presentations of duct-dependent congenital heart disease are cyanosis and/or shock.
7. Prostaglandin E_1 is the life-saving treatment in duct-dependent congenital heart disease.
8. Supraventricular tachycardia (SVT) should be considered when the heart rate is > 220 bpm.

Skills

- Blood pressure measurement
- Cardiorespiratory monitoring
- Chest radiograph interpretation
- Prostaglandin E_1 (PGE$_1$)
- Dopamine

Introduction

Failure of ventilation and/or oxygenation is a critical cause of cardiovascular instability in newborns. The Resuscitation and Respiratory Sequences address these problems.

Once effective ventilation and oxygenation are established, cardiovascular instability is most commonly due to decreased oxygen delivery to the tissues due to one or more of the following:

- insufficient circulating blood volume
- poor heart muscle function (myocardial dysfunction)
- anatomical abnormalities of the heart and great vessels (cyanotic and acyanotic congenital heart disease)
- abnormality of heart rhythm (tachyarrhythmia or bradyarrhythmia)
  - bradyarrhythmias are uncommon in newborns and are outside the scope of ACoRN

Alerting Signs

A baby who demonstrates one or more of the following Alerting Signs enters the Cardiovascular Sequence:

> **Cardiovascular**
> ☐ Pale, mottled, or grey*
> ☐ Weak pulses or low BP*
> ☐ Cyanosis unresponsive to O_2
> ☐ Heart rate > 220 bpm

Pale, mottled or grey

A pale, mottled, or grey appearance is a manifestation of poor skin perfusion, which should alert one to conditions that result in redistribution of blood flow to the vital organs. This appearance is more pronounced when there is decreased cardiac output, such as in hypovolemia or impaired cardiac function, and less pronounced when skin perfusion is decreased due to cold stress, acidosis, and/or pain. This Alerting Sign may also be present in babies on vasopressor medications (dopamine and epinephrine).

Pulse oximetry can usually distinguish between poor skin perfusion (SpO_2 is normal) and central cyanosis, however, pulse oximetry may not function reliably in very low cardiac output states or when there is marked edema.

Weak pulses or low blood pressure

Radial, posterior tibial, brachial, and femoral arterial pulses are usually palpable in healthy babies. In cardiovascular instability, some or all of the peripheral pulses (particularly the more distal radial and posterior tibial pulses) may be diminished or absent, and therefore difficult to palpate.

The normal range of blood pressure varies with gestational age, weight, postnatal age, and status as small for gestational age (SGA) or large for gestational age (LGA). No single blood pressure chart addresses all conditions and all babies. A practical estimate of the normal lower limit of mean arterial blood pressure in mmHg at birth is the baby's gestational age in completed weeks. It is important to note that 10% of healthy term newborns and a higher percentage of extremely preterm newborns may have a low mean arterial blood pressure using this criterion. In an otherwise well baby, treatment should not be guided by blood pressure measurement alone.

Low blood pressure may reflect low circulating blood volume, low cardiac output, or peripheral vasodilatation.

 Blood pressure measurement

Cyanosis unresponsive to oxygen therapy
Central cyanosis is always abnormal. It is clinically observed as a bluish discoloration (duskiness) of the body, lips, and mucous membranes. It occurs due to the presence in the arterial and capillary blood of a larger proportion of darker, oxygen-depleted blood when,
- the lungs fail to oxygenate the blood passing through them,
- part of the blood pumped by the right side of the heart bypasses the lungs, or
- oxygenated blood coming from the lungs mixes with deoxygenated blood before it is pumped by the left side of the heart.

Generally cyanosis is only detectable by the eye when ≥ 50 g/L of deoxygenated hemoglobin is present in the capillary blood. This usually occurs when the SaO_2 is in the 73 to 78% range in babies with normal hemoglobin levels.
- In the presence of marked anemia, hypoxia may not be observed as cyanosis.
- Cyanosis may be more difficult to detect despite hypoxia in babies with dark skin, or when lighting is poor.

Slow capillary circulation (hyperviscosity due to high hemoglobin levels, or conditions with low cardiac output) leads to peripheral cyanosis, which may be confused with central cyanosis.

A low saturation reading by pulse oximetry or a low PaO_2 value confirms the presence of cyanosis.

Heart rate > 220 bpm
Babies show great variation in heart rate depending on their baseline heart rate and level of arousal. The normal heart rate range is from 100 to 160 bpm, but some term babies may have a resting heart rate as low as 80 bpm. Heart rates between 160 and 220 may be seen when a baby is agitated or sick (sinus tachycardia).

A heart rate > 220 almost always indicates an abnormal fast rhythm or tachyarrhythmia. It is important to confirm by auscultation or palpation to rule out double counting by the cardiorespiratory monitor. Supraventricular tachycardia (SVT) is the most common tachyarrhythmia in babies.

Babies with a tachyarrhythmia may be stable or may show decreased level of consciousness and activity, low tone, and other cardiovascular or respiratory signs of instability.

The Cardiovascular Sequence

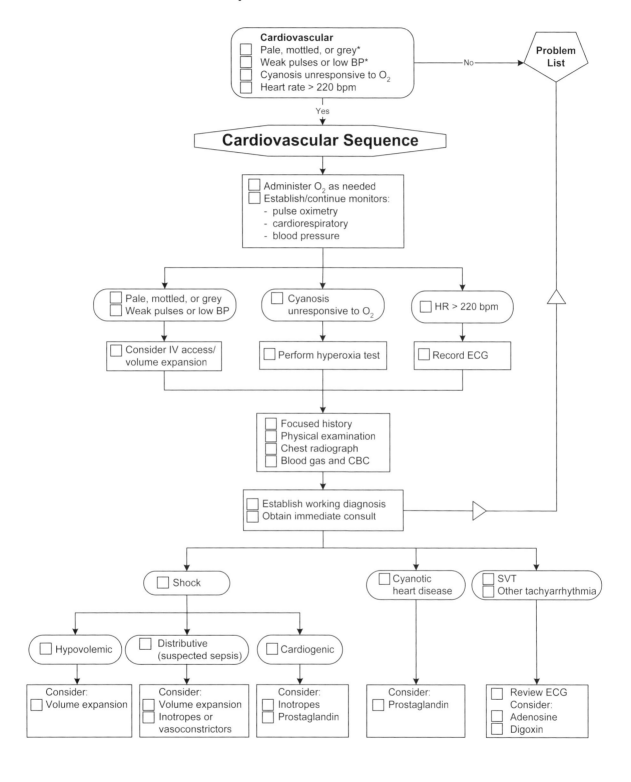

Most babies with SVT can sustain heart rates of up to 250 bpm for several hours, allowing time for consultation prior to initiation of medical treatment. Babies with sustained tachyarrhythmia will eventually develop signs of heart failure.

Core Steps

These are the interventions and monitoring activities applicable to all babies who enter the Cardiovascular Sequence. These include:

- administer oxygen as needed
- establish/continue pulse oximetry, cardiorespiratory, and blood pressure monitors.

 Cardiorespiratory monitoring

Organization of Care

The course of action for babies with cardiovascular compromise depends on whether the baby has poor circulation, cyanosis, or tachycardia.

When there is an overlap of these categories, the organization of care should be prioritized using the following considerations:

- A baby with tachycardia can also be pale, mottled, or grey.
  - o   If the heart rate is > 220 bpm the rhythm is most likely to be SVT, and evaluation and treatment of the tachyarrhythmia takes priority.
  - o   If the heart rate is 160 to 220 bpm, then low perfusion or congenital heart disease are the more likely causes of the tachycardia.
- A baby with cyanosis can also have poor circulation. The underlying cause is likely cyanotic congenital heart disease with poor cardiac output. This is a medical emergency requiring immediate consultation and treatment (for example, prostaglandin infusion).

Clinical assessment of circulation

Assessment of the adequacy of circulation (circulatory stability) involves checking,

- level of consciousness (LOC), activity, and tone
- skin color
- capillary refill time
- temperature of extremities
- pulses
- blood pressure
- heart rate.

To understand the significance of these findings in terms of cardiovascular status, they must be interpreted in conjunction with each other, and with a focused history and physical examination.

LOC, activity and tone   A baby with inadequate circulation or oxygenation becomes lethargic, and shows a decreased level of activity and low tone. These signs are important when trying to determine if a baby is coping with cardiovasculr distress due to shock, cyanosis or prolonged tachycardia.

Skin color   Observing a baby's skin color provides an opportunity to gain a sense of the amount of blood flowing to the skin, the amount of hemoglobin contained in that blood, and the degree of oxygenation of the hemoglobin. These observations are described using words like "pink", "pale", "mottled", "grey", "blue", "dusky", "plethoric" (ruddy), "centrally cyanotic" and "acrocyanotic".

"Pink" implies oxygenated blood and well-perfused skin. "Pale, mottled, or grey" implies poor skin perfusion due to decreased cardiac output and/or hypovolemia, or peripheral vasoconstriction. "Pallor" may also indicate low blood hemoglobin content. "Plethora" implies a high hemoglobin level, and may also be associated with sluggish circulation due to high blood viscosity.

Capillary refill time   The capillary refill time is estimated by pressing the skin in a central location (sternum or forehead) for 2 seconds, and then counting the number of seconds for the blanched skin to refill with capillary blood. This is repeated in a peripheral location (distal limb).
- the normal capillary refill time is ≤3 seconds in a central and peripheral location
- a longer capillary refill time or widening between central and peripheral locations indicates decreased peripheral perfusion. This may be due to hypovolemia, decreased cardiac output, or when blood is being diverted from the skin (for example, vasoconstriction due to cold stress, or inotropic medication).

Temperature of extremities   The temperature of feet and hands are felt and subjectively compared to the temperature over the trunk. Normally, the temperature of all three areas feels similar.

Cool feet and hands in comparison with the trunk suggest poor peripheral perfusion, however this sign may be partially masked in babies nursed under radiant warmers.

Pulses   Pulses are palpated in order to determine if they feel normal, increased or decreased. Upper and lower limb pulses need to be compared.

Pulses may be weak globally, or weaker or absent distally when compared to proximal pulses if the baby is hypovolemic, peripherally vasoconstricted or when cardiac output is decreased such as in hypoplastic left heart syndrome or critical aortic stenosis. In coarctation of the aorta, the lower extremity pulses (femoral, popliteal, posterior tibial and pedal) are markedly decreased compared to the upper extremity (brachial, ulnar and radial) pulses.

Palpating pulses is an acquired skill. Routinely checking pulses in healthy babies will help you become familiar with their characteristics.

Blood pressure   It is normal for the systolic blood pressure in the legs to be slightly higher than systolic blood pressure in the arms, but the mean blood pressure should be the same.

Upper and lower limb, and right and left arm blood pressure should be compared, as the left subclavian artery may take off before, at, or after the ductus. A pre-ductal right arm systolic blood pressure ≥ 15 mmHg above the post-ductal lower limb systolic blood pressure is abnormal. A difference of ≥ 10 mmHg in systolic blood pressure between arms is also abnormal. Both may indicate coarctation of the aorta or related aortic abnormalities.

It is rare to find a significant difference in blood pressure in the absence of a palpable difference in pulses. If there is a difference in limb blood pressure measurements, recheck the pulses.

Clinical assessment of cyanosis

Cyanosis of respiratory origin   Central cyanosis may be of respiratory or cardiac origin.

Cyanosis of respiratory origin is associated with respiratory distress and usually responds to oxygen therapy. In cyanosis of respiratory origin all of the blood pumped by the right ventricle goes through the lungs before being pumped by the left ventricle to the body.

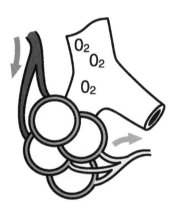

Healthy lung (alveoli well inflated), room air, blood oxygenated in the lung is "pink" (light color).

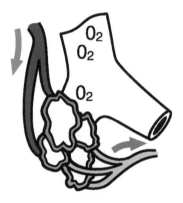

Alveoli poorly inflated, room air, blood oxygenated in the lung is cyanotic (dark).

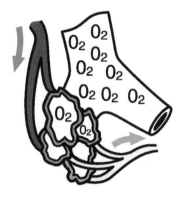

Alveoli poorly inflated, on supplemental oxygen, blood oxygenated in the lung is "pink (light color).

Cyanosis of cardiac origin   Cyanosis of cardiac origin is strongly suggested when it occurs in the absence of respiratory distress and is unresponsive to 100% oxygen therapy.

Cyanosis of cardiac origin occurs when blood that has been oxygenated in the lungs mixes with oxygen-depleted blood via a structural abnormality in the heart or great vessels. A "right-to-left shunt" is said to occur when venous blood is recirculated to the body without having reached the lungs to become oxygenated. Since the blood that passes through the lungs is already being oxygenated and the blood shunted away from the lungs cannot be oxygenated, providing supplemental oxygen does not substantially improve the oxygen saturation in the mixture or the central cyanosis.

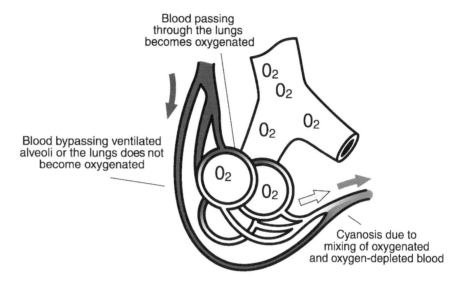

The blood that passes through the lungs is already being oxygenated and the blood shunted away from the lungs cannot be oxygenated. Providing supplemental oxygen does not substantially improve the oxygen saturation in the mixture or the central cyanosis.

Babies with cyanotic congenital heart disease often have minimal respiratory distress, presenting with a slightly elevated respiratory rate and easy breathing. Many of these babies have so-called ductus-dependent cyanosis which becomes more evident as the ductus arteriosus begins to close. In these babies, maintaining the ductus open is a critical part of stabilization.

A baby who has a documented $PaO_2 > 150$ mmHg is not likely to have cyanotic heart disease.

Response

The immediate response depends on the main manifestation identified during the organization of care.

Shock

A pale, mottled, or grey appearance, with weak pulses, and/or low blood pressure is characteristic of low cardiac output states or shock. Shock is an unstable cardiovascular state in which cardiac output is insufficient to meet the oxygen and energy demands of the vital organs, resulting in deteriorating organ function and the build-up of metabolic by-products. If untreated, shock is usually fatal.

The cause of shock may not be obvious, but regardless of the cause, it is a condition characterized by underperfusion of the vital organs.

Initial management, instituted in advance of developing a working diagnosis, includes immediate establishment of venous access and administration of an intravascular volume expander (0.9% NaCl) at an initial dose of 10 mL/kg.

Cyanosis The hyperoxia test is useful for distinguishing cyanotic disorders of respiratory origin from those of cardiovascular origin with a fixed right to left shunt, on the basis that oxygen administration improves oxygenation in lung disease.

Tachyarrhythmia In babies with a heart rate > 220 bpm, an electrocardiogram (ECG) should be obtained promptly. The ECG will be needed by an immediately consulted specialist for advice on management, and may need to be faxed if this is an external resource. Therapeutic intervention is rarely required within minutes or prior to completing the ACoRN Next Steps, and should await the immediately obtained specialist advice.

Next Steps

The Next Steps are to obtain a focused history, conduct a physical examination, order diagnostic tests, and establish a working diagnosis.

Focused cardiovascular history

Information obtained during the focused cardiovascular history that may be helpful in reaching a working diagnosis includes:

Antepartum
- a family history of congenital heart disease or genetic syndromes that may be associated with cardiac disease (for example, Marfan's syndrome, Noonan's syndrome)
- maternal medical conditions such as diabetes or collagen vascular disease (for example, lupus)
- infections or exposure to teratogens (for example, alcohol, cocaine, phenytoin, or lithium) in early pregnancy
- antenatal ultrasound diagnosis of cardiac abnormalities
- rapid or slow fetal heart rate in utero

Intrapartum
- indicators of fetal compromise during labour (non-reassuring or ominous fetal surveillance and/or fetal acidosis) and delivery
- excessive blood loss (for example, abruption) or other complications encountered during delivery
- abnormal cord insertion on examination of the placenta
- risk factors for sepsis

Neonatal
- onset of symptoms (at birth or during the first week of life)
- disinterest in, or fatigue with, feeding
- excessive weight gain or loss
- diaphoresis

Physical examination In addition to the examination conducted during the Primary Survey, a focused cardiovascular physical examination should include:

Observation
- color
- dysmorphic features – chromosomal abnormalities such as trisomy 21, 13 or 18, and genetic syndromes markedly increase the risk of congenital heart disease

Measurement of vital signs: respiratory rate, heart rate, temperature, oxygen saturation, and 4-limb blood pressure.

Examination
- level of consciousness and activity, and tone
- peripheral edema
- increased respiratory rate due to pulmonary congestion
- capillary refill time, evaluated centrally and peripherally
- temperature of feet and hands, subjectively compared to the temperature over the trunk
- pulses palpated in the upper and lower extremities, described and compared
- an observable active precordium or palpation of an increased cardiac impulse over the sternum (right ventricle) or apex (left ventricle) is suspicious of cardiac disease; less common are a palpable second heart sound or a thrill (a palpable murmur, which is always abnormal but very rare in the newborn)
- auscultation of abnormal heart sounds and murmurs
  - a murmur in the presence of cardiac instability is a strong indicator of cardiac disease; murmurs heard away from the heart (in the chest or back) are abnormal
  - a gallop rhythm (three consecutive heart sounds instead of two) may be heard in babies with heart failure
  - soft, flow murmurs at the apex or over the large vessels are common in the newborn
- the presence of hepatomegaly is suggested when the edge of the liver is palpable ≥ 3 cm below the costal margin; in lung disease with hyperinflation the liver may be displaced downwards

Diagnostic tests Four diagnostic tests that can assist in reaching a working diagnosis for cardiovascular conditions include:

1. **Chest radiograph**
    *   The most helpful view is supine and antero-posterior (AP), preferably including the upper abdomen to determine the position of the stomach.
    *   Four questions are asked when reviewing chest radiograph during a cardiovascular assessment:
        o   is the heart size normal, large or small?
        o   is the heart shape normal or abnormal?
        o   are the lung vascular markings normal, increased or decreased?
        o   is the stomach in the normal position?

 Chest radiograph interpretation

Normal chest radiograph

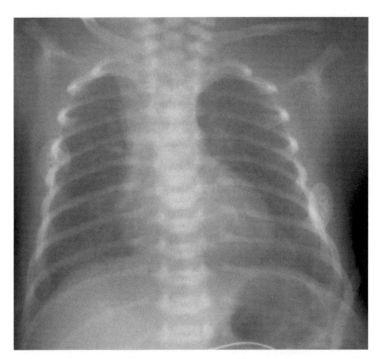

Normal heart size and shape, normal vascular markings, and stomach in the normal position.

**Transposition of
the great arteries
(TGA)**

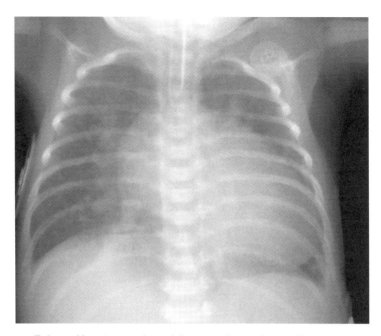

Enlarged heart, egg-shaped, increased vascular markings.
The stomach is not visible in this particular view.

**Left-to-right shunt
due to PDA**

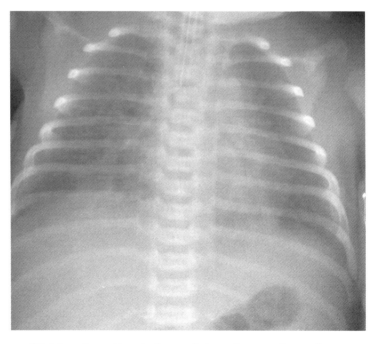

Slightly enlarged heart of normal shape, increased vascular
markings, and stomach in the normal position.

2. **Hemoglobin and hematocrit level**
   - normal hemoglobin range in term babies at birth is 150 to 220 g/L, and the normal hematocrit 0.45 to 0.66
   - a low hemoglobin at birth may be an indicator of blood loss
     - when the blood loss is acute there are signs of shock
     - when the blood loss is chronic, there is anemia without shock

3. **Blood gases**
   - metabolic acidosis (low pH and high base deficit) may indicate that the tissues are not receiving enough oxygen (tissue hypoxia), as a result of:
     - inadequate circulation (shock)
     - insufficient oxygen in the blood (extreme cyanosis)
   - metabolic acidosis can be detected and quantified by analysis of venous, arterial or capillary blood

4. **Electrocardiogram (ECG)**
   - is helpful in the evaluation of babies suspected of having congenital heart disease, and is essential in babies with tachyarrhythmias or other disturbances of cardiac rhythm,
     - a baby with cardiac rhythm abnormality should not receive medication until after a ECG has been done and reviewed by a specialist where possible

Establish a Working Diagnosis

Working diagnoses in the Cardiovascular Sequence are:

Shock
- hypovolemic (due to low circulating blood volume, typically found in acute blood loss)
- distributive (due to vascular dilatation, as may occur in bacterial sepsis)
- cardiogenic (due to impaired myocardial function, as seen in left ventricular outflow tract obstruction or cardiomyopathy)

Cyanotic congenital heart disease

Tachyarrhythmia

Specific Management

Because of the complexity of cardiovascular conditions contained in these categories, care should be guided by specialist consultation.

The key interventions are:
- volume expansion
- inotropic drugs, such as dopamine infusion or vasoconstrictors
- PGE_1 infusion
- antiarrhythmic therapy.

Cardiovascular Case # 1 – The baby presenting with shock

You are called to attend a baby who was born at 36 weeks gestation by emergency Cesarean. The mother was admitted in early labor with decreased fetal movements. The fetal heart tracing showed a sinusoidal pattern.

The baby was depressed at birth, with low tone, irregular respiration and heart rate < 100 bpm. She was given two minutes of bag-and-mask ventilation followed by free-flow oxygen.

The baby is now 10 minutes old, she is breathing spontaneously and regularly and her heart rate is 180 bpm. She is markedly pale. You have difficulty finding the brachial or femoral pulses.

Marked pallor and weak pulses indicate that the baby is unwell and needs stabilization using ACoRN.

The baby now shows none of Resuscitation Signs.

You begin an ACoRN Primary Survey.

Resuscitation
- [ ] Ineffective breathing
- [ ] Heart rate < 100 bpm
- [ ] Central cyanosis

The baby is lying quietly on a radiant warmer.

She is breathing quickly but easily with a respiratory rate of 54/minute. Her heart rate is 180 bpm by auscultation.

Free flow oxygen continues by mask. She is neither cyanotic nor pink; the most striking feature is her marked pallor. Peripheral pulses are difficult to palpate. Her tone remains low.

The heel is being warmed to enable blood sampling for glucose determination.

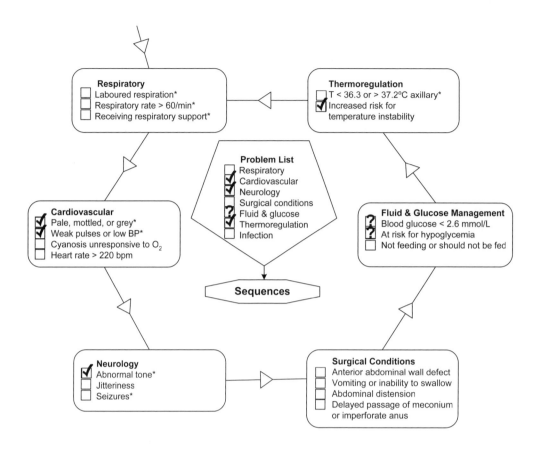

The first area of concern on the Problem List is Cardiovascular. The baby exhibits two Alerting Signs for the Cardiovascular Sequence. You enter the Sequence and carry out the remaining Core Steps.

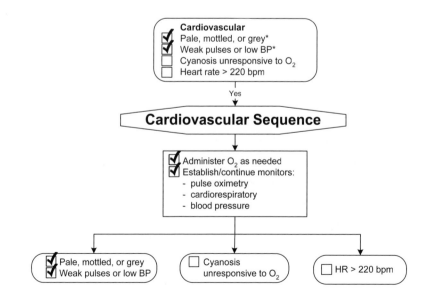

> Oxygen saturation is 100% in free-flow oxygen. Respiratory rate is 60/minute and heart rate is 184 bpm on the cardiorespiratory monitor. Mean blood pressure is 28 mmHg. You connect the servocontrol probe. Axillary temperature is 37.1°C.

I.   Is the blood pressure of this baby in the normal range or not? What is a quick way to determine this?

_____

_____

> In organizing your care, you note that the baby is pale, has weak pulses, and the capillary refill is 4 to 5 seconds.
>
> She is not cyanotic and her heart rate is not > 220 bpm.

II.   Complete the following table for clinical assessment of circulation, comparing normal findings and the abnormal findings in this baby.

Observation	Normal findings	Abnormal findings in this baby
Skin color		
Temperature of the extremities		
Peripheral pulses		
Capillary refill		
Mean blood pressure		
Heart rate		

The baby exhibits several findings indicative of inadequate circulation. Following the course of action indicated by the pallor and weak pulses, you proceed to obtain emergency vascular access with an umbilical venous catheter in order to administer volume expansion. You consider the information already obtained through the history and physical examination, and obtain blood samples for a stat CBC and venous blood gas immediately upon insertion of the UVC. You estimate the weight of the baby to be 3000 grams.

III. **Calculate the type and amount of volume expander you will administer to this baby.**

_____

_____

You administer the bolus of volume expander over 5 minutes.

What is shock? Shock is an unstable cardiovascular state in which cardiac output is insufficient to meet the oxygen and energy demands of vital organs, resulting in deteriorating organ function and build-up of chemical by-products of metabolism such as lactic acid. If untreated, shock is usually fatal.

Types of shock There are three main categories for shock:

1. **Hypovolemic shock** occurs when there is reduced circulating blood volume due to hemorrhage or to leaking of intravascular fluid into the tissues ("third-spacing"). Blood loss may occur:
   - Antepartum/intrapartum. These babies present at birth. Causes include, bleeding into the mother's circulation (fetal-maternal hemorrhage), into a twin, or due to rupture of a vasa previa. The blood loss seen in placental abruption or placenta previa is almost exclusively maternal.
   - After delivery. These babies present several minutes or hours after birth. Causes include, bleeding from the umbilical cord, or into the scalp in a subgaleal hemorrhage (may occur following vacuum or forceps delivery).

   A major feto-maternal hemorrhage may be suspected antenatally when the mother presents with decreased fetal movements and a non-reassuring fetal heart tracing, including a sinusoidal pattern, as in this case. However, milder cases are not detected until the baby is born. A maternal blood smear stained for detection of fetal cells (Kleihauer-Betke) should be requested in all cases of unexplained neonatal shock or anemia.

ACoRN

In hypovolemic shock, the chest radiograph may show a normal-sized or small heart.

The hemoglobin concentration will be low. However, immediately following an acute blood loss, before hemodilution occurs, the drop in hemoglobin concentration may underestimate the magnitude of the hemorrhage.

2. **Cardiogenic shock** occurs when the heart pumps inadequately. It may be due to functional or structural impairment of heart function.

Functional impairment occurs in perinatal asphyxia (due to myocardial ischemia), severe respiratory failure, septicemia, and cardiomyopathies. It may also be secondary to dysrhythmia. Many of these babies respond to the basic interventions provided during resuscitation and stabilization, but may require circulatory support with inotropic drugs such as dopamine.

Structural impairment occurs in congenital heart disease (cyanotic or acyanotic). These conditions ultimately require surgical intervention.

Cardiogenic shock due to congenital heart disease should be suspected when,
- there is no history of adverse perinatal events
- symptoms worsen during the time the ductus arteriosus closes, hours to days after birth ("duct dependence")
- shock co-exists with absent lower limb pulses or signs of heart failure (cardiomegaly, pulmonary edema, and hepatomegaly).

The left heart obstructive lesions that most commonly present with shock in a previously acyanotic baby are:
- Hypoplastic left heart syndrome. Has the earliest onset of symptoms (shortly after birth): pallor, some cyanosis (pulmonary and systemic venous blood mixes in the right ventricle), poor peripheral pulses, single second sound, ± murmur, cardiomegaly on chest radiograph, right ventricular hypertrophy on ECG
- Coarctation of the aorta (including interrupted aortic arch). Has onset of symptoms a few hours to days after birth: femoral pulses present but diminished or delayed, ± murmur, cardiomegaly on chest radiograph, right ventricular hypertrophy on ECG. Differential cyanosis occurs when the coarctation is preductal, and the lower part of the body is supplied by the right ventricle via the PDA.

In "duct-dependent" congenital heart disease cases, the closure of the ductus is fatal if not prevented by the administration of prostaglandin E_1 prior to surgical treatment.

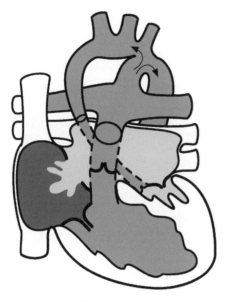

Hypoplastic left heart: when the ductus arteriosus is open, systemic cardiac output can be supported by the right ventricle.

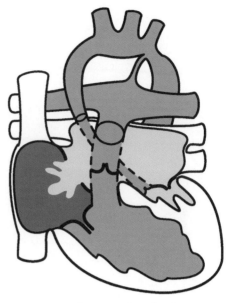

Hypoplastic left heart: when the ductus arteriosus starts closing, the systemic cardiac output can no longer be supported by the right ventricle.

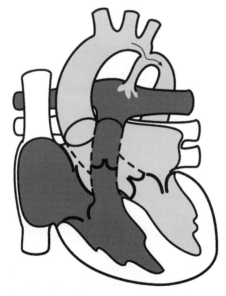

Coarctation of the aorta: when the ductus arteriosus is open, blood is able to flow in the aortic arch and descending aorta despite the coarctation.

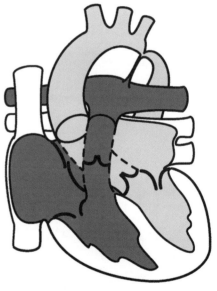

Coarctation of the aorta: when the ductus arteriosus is closed, the obstruction at the level of the coarctation is further narrowed. This markedly decreases blood flow to the descending aortal (lower extremities ± left arm).

Prostaglandin E₁ (PGE₁)

3. **Distributive shock** occurs when blood vessels in the body do not maintain normal vascular tone and permeability. In early distributive shock, the over-riding feature is vasodilatation associated with hypotension ("warm phase") and the baby appears pink. This clinical presentation can be deceptive and may lead to delayed diagnosis of shock. In a later stage, blood is redirected away from the periphery toward the vital organs and the baby appears grey and mottled ("cold phase").

   An example of distributive shock is septic shock. There may be a history of preterm labor, prolonged rupture of membranes, or maternal fever. Babies with septic shock are globally ill, and have multisystem failure and high mortality. In septic shock, abnormal blood vessel tone and loss of intravascular fluid into the tissues results in inadequate circulatory volume. Urgent management includes antibiotics, volume expansion and dopamine. Dopamine is an inotrope that increases the force of contraction of the heart, and a pressor that vasoconstricts peripheral blood vessels.

   Distributive shock has become rare since antepartum/intrapartum group B streptococcus (GBS) prophylaxis became common.

 Dopamine

Given the multiple causes of shock, and the complex relationship between circulating volume, blood vessel tone, and heart function following initial resuscitation, the immediate management should include rapid intravascular volume expansion and a clinical evaluation of the response.

The nurse and doctor who delivered the baby provide you with a focused interim history. The mother was a 42-year-old in her sixth pregnancy, and has five living children. She arrived at the hospital in early labour, with intact membranes. The pregnancy had been uneventful until she noticed decreased fetal movements and contractions on the day of admission to hospital. The obstetrician was called immediately as the nurse noted a sinusoidal pattern on the fetal heart tracing. Concerned about the well-being of the fetus, the obstetrician proceeded with a Cesarean section.

The remainder of the physical examination reveals no further information. After receiving 10 mL/kg of 0.9% NaCl over 5 minutes, the baby remains pale and mottled, with cool extremities and weak pulses in the upper and lower extremities. The capillary refill is 4 to 5 seconds, and the blood pressure by cuff is 44/20, mean of 32 mmHg. The heart rate is 180 bpm.

IV.   What do you think is the cause of this baby's shock and what do you do next?

_____

_____

In response to your actions, the mean blood pressure increases to 35 mmHg and the heart rate decreases to 160 bpm.

The first laboratory results show that the hemoglobin is 65 g/L. The venous blood gas shows pH 7.22, P_{CO_2} 32 mmHg, and BD 12.

The blood pressure has increased and the heart rate decreased in response to volume expansion with 0.9% NaCl IV, but these have not returned to the normal range.

You recognize that this baby is still hypovolemic and has metabolic acidosis.

You decide that a third bolus of IV fluid is indicated. Given the presence of marked anemia and metabolic acidosis, you opt to administer O-negative uncross-matched packed red cells.

When do you administer blood?

The choice between uncross-matched O-negative blood or cross-matched type-specific red cells depends on the urgency of the transfusion.

The decision to give blood must take into consideration the clinical condition of the baby (in this case, refractory hypovolemic shock with anemia), the potential complications associated with blood products, and ability to obtain parental consent. A current policy should be in place at every institution describing the procedure to access blood products urgently and defining circumstances for use of uncross-matched blood, and for when there is parental refusal.

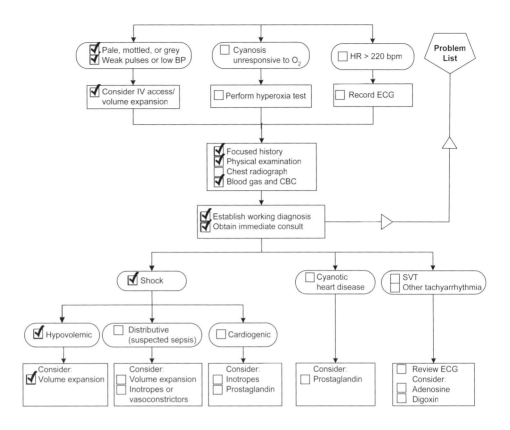

The baby weighs 2940 grams. You draw the blood up into a syringe, and give 44 mL (15 mL/kg) over the next 15 minutes.

You exit the Cardiovascular Sequence and return to the ACoRN Problem List.

Having formulated a working diagnosis and management plan, you exit the Cardiovascular Sequence and continue with Neurology, Fluid & Glucose Management and Thermoregulation Sequences as identified in the Problem List.

Toward the end of the transfusion, there is a prompt rise in the mean arterial pressure to over 40 mmHg, and a fall in heart rate to 152 bpm. The baby is less pale, and the circulation is improved. The capillary refill time is 3 seconds, the hemoglobin is 100 g/L and the venous gas has normalized.

Cardiovascular Case # 2 – Baby with persistent cyanosis

> You are changing the diaper of a 3500 gram term baby after helping a mother successfully initiate breastfeeding in the birthing suite. Labour and birth were uncomplicated. As you do this, you notice that the baby's color is dusky and his lips are bluish.
>
> Because the baby is cyanotic, a Resuscitation Sign, you initiate the Core Steps of the Resuscitation Sequence.

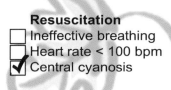

Resuscitation
- ☐ Ineffective breathing
- ☐ Heart rate < 100 bpm
- ☑ Central cyanosis

> You call for assistance, take the baby to the radiant warmer, attach the servocontrol probe, provide free-flow oxygen and perform the other core steps of the Resuscitation Sequence.

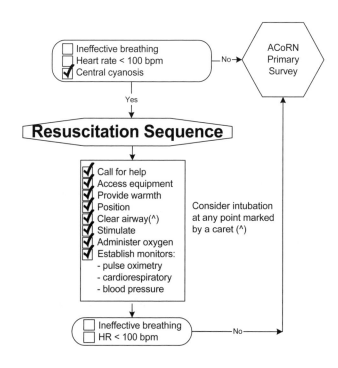

The baby does not appear distressed, is active and alert, and breathing rapidly at a rate of 60/minute. On auscultation, breath sounds are heard bilaterally, and the heart rate is 140 bpm. His skin is warm to touch.

He remains centrally cyanotic, despite receiving 100% oxygen by face mask.

Cyanosis unresponsive to oxygen therapy, as an isolated sign, requires no further immediate resuscitative efforts.

You leave the Resuscitation Sequence and proceed to the ACoRN Primary Survey.

The mean blood pressure is 38 mmHg and axillary temperature is 36.8ºC. Oxygen saturation is 70%. The baby begins to cry, and the cyanosis deepens.

The physician arrives and you review the findings of the Primary Survey.

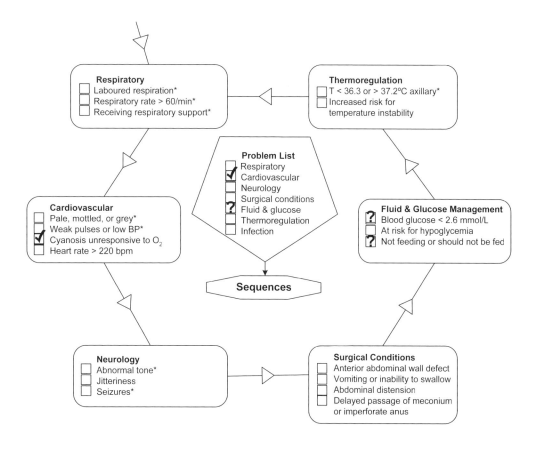

This baby exhibits one of the Alerting Signs for the Cardiovascular Sequence. You enter the Sequence and carry out the remaining Core Steps.

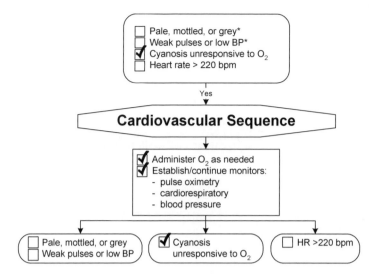

The baby remains alert and active. His vital signs are stable. He remains cyanotic despite oxygen therapy.

Review of transition from fetal to neonatal circulation and breathing

In-utero, fetal blood is oxygenated in the placenta and returned via the umbilical vein and the inferior vena cava to the right atrium. Most of this oxygenated blood then crosses to the left atrium via the foramen ovale, and is pumped by the left ventricle. The deoxygenated blood returning to the right atrium via the superior vena cava mostly enters the right ventricle, crossing to the aorta via the ductus arteriosus. Thus, the blood pumped into the aortic arch and the brain is less mixed and better oxygenated than the blood distal to the ductus arteriosus. Approximately 90% of the bi-ventricular cardiac output bypasses the lungs which are filled with lung fluid.

Shortly after birth, during the transition from fetal to neonatal circulation, the lungs become the organ in which oxygenation and ventilation takes place, and the foramen ovale and ductus arteriosus close.

Under normal circumstances, adult circulation is established within the first few breaths. Once that occurs, the right and left side of the heart work in series; that is, blood travels in one direction only, and venous and arterial blood do not mix. Venous blood travels from the right side of the heart to the lungs, gains oxygen and loses carbon dioxide, and returns to the left side of the heart as oxygenated blood.

Post-natal gas exchange is most effective when,
- all the alveoli are open, and cycle with breathing (ventilation) and contain oxygen (oxygenation), and
- all the blood circulates around open alveoli (perfusion).

What are the mechanisms of cyanosis in a newborn?

Intrapulmonary shunt of respiratory disease

A portion of the blood passing through the lungs circulates around alveoli that are not ventilated or are poorly ventilated, due to lung disease. This blood then mixes with blood that has circulated around fully ventilated alveoli, reducing the overall oxygen content by dilution.

This form of cyanosis responds to oxygenation and ventilation (Page 4-8).

Persistent pulmonary hypertension (PPHN)

The small muscular branches of the pulmonary arteries fail to relax or increase their resistance to flow after birth causing the pressure in the pulmonary artery, the right ventricle and the right atrium to remain high. As a result, some of the blood being pumped to the lungs by the right side of the heart may be diverted (shunted) through the ductus arteriosus to the post-ductal aorta and across the foramen ovale to the left atrium. When these shunts are present, the oxygen content of the blood returning from the lungs to the left side of the heart is diluted in the left atrium and again in the post-ductal aorta.

Persistent pulmonary hypertension of the newborn (PPHN) usually occurs in association with lung disease and can occur as a primary condition.

Oxygenation and ventilation decrease the resistance to flow in the pulmonary circuit, therefore this form of cyanosis responds to oxygenation and ventilation, and may further respond to a short period of hyperventilation. However, hyperventilation is not recommended as a form of therapy as the response is transient, it results in increased lung injury and may decrease oxygen delivery to the brain.

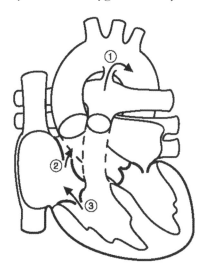

PPHN: (1) right to left shunt via the ductus arteriosus, (2) right to left shunt via patent foramen ovale, (3) functional tricuspid insufficiency and regurgitation due to right ventricular dysfunction

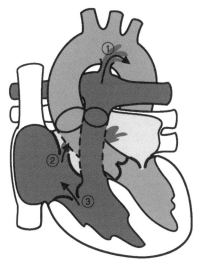

Oxygenated blood returning from the lungs to the left atrium is mixed with blood shunted from the right atrium. Further shunting occurs via the PDA, from the pulmonary artery to the aorta.

The responsiveness to oxygen and ventilation in respiratory disease and PPHN indicates that the mechanism of cyanosis is functional rather than anatomic and responsive to management strategies aimed at,

- expanding collapsed alveoli (ventilation)
- increasing the concentration of inspired oxygen in order to better oxygenate the alveoli that are partially ventilated (oxygenation)
- avoiding low Pa_{O_2} or acidosis which cause pulmonary vasoconstriction and increase the resistance to flow in the pulmonary circuit resulting in,
  - decreased pulmonary blood flow and
  - mixing of deoxygenated blood with oxygenated blood (right to left shunt) via the foramen ovale or the ductus arteriosus.

Cyanotic congenital heart disease

Certain structural abnormalities of the heart or large blood vessels result in cyanosis because there is,

- separation between the right and left sided circuits, or
- right to left shunt of deoxygenated blood away from the lungs, or
- mixing of already oxygenated blood with deoxygenated blood.

The more common examples of each of these three mechanisms are: transposition of the great arteries, tricuspid atresia, and total anomalous pulmonary venous return into the right side circulation.

In general, the cyanosis present in this group of disorders is not responsive to oxygenation and ventilation as the presence of cyanosis is not due to poor oxygenation at the level of the lung.

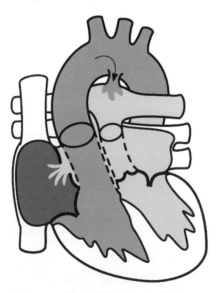

In transposition of the great arteries, the right and left circulations are separated. The ability to mix blood at the atrial level is essential for survival. Keeping the ductus arteriosus open increases blood flow to the lungs, improving oxygenation.

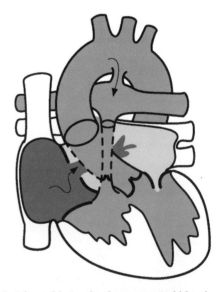

In tricuspid atresia, deoxygenated blood from the right atrium flows into the left atrium via the foramen ovale, mixing with oxygenated blood. Keeping the ductus arteriosus open increases blood flow to the lungs, improving oxygenation.

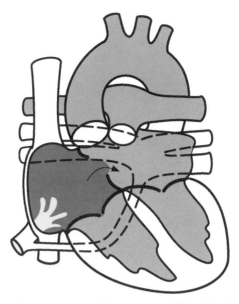

Mixing of oxygenated and deoxygenated blood in the right atrium in total anomalous pulmonary venous return. This condition is difficult to differentiate clinically from PPHN.

Cyanotic congenital heart disease should be suspected when a $Pa_{O_2} > 150$ mmHg or $Sp_{O_2} > 95\%$ have never been documented during the baby's clinical course.

The Hyperoxia Test

The hyperoxia test is useful for distinguishing cyanotic disorders of respiratory origin from those of cardiovascular origin with a fixed right to left shunt, on the basis that oxygen administration improves oxygenation in lung disease.

As close to 100% oxygen as possible is administered for 15 to 20 minutes. This washes out all the nitrogen from even poorly ventilated alveoli and equalizes the partial pressure of oxygen throughout the lungs.

The response to a hyperoxia test may be measured using either a pulse oximeter or an arterial blood sample. Failure to achieve a significant rise in $Sp_{O_2} > 10\%$ or $Pa_{O_2} > 20$ to 30 mmHg after 20 minutes in 100% oxygen is suggestive of cyanotic congenital heart disease with a fixed right to left shunt.

- The hyperoxia test may be abnormal in severe respiratory disease, however, severe respiratory distress and hypercarbia will also be present in those cases.
- The hyperoxia test may result in increased oxygenation despite cyanotic heart disease when the right to left shunt is not fixed and oxygen administration increases the pulmonary blood flow, mixing more oxygenated into deoxygenated blood (anomalous venous return without obstruction, or transposition of great arteries with PPHN).

Measurements of Sp_{O_2} can be obtained from the right hand (preductal) and from a foot (postductal) to provide information about ductal flow patterns.

After the hyperoxia test is completed, the administered oxygen concentration should be decreased to achieve Sp_{O_2} levels advised by the consultant. The baby's Sp_{O_2} may drop while the oxygen concentration is decreased if there is an element of respiratory disease, lung congestion, or pulmonary hypertension in addition to the cardiac abnormality. In this case,

- the oxygen concentration should be increased until the Sp_{O_2} improves
- CPAP may need to be provided if there is extensive alveolar collapse or lung congestion, or mechanical ventilation if there is respiratory acidosis
- metabolic acidosis should be corrected to prevent pulmonary hypertension.

Prevention or lessening of pulmonary hypertension improves blood flow to the lungs, reduces the magnitude of right to left shunting, and improves oxygenation.

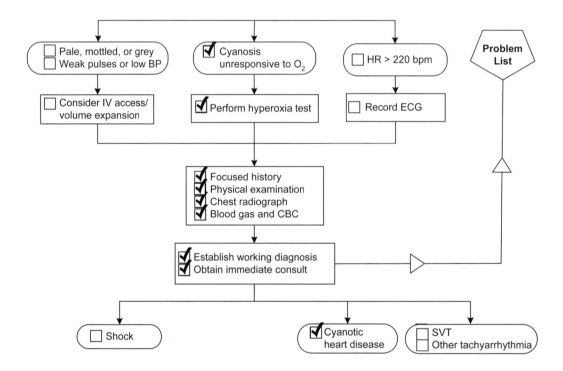

Following the Response indicated by the finding of cyanosis unresponsive to oxygen therapy, you and the respiratory therapist prepare to conduct a hyperoxia test while the physician speaks with the mother and reviews the chart in order to obtain a focused history.

The physician returns, remarking that the focused history does not contribute any additional information toward establishing a working diagnosis. Other than the cyanosis, the only significant cardiac finding on physical examination is an active precordium (sternal heave). The baby's liver is not enlarged and there is no heart murmur.

The saturation prior and during the hyperoxia test remained at 65 to 70%.

A chest radiograph is ordered, and you gradually decrease the oxygen concentration in the oxygen hood.

The physical findings and the result of the hyperoxia test are suggestive of cyanotic congenital heart disease.

The chest radiograph is shown below:

Transposition of the great arteries with a right-sided aortic arch

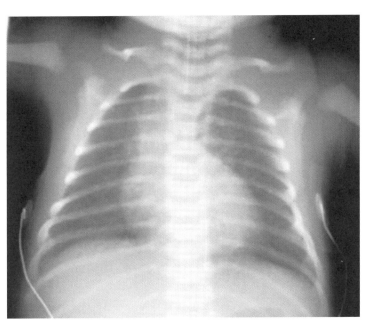

- o the lung fields are clear allowing for the silhouette of the heart and the diaphragm to be clearly seen throughout
- o the pulmonary vessels are somewhat increased (the radial markings seen entering the lung on both sides of the heart)
- o the size of the heart is slightly enlarged (right atrium and right ventricle) and the mediastinum (above the heart) is narrow, giving the heart the shape of an egg
- o the antero-posterior arrangement of the aorta and pulmonary artery projects as a narrow cardiac pedicle

The radiological findings are suggestive of transposition of the great arteries (TGA) with an intact ventricular septum where,

- blood from the two separate circuits mixes through the foramen ovale at the atrial level and through the ductus arteriosus
- the distribution of blood between the pulmonary and systemic circuits is variable, but tends to be greater in the pulmonary side (because of falling pulmonary resistance), giving rise to increased pulmonary vascular markings
- the aorta is anterior and is supplied by the right ventricle and the main pulmonary artery is posterior and supplied by the left ventricle; this anterio-posterior (AP) alignment projects as a narrow mediastinum and "hides" the arch of the aorta.

Depending on the degree of mixing through the foramen ovale and ductus arteriosus, the baby may be moderately cyanotic or intensely blue.

TGA is the most common cyanotic congenital heart condition. Other structural heart defects with right-to-left shunt include the other 4 Ts,

- tricuspid atresia/pulmonary atresia
- total anomalous venous return
- truncus arteriosus
- tetralogy of Fallot with marked pulmonary stenosis.

Prostaglandin E$_1$ (PGE$_1$)

In all these conditions, oxygenation may be improved by initiating a prostaglandin infusion to maintain a patent ductus arteriosus. In TGA it is essential that there be at least some atrial mixing in addition to a patent ductus arteriosus.

When PGE$_1$ treatment is effective, the SpO$_2$ and PaO$_2$ rise and the acidosis resolves.

The clinical response to prostaglandin must be monitored, documented and communicated to the consultant.

Adverse reactions to PGE$_1$ include apnea, and vasodilation leading to hypotension and hyperthermia. The need for intubation should be anticipated; volume expansion may be needed.

The absence of response to PGE$_1$ indicates a critically ill baby, with minimal or no atrial mixing. These babies are at risk of dying and need urgent cardiac assessment and intervention at a referral centre. In TGA, metabolic acidosis or lack of response to PGE$_1$ indicate insufficient atrial mixing requiring an emergency atrial septostomy.

Prostaglandin E$_1$ (PGE$_1$)

The blood gas shows: pH 7.28, P$_{CO_2}$ 32 mmHg, P$_{O_2}$ 35 mmHg, and BD 9.
The SpO$_2$ remains 65 to 70%. The Hb is 11.5 g/L.
The physician places a call to the referral centre.

Having formulated a working diagnosis and management plan, you exit the Cardiovascular Sequence and continue with the Fluid & Glucose Management Sequence as identified in the Problem List.

What is the significance of this baby's oximetry and blood gas result?

When there is marked arterial desaturation, the delivery of oxygen to the tissues becomes compromised and metabolic acidosis develops. The table below indicates how different levels of SpO_2 are usually tolerated.

SpO_2	Degree of desaturation	Tolerance
> 75%	mild to moderate	usually well tolerated
65 to 75%	marked	may be less well tolerated if baby otherwise sick
< 65%	severe	poorly tolerated

In addition to SpO_2, two other factors determine the delivery of oxygen to the tissues,
- hemoglobin level
- cardiac output.

A metabolic acidosis with a base deficit > 5 to 8 or increased lactic acid indicates insufficient tissue oxygenation requiring immediate action to ensure that,
- the ductus arteriosus remains patent
  - initiate a PGE_1 infusion
- the hemoglobin concentration is in the normal level (approximately 140 g/L) to provide sufficient oxygen carrying capacity
  - transfuse if necessary
- the baby is immediately transferred to a center able to treat or palliate the primary problem.

The arterial PO_2 of 35 mmHg is in the hypoxemic range (< 50 mmHg) and the SpO_2, of 65 to 70% indicates marked desaturation.

The low Hb of 115 g/L indicates there are not enough red cells to carry oxygen to the tissues (insufficient oxygen carrying capacity). The cause of the low hemoglobin concentration is unclear at this point.

The BD of 9 most likely indicates significant metabolic acidosis due to insufficient tissue oxygenation.

The PCO_2 of 32 mmHg indicates the baby is hyperventilating (respiratory alkalosis) to compensate for the metabolic acidosis.

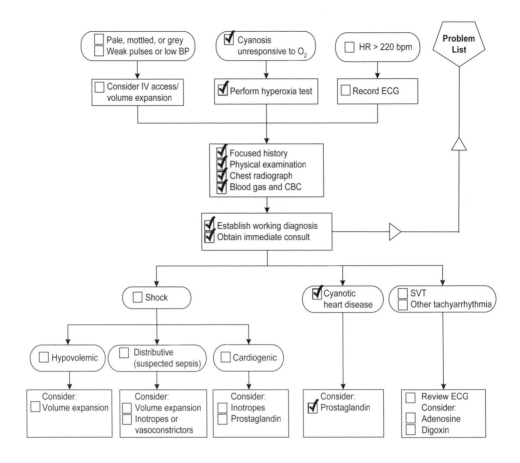

The baby's physician discusses the baby's condition and assessment with the consultant at the referral centre. The consultant agrees with the working diagnosis of cyanotic congenital heart disease and concurs with the need for immediate initiation of PGE_1 infusion. He also recommends a red cell transfusion of 10 to 15 mL/kg of packed red cells to increase oxygen carrying capacity. You proceed to start intravenous access.

The baby was started on a PGE_1 infusion and transferred to the referral centre. Arrangements were made to transfer the mother as soon as possible to allow her to be close to her baby.

On arrival to the referral center, an echocardiogram confirmed the diagnosis of transposition of the great arteries. Due to persistent desaturation and acidosis despite PGE_1, an atrial septostomy was performed shortly after admission.

A few days later, an arterial switch procedure was performed.

The baby was discharged home after two weeks.

Cardiovascular Case # 3 – Baby with supraventricular tachycardia

As you do the pre-discharge examination of a 48-hour old term newborn, you note her heart rate on auscultation is very fast, making it very difficult to count. The baby appears otherwise well. Her color is pink and breathing is regular.

The baby's marked tachycardia indicates she needs stabilization using ACoRN. She shows none of the Resuscitation Signs and you proceed with an ACoRN Primary Survey.

Resuscitation
- [ ] Ineffective breathing
- [ ] Heart rate < 100 bpm
- [ ] Central cyanosis

The respiratory rate is 60/minute. There are no signs of respiratory distress. The heart rate is so fast that it cannot be counted. The pulses are decreased in amplitude. You request a cardiorespiratory monitor be attached and her blood pressure be measured. The baby is alert and active. Her movements are symmetrical and age-appropriate. According to the mother and nurse, the baby was fussy during the night, but she has been breastfeeding well every 2 to 3 hours since birth. A glucose measurement has not been done because the baby was low risk and had a good feeding history.

While performing a clinical assessment of the cardiovascular system, it is important to know that,
- the highest heart rate that can be clinically counted is in the range of 200 to 220 bpm
- non-invasive blood pressure monitors are less accurate when the heart rate exceeds 200 to 220 bpm.

The baby exhibits two of the Alerting Signs for the Cardiovascular Sequence. You know you will need to also consider the baby's needs for Fluid & Glucose Management and Thermoregulation.

You enter the Cardiovascular Sequence and carry out the remaining Core Steps. The baby is not pale, mottled or grey, and the capillary refill is 3 seconds. The mean blood pressure is 42 mmHg. The oxygen saturation by pulse oximetry is 93% in room air. The cardiorespiratory monitor shows a heart rate of 260 bpm. The axillary temperature is 36.8°C.

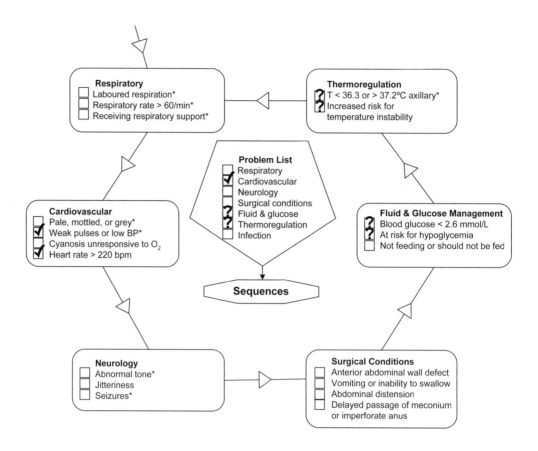

The significant findings of the cardiovascular assessment so far are:
1. the baby is not pale, mottled or grey and the capillary refill is within the normal range
2. pulses are fast and somewhat difficult to palpate
3. the mean blood pressure is similar to her gestational age
4. is pink in room air
5. has a heart > 220 bpm.

I.   How would you organize your care if the baby had a heart rate > 220 and poor peripheral perfusion or low blood pressure?

_____

_____

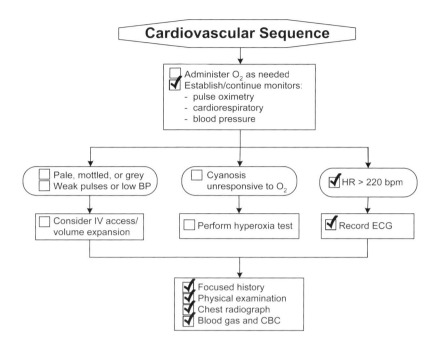

The immediate Response under Tachyarrhythmia is to obtain a rhythm strip and a 12-lead ECG as soon as possible, and to proceed to the Next Steps.

A baby with tachycardia who is unstable requires urgent intervention.

You request a rhythm strip and a 12-lead ECG.

In some cardiorespiratory monitors, a rhythm strip may be obtained by pressing a "print" button. A rhythm strip is helpful if the P wave, the QRS complex and the T wave are all visible, but does not replace a full ECG.

You complete a focused history and physical examination.

There were no concerns at, or prior, to the spontaneous, vaginal vertex birth of this term baby. The Apgar scores were 9 and 9, at 1 and 5 minutes respectively.

The mother tells you her baby looked healthy at birth, but that over the last several hours the baby has been a bit fussy with feeds and not as interested in sucking from the breast.

The baby is active, looks well, and appears well hydrated. Perfusion is good with a capillary refill time of 2 to 3 seconds on the trunk and extremities. The limbs and trunk are equally warm. Femoral and brachial pulses are palpable. There are no signs of respiratory distress and the lungs sound clear. The heart sounds are normal but the fast rate makes it difficult to count the rate and to determine if there are abnormal heart sounds or a murmur. There is slight edema in the hands, feet, sacrum, and scalp. She has lost 300 grams since birth.

How do you determine if this baby is unstable?

Babies with sustained tachyarrhythmia may develop heart failure, but it usually takes hours of sustained tachycardia before they decompensate.

The following table can be used to differentiate a baby with tachyarrhythmia who is stable from one who is unstable.

Stable	Unstable
alert, active and looking well, normal tone	listless or lethargic and/or distressed, decreased tone
capillary refill < 3 seconds centrally and peripherally	capillary refill > 3 seconds
pulses palpable and full	pulses weak
heart sounds normal	gallop
no edema or signs of third space fluid	edema or signs of other third space fluid
clear lungs and normal-sized heart on chest radiograph	congested lungs or pleural effusions, and/or enlarged heart on chest radiograph

You decide that the most important finding in the physical examination of this baby, other than the tachycardia, is that the baby is alert, active and looks well. This is consistent with a baby who is stable from a cardiovascular point of view.

The fact that the baby has peripheral edema despite having lost weight since birth, suggests that she may have been more edematous at birth and that this went unnoticed.

Despite clinical stability, babies with tachyarrhythmia require immediate consultation, close observation and venous access for possible administration of medications. If they decompensate they may require mechanical ventilation, and cardioversion under the guidance of a specialist.

How do you assess a baby with a tachyarrhythmia?

Auscultation Determine if the heart rate by precordial auscultation corresponds to the number showing on the cardiorespiratory monitor.

Cardiorespiratory monitor Obtain and print a rhythm strip from the cardiorespiratory monitor once a robust signal is obtained.
- ensure the ECG electrodes are adherent to the skin and that the ECG signal on the monitor is as free as possible of motion and other artifacts
- choose the lead (I, II, or III) that best demonstrates the distinctive pattern with P, QRS, and T waves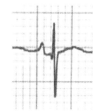
- the QRS complex should be taller than the T wave to avoid erroneous 'double-counting' by the monitor.

If the tachyarrhthmia is intermittent, strips should be obtained while the rhythm is tachycardic and normal, especially at the time of transition.

12-lead ECG For babies with cardiac arrhythmias, including tachyarrhythmia, it is critical to do a 12-lead ECG with a rhythm strip, and have it reviewed by a cardiology consultant before initiating therapy.

If no cardiology specialist is on site, the ECG and rhythm strip should be faxed to the referral center. Management and prognosis will depend on the origin of the electrophysiological disturbance.

What do you look for in a rhythm strip?

Heart rate Count the number of millimeters (small squares) between R waves (R-R interval). Next, divide 1500 by the number of millimeters counted when the paper in the ECG strip is running at a standard 25 mm/second.

For example:
$$\frac{1500}{5 \text{ mm}} = 300 \text{ bpm}$$

The heart rate calculated above is the ventricular heart rate. You can repeat the same procedure using the distance between the P waves to calculate the atrial rate.

If the rhythm is irregular, one cannot rely on the R-R interval to calculate the ventricular heart rate. In that case, count the number of QRS complexes over 6 seconds (15 cm if the ECG strip is running at a standard 25 mm/seconds) and multiply by 10.

Rhythm   Observe if the rhythm is regular or irregular.

P, QRS and   Observe if,
T wave   • every QRS complex is preceded by a P wave
morphology   • all P waves have similar shape and point in the same direction
      • all QRS complexes have similar shape and point in the same direction
      • the distance between the P wave and the Q or R waves is constant
      • the P waves are equally spaced from each other
      • the R waves are equally spaced from each other
      • the QRS is narrow or wide.

Examples:

Normal sinus rhythm in a term newborn

• the heart rate is in the usual range with intact conduction pathways
• accelerates or decelerates in response to physiologic changes such as breathing, maintains normal beat to beat variability

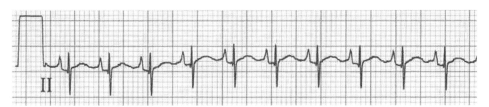

The rhythm is regular, and all P wave and QRS complexes look normal and alike. The heart rate is around 167 bpm (1500 divided by an R-R interval of approximately 9 mm). P waves are present and each is followed by a QRS complex after a similar interval. It cannot be determined if there is beat to beat variability in this type of tracing.

Sinus tachycardia:

- the heart rate is above the usual range with intact conduction pathways
- accelerates or decelerates in response to physiologic changes such as breathing
- seldom exceeds 200 to 220 bpm
- occurs with conditions such as crying and pain, but may be associated with pathology, including hypovolemia, anemia, stimulant medications (methylxanthines such as aminophylline and caffeine), sepsis, and hyperthermia or in babies of mothers with hyperthyroidism
- is benign, requires no specific treatment, and responds to treatment of the underlying condition.

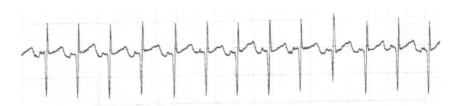

In this strip, the heart rate is 188 bpm (1500 / 8 mm), exceeding the normal range but remaining < 220 bpm. The rhythm is regular and all P wave and QRS complexes look normal and alike. P waves are present and each is followed by a QRS complex after a similar interval. It cannot be determined if there is beat-to-beat variability in this type of tracing.

Supraventricular tachycardia

- the heart rate is above the usual range (usually > 220 bpm) and the conduction pathway is abnormal
- while in SVT, the heart rate does not vary with physiologic changes such as breathing, and there is no beat to beat variability
- sudden onset not triggered by external events; conversion back to sinus is also sudden, whether spontaneous or in response to therapy
- may occur in "runs" lasting minutes to hours; the main concern is heart failure, which does not usually develop until after several hours
- the cardiac anatomy is usually normal in babies with SVT; sometimes a specific electrophysiologic diagnosis is made (for example, Wolff-Parkinson-White syndrome) or congenital heart disease is present (for example, Ebstein's anomaly)
- the episodes of SVT usually become less frequent or cease by 6 to 12 months of age
- SVT needs to be differentiated electrophysiologically from other tachyarrhythmias, which may be even more serious or life threatening
- SVT may occur in utero leading to fetal heart failure; when hydrops fetalis occurs, there is high fetal mortality and morbidity
  - the mother requires specialized prenatal assessment and monitoring, and may need to receive treatment to control the fetal heart rate with the aim of prolonging gestation
  - the fetal cardiac anatomy and physiology requires careful evaluation

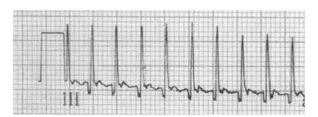

The strip above shows a tachycardia of 300 bpm.

Atrial flutter

Babies with atrial flutter have a characteristic "saw tooth" undulating baseline representing the "flutter waves". The atrial rate is around 300 bpm. In these babies the ventricular rhythm is irregular, and the ventricular rate tends to be < 220 bpm, as they have a variable heart block, meaning that not all atrial contractions generate a ventricular contraction.

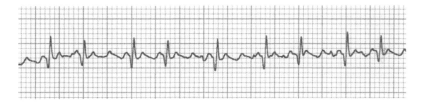

In the strip above, the "saw tooth" undulating baseline represents the "flutter-waves". The atrial rate is approximately 300 bpm. There are two to three flutter waves for each QRS complex, indicating a 2:1 to 3:1 block. As a consequence of the variable heart block, the rhythm is irregular.

Summary of key features in conditions where the heart rate is > normal

Sinus tachycardia	Supraventricular tachycardia (SVT)	Atrial flutter
heart rate < 220 bpm	heart rate 220 to 300 bpm	atrial rate 300 to 500 bpm
gradual onset and cessation	sudden onset and cessation	heart rate varies with AV conduction block (heart rate can half suddenly if 1:1 becomes 2:1 block)
preserved beat to beat variability	no beat to beat variability	no atrial beat to beat variability
narrow QRS	narrow QRS in ~ 90% of cases	narrow QRS
P waves precede each QRS	P wave relationship to QRS complex is variable. P waves are often not visible during SVT	P-waves with sawtooth pattern better seen in the inferior and right precordial leads on a 12-lead ECG AV conduction is variable

Below is the rhythm strip printed from the baby's cardiac monitor. The strip shows a heart rate of 300 bpm.

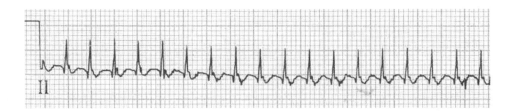

You establish a working diagnosis of SVT.

The baby's chest radiograph shows increased lung markings and minimal pleural effusions. The heart size appears slightly enlarged.

The capillary blood gas shows: pH 7.40, P_{CO_2} 36 mmHg, P_{O_2} 45 mmHg, BD 4.

You determine the baby is clinically stable and the capillary blood gas is within the normal range.

Babies with an unstable cardiovascular status accumulate metabolic acids in the circulation. This is noted as an increase in the base deficit. A base deficit > 6 to 8 would be of concern in this situation.

Babies in heart failure also show difficulty with gas exchange, because they have congested lungs. This is noted as an increased P_{CO_2}.
A P_{CO_2} > 55 mmHg would be of concern in this situation.

You proceed to address the Fluid & Glucose Management and Thermoregulation Sequences as identified in the Problem List.

You call the neonatologist at the referral center.

You describe the baby's present condition and supply the following additional information,
- fetal tachycardia was never noted during prenatal visits or labor
- tachycardia was not noted at birth or on auscultation since birth
- the baby fed well in the first 2 days of life but, over the last several hours, has been described by the mother as "a bit fussy and not as interested in sucking form the breast"
- the baby shows mild edema which had not been observed before.

In consultation, a decision is made to,
- transport the baby to the referral centre for further assessment
- fax a 12-lead ECG for review by the cardiologist and send the original or clear copy with the transport team.

The neonatologist tells you there is no urgency for cardioversion using vagal maneuvers or medication at this time as the baby is stable and definitive treatment can await specific diagnosis.

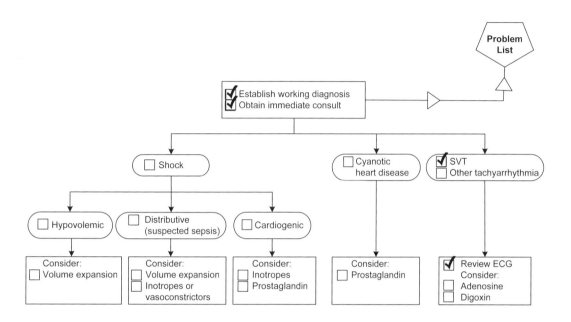

Shortly before the arrival of the transport team, the baby spontaneously converted to sinus rhythm.

Assessment at the referral hospital confirmed the diagnosis of SVT.

The baby was started on a Class 1A antiarrhythmic agent. A repeat ECG was satisfactory. An echocardiogram confirmed the clinical impression there was no structural congenital heart disease.

He was discharged in good condition at 8 days of age, with an indication to remain on medication until reassessment at the cardiology clinic at 3 months of age.

Answers to the questions in Chapter 4

Case # 1:

I.   Is the blood pressure of this baby in the normal range or not? What is a quick way to determine this?

The blood pressure of this baby is low, at 28 mmHg.

A practical estimate of the lower limit of the mean blood pressure is 36 mmHg for a baby of 36 weeks gestational age.

II.   Complete the following table for clinical assessment of circulation, comparing normal findings and the abnormal findings in this baby.

Observation	Normal findings	Abnormal findings in this baby
Skin color	Uniformly pink	Marked pallor
Temperature of the extremities	Warm trunk and extremities	?
Peripheral pulses	Normal 4 extremities	Decreased
Capillary refill	≤ 3 sec	> 3 sec
Mean blood pressure	≥ gestational age	< gestational age
Heart rate	140 to 160 bpm	>160 bpm

III.   Calculate the type and amount of volume expander you will administer to this baby.

0.9% NaCl

Estimated weight of 3 kg x 10 mL/kg = 30 mL

IV.   What do you think is the cause of this baby's shock and what do you do next?

Hypovolemic shock, likely due to acute blood loss in utero.

Give a second bolus of 0.9% NaCl IV and request urgent blood for transfusion

Case # 3

I.   **How would you organize your care if the baby had a heart rate > 220 and poor peripheral perfusion or low blood pressure?**

According to the Introduction section (page 4-6), whether the baby has good perfusion and blood

pressure or not, if the HR > 220 bpm you will organize care under Tachyarrhythmia

Bibliography

Behrman: Nelson Textbook of Pediatrics, 16th ed., Part XIX (The Cardiovascular System). Philadelphia, PA: W. B. Saunders Company, 2000.

Carcillo JA, Fields AI; American College of Critical Care Medicine Task Force Committee Members. Clinical practice parameters for hemodynamic support of pediatric and neonatal patients in septic shock. Critical Care Medicine, Jun 2002; 30(6): 1365-78.

Guidelines for good practice in the management of neonatal respiratory distress syndrome. Report of the second working group of the British Association of Perinatal Medicine. Nov 1998.

Kattwinkel J, Cook LJ, Hurt H, Nowacek GA, Short G. Perinatal Continuing Education program. Charlottesville: University of Virginia, 2002.

Klaus MH Fanaroff AA (Eds). Care of the High Risk Neonate. 6th edition. Philadelphia, PA: W.B. Saunders, 2001.

Park: Pediatric Cardiology for Practitioners, 4th ed., Part VII (Neonatal Cardiac Problems) Mosby, Inc. 2002.

Richmond S and Wren C. Early diagnosis of congenital heart disease. Seminars in Neonatology. 2001;6(1):27-35.

Chapter 5
Neurology

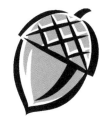

Objectives

Upon completion of this chapter, you should be able to:
1. Identify babies who require neurologic stabilization.
2. Apply the Neurology Sequence.
3. Assess and recognize abnormal tone.
4. Recognize and manage abnormal neurologic activity.
5. Recognize and manage neonatal encephalopathy.
6. Recognize when to exit to the other ACoRN Sequences.

Key Concepts

1. Abnormal tone can occur in many neonatal conditions, some of which may require immediate intervention.
2. Jitteriness must be distinguished from seizure activity because their significance and management is different.
3. Seizures in the neonate may present as a subtle change in activity.
4. Anticonvulsant therapy should be instituted even if the underlying cause of seizures has not been determined.
5. Hypoglycemic seizures may have long term neurodevelopmental consequences. Hypoglycemia must be treated as an emergency, particularly when associated with seizures.
6. Neonatal encephalopathy has multiple etiologies.
7. Neonatal encephalopathy may or may not result in permanent neurologic impairment.
8. Neonatal encephalopathy due to hypoxic ischemic injury may be associated with pathology in other organs or systems, particularly the kidney, liver, heart or respiratory system.
9. Neonatal abstinence syndrome must be considered in babies who present with unexplained irritability, jitteriness or seizures.

Skills

- Anticonvulsants: phenobarbital and phenytoin
- Morphine

Introduction

Abnormal neurological signs may be due to neurological, neuromuscular, or systemic conditions. Some of these conditions are reversible and/or treatable. Prompt management may prevent or minimize long-term morbidity.

The baby usually presents with abnormalities of tone or activity, and often has poor suck or swallow reflexes. These abnormalities may be transient; however, they may predict a more serious and long-term disability.

Alerting Signs

A baby who demonstrates one or more of the following Alerting Signs enters the Neurology Sequence:

> **Neurology**
> ☐ Abnormal tone*
> ☐ Jitteriness
> ☐ Seizures*

Abnormal tone

Tone is the normal tension or resistance to stretch of a healthy muscle. It is assessed by checking resting posture and resistance to movement. There is a natural increase in tone with increasing gestational age. A term baby with normal tone has flexion of arms and legs at rest.

Abnormal tone is described as either decreased (hypotonia) or increased (hypertonia).
- The hypotonic baby may be described as floppy (low tone) or flaccid (very low tone) and may or may not have decreased activity.
- The hypertonic baby may be described as having high tone or being rigid or spastic (very high tone),
  - excessive tone usually manifests in the flexor or extensor muscles of the extremities although, in certain conditions, truncal tone is also increased
  - in severe circumstances, there may be neck stiffness or posturing.

Jitteriness

Jitteriness may be confused with seizures. It is characterized by symmetrical, rapid movements of the hands and feet. It can also be described as tremulousness. These movements stop when the limb is held.

The most common causes of jitteriness are,
- hypoglycemia
- hypocalcemia
- drug withdrawal
- neonatal encephalopathy.

Jitteriness in the absence of the above causes is a benign sign.

Seizures   Seizures in newborns usually present as subtle changes in activity, clonic movements, or tonic posturing. These movements do not stop when the limb is held. Classic tonic-clonic seizures are not usually seen in the neonate.

Seizures are important to identify because they may,
- be related to a condition that requires urgent specific therapy, such as hypoglycemia
- interfere with important physiologic functions such as breathing
- be a manifestation of a pre-existing brain injury, and/or aggravate a pre-existing brain injury.

The table below indicates how to differentiate between jitteriness and seizures.

Observation	Jitteriness	Seizures
Abnormal gaze or eye movement	no	yes
Movements exquisitely sensitive to stimuli	yes	no
Predominant movement	tremor	clonic jerking
Movements cease with passive flexion	yes	no
Autonomic changes (e.g., tachycardia, increase in blood pressure, or apnea)	no	yes

Adapted from Volpe JJ. Neurology of the Newborn. 4th Edition. Philadelphia: WB Saunders Company, 2001

Core Steps   The interventions and monitoring activities applicable to all babies who enter the Neurology Sequence include,
- recheck the airway and breathing
- administer oxygen therapy as needed
- check blood glucose
- establish/continue pulse oximetry and cardiorespiratory monitoring.

Organization of Care   The course of action for babies with neurologic compromise depends on
- whether the baby presents with abnormal tone, jitteriness, or seizures, and
- the blood glucose level.

The Neurology Sequence

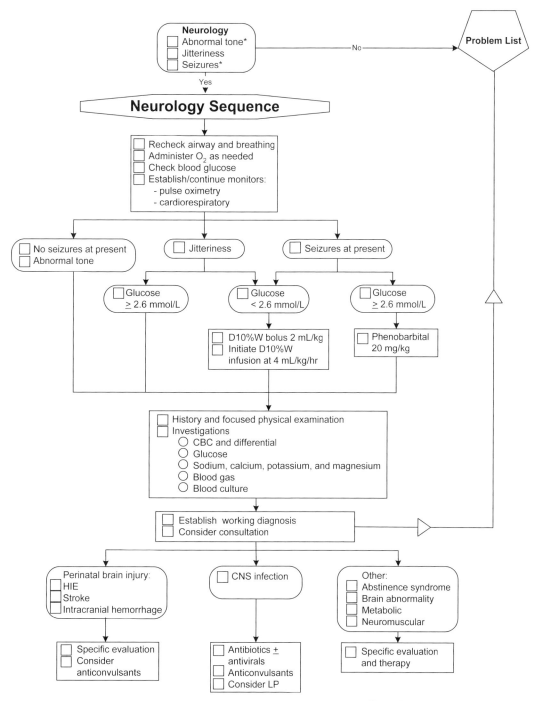

Blood glucose conversion: 2.6 mmol/L is equivalent to 47 mg/dL

Babies with hypoglycemia may be asymptomatic or may present with non-specific signs such as,

- jitteriness, tremor, seizure, or coma
- irritability, lethargy, or stupor
- hypotonia or limpness

- apnea or cyanotic spells
- poor feeding, having previously fed well
- hypothermia

Symptomatic hypoglycemia is assumed in babies who have any of the non-specific signs associated with hypoglycemia and have a blood glucose < 2.6 mmol/L (47 mg/dL). Symptomatic hypoglycemia is an emergency because it is associated with an increased risk for neurodevelopmental sequelae.

Response

The Response and the urgency of the Response is different for each of the Alerting Signs, and is dependent on the blood glucose level.

Abnormal tone

No urgent interventions are required if the baby exhibits the isolated finding of abnormal tone. In this instance, proceed directly to Next Steps.

Jitteriness

Symptomatic hypoglycemia requires immediate treatment. If jitteriness is associated with a blood glucose ≥ 2.6 mmol/L (47 mg/dL), proceed directly to Next Steps.

Seizures

If hypoglycemia is not present, phenobarbital is the first line therapy in a baby who is having seizures.

Symptomatic hypoglycemia

Babies with presumed symptomatic hypoglycemia require immediate intravenous dextrose.

A mini bolus of 2 mL/kg of D10%W should be considered, however the administration of a bolus of D10%W is controversial.

- It may reduce the time to normalization of the blood glucose level.
- It may stimulate insulin secretion and suppress glucagon secretion, resulting in rebound hypoglycemia.
- It remains in circulation for 20 minutes or less.

The key to the management of a baby with symptomatic hypoglycemia is to,

- start a D10%W infusion at 4 ml/kg/hour
- monitor blood glucose every 30 minutes until ≥ 2.6 mmol/L (47 mg/dL)
- adjust the hourly rate and/or concentration of the infusion as needed.

The management of babies with symptomatic hypoglycemia is continued in the Fluid & Glucose Management Sequence.

Next Steps   The Next Steps are to obtain a focused history, conduct a physical examination, order diagnostic tests, and establish a working diagnosis.

Focused history   Essential information to gather during the focused neurology history includes:

Antepartum
- maternal health before and during pregnancy, including nutrition and specific illnesses related to, or complicated by, pregnancy
- dosage and duration of medications taken during pregnancy
- substance use (illicit drugs, alcohol, and tobacco)
- congenital or hereditary disorders in the family
- family history of sleep myoclonus
- perception of fetal movements

Intrapartum
- nature of labour, analgesia used, type of delivery, including degree of difficulty, and complications encountered
- indicators of fetal compromise such as non-reassuring fetal heart rate or acidosis noted on a fetal scalp sampling

Neonatal
- umbilical cord blood gas (arterial and venous) obtained at birth
  - arterial cord gases reflect the degree of acidosis in the fetus, and venous blood gases the degree of acidosis in the blood coming from the placenta
  - in a fetus with malfunctioning placenta, the acidosis is present in both arterial and venous gases and the arterio-venous difference tends to be small
  - in a fetus with an acute interruption of umbilical circulation, the acidosis is mostly in the arterial cord blood and the arterio-venous difference is large
- condition at birth and time of onset of respiration
- need for resuscitation at birth and extent of the resuscitative efforts
- Apgar scores (including extended scores at 10 and 20 minutes)
- gestational age
- feeding history

Focused physical examination   In addition to the examination conducted during the Primary Survey, a focused neurology physical examination should include:

Observation
- level of consciousness (LOC) and activity
- posture
- spontaneous movements

Measurement of vital signs: respiratory rate, heart rate, temperature, and blood pressure.

Examination
- head circumference (must be measured and plotted in a chart)
- evidence of external injury (for example, a fracture or cephalohematoma)
- abnormal movements
- posture and tone (popliteal angle, raise to sit manoeuvre, and ventral suspension)
- fullness/tension of fontanels and measurement of suture separation
- primary reflexes (such as suck–swallow, Moro's, palmar grasp, and response to traction)
- brain stem reflexes (gag, corneal, pupillary size and reaction to light, oculo-vestibular)
- deep tendon reflexes (biceps and patellar)
- examination of spontaneous extraocular movements
- fundoscopic appearance (such as retinal hemorrhage or chorioretinitis)

Diagnostic tests

Many of the diagnostic tests used to differentiate neurologic disorders are specialized, but a few simple blood tests can assist in reaching a working diagnosis:

1. **CBC and differential**
   - assists in the diagnosis of acute anemia from blood loss, polycythemia or sepsis

2. **Blood chemistry**
   - to rule out hypoglycemia and electrolyte abnormalities (sodium, calcium and magnesium levels)

3. **Blood gas**
   - to rule out metabolic acidosis

4. **Blood culture if sepsis is suspected**
   - although this will not affect your immediate management, the specimen must be drawn before antibiotics are administered

Establish a Working Diagnosis

The actual diagnosis of a neurologic condition may be time-consuming and requires specialized investigations. Sometimes the etiology may be obscure. In the interim, a working diagnosis based on groups of symptoms provides direction for planning ongoing investigation and management.

Specific Management

In this sequence, the working diagnosis that requires urgent Specific Management is persistent hypoglycemia (guidelines are provided in the Fluid & Glucose Management Sequence).

Specific Management for perinatal brain injury, central nervous system infection, and other neonatal neurological disorders needs to be individualized and based on the actual diagnosis. For the purposes of ACoRN, perinatal brain injury comprises hypoxic ischemic encephalopathy (HIE), perinatal stroke, and intracranial hemorrhage.

Because of the complexity of neurological conditions contained in these categories, ongoing consultation is recommended.

Neurology Case # 1 – The floppy baby

> You are a family physician who has just been informed that your patient, a mother in her second pregnancy, has delivered a baby by urgent Cesarean section at 37 weeks gestation following a motor vehicle accident.
>
> The mother has awakened from her anesthetic and is doing well. She has no injuries related to the accident but her baby required resuscitation.
>
> You arrive when the baby is one hour of age. She is on a radiant warmer in the observation nursery area. She is breathing regularly and without difficulty, her vital signs (HR, RR, BP) are normal, and she is pink in room air.

Resuscitation
- [ ] Ineffective breathing
- [ ] Heart rate < 100 bpm
- [ ] Central cyanosis

> You determine that the baby shows none of the Resuscitation Signs and begin the Primary Survey.
>
> Skin color, perfusion and peripheral pulses are normal. The nurse tells you the baby's tone appears low. You observe the baby is lying with arms and legs extended. The temperature probe on the radiant heater reads 36.7°C; an axillary temperature is being taken. The baby's weight is 3500 grams.

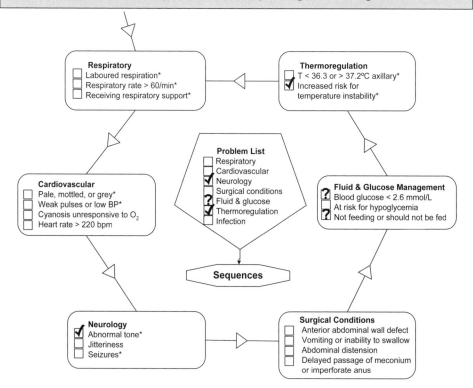

Respiratory
- [ ] Laboured respiration*
- [ ] Respiratory rate > 60/min*
- [ ] Receiving respiratory support*

Thermoregulation
- [ ] T < 36.3 or > 37.2°C axillary*
- [x] Increased risk for temperature instability*

Problem List
- [ ] Respiratory
- [ ] Cardiovascular
- [x] Neurology
- [ ] Surgical conditions
- [?] Fluid & glucose
- [x] Thermoregulation
- [ ] Infection

Cardiovascular
- [ ] Pale, mottled, or grey*
- [ ] Weak pulses or low BP*
- [ ] Cyanosis unresponsive to O_2
- [ ] Heart rate > 220 bpm

Fluid & Glucose Management
- [?] Blood glucose < 2.6 mmol/L
- [?] At risk for hypoglycemia
- [?] Not feeding or should not be fed

Sequences

Neurology
- [x] Abnormal tone*
- [ ] Jitteriness
- [ ] Seizures*

Surgical Conditions
- [ ] Anterior abdominal wall defect
- [ ] Vomiting or inability to swallow
- [ ] Abdominal distension
- [ ] Delayed passage of meconium or imperforate anus

The first area of concern on the Problem List is Neurology. You enter the Neurology Sequence and carry out the Core Steps.

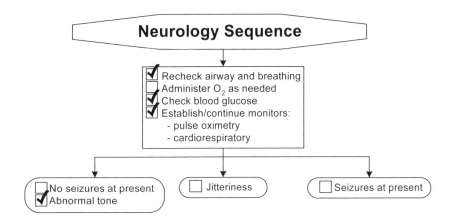

The baby's airway is patent. There is no respiratory difficulty or abnormalities on auscultation. The respiratory rate is 54/minute and the heart rate 160 bpm. Oximetry saturation is 93% in room air.

Oxygen does not need to be administered, therefore is not ticked with a check mark.

Why do you check the airway and breathing as part of the Core Steps?

Conditions that cause abnormal tone, jitteriness or seizures may also compromise breathing, either due to abnormal respiratory muscle activity or poor central respiratory drive. During seizures, a baby may have periods of apnea, difficulty protecting the airway, or may not have a coordinated suck/swallow reflex thus risking aspiration of milk or secretions.

In organizing your care, your attention is drawn to the baby's low tone.

Clinical assessment of tone

Tone is evaluated in a baby at rest by observing and examining,
- resting posture
- range of motion of several joints such as the knee, elbow or shoulder joints
- extensor and flexor tone of the neck while being pulled to sit
- posture while being suspended ventrally.

You may decide not to examine the last two components of the assessment of tone in unstable babies or babies in whom birth injury is suspected.

Resting Posture Resting posture is evaluated by observation when the baby is supine and at rest. The degree of flexion at rest decreases with gestational age. The arms and legs of a term baby should be flexed (right panel). A term baby with decreased tone adopts a less flexed position.

This may indicate neurological compromise.

Flaccid 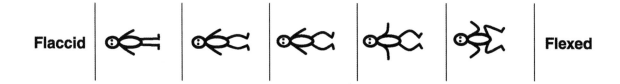 **Flexed**

Popliteal angle The baby is placed in the supine position with the pelvis flat on the examination surface. One hand is used to fully flex the hip joint. The other hand is used to extend the lower leg, feeling the resistance to passive movement. The angle obtained at the knee is measured.

A term baby with good tone will have a popliteal angle $\leq 90°$ while a hypotonic or preterm baby will have an angle $> 90°$.

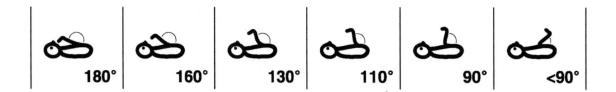

180° 160° 130° 110° 90° <90°

Pull to sit maneuver This test demonstrates active neck flexor and extensor tone, and is intended for the assessment of the term baby.

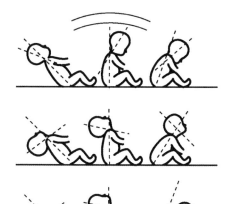

In the term baby with normal tone, the head is balanced over the torso in the sitting position.

In the term baby with increased extensor tone, the head is hyperextended and cannot drop forward.

In the term baby with decreased tone, the head lags in extension and then drops forward.

Ventral suspension The baby is placed in the prone position with the chest resting on the examiner's palm. The posture is observed as the baby is lifted off the examining surface.

The continuum of tone in a term baby, from poor (left) to normal (3rd and 4th panel) to increased (right) is illustrated in the diagram below.

| Head droops, back greatly arched, limbs dangle | Head slightly raised, back less curved | Head raised but not to body axis, back slightly curved | Head in line with body axis, back straight | Head raised above body axis, back straight |

Further to lying with arms and legs extended, you note on examination that the popliteal angle is 130°. In addition, the raise to sit maneuver shows the head has a moderate lag in extension. On ventral suspension, the head is raised but not to the body axis and the back is slightly curved.

There are no abnormal movements suggestive of seizures and the baby is not jittery at this time.

> You proceed to the Next Steps.
>
> The nurse tells you that the mother was involved in a head-on collision and noticed contractions on arrival to the emergency room. The initial fetal heart-rate tracing showed late decelerations and minimal variability. A scalp pH was unobtainable as the cervix was closed and the presenting part had not descended. The obstetrician opted to proceed with a Cesarean section. A cord blood gas was obtained at the time of birth.
>
> You know from your prenatal care of the mother that she is healthy.
>
> Apgar scores were 1 at 1 minute and 3 at 5 minutes. The baby required bag-and-mask ventilation for several minutes, following which she began to breathe spontaneously.

I.   **What four key pieces of information have you obtained so far that may assist you in obtaining a focused history to arrive at a working diagnosis?**

_____

_____

_____

_____

> You go to the post-operative recovery room to inform the parents of their baby's condition and seek additional information. The mother tells you that her other child is healthy, and there is no family history of any neurologic or muscular disorder. She hasn't had any recent colds or flu-like illness.
>
> The obstetrician mentions that the Cesarean section was uneventful except for the presence of a placental abruption.
>
> You perform a focused physical examination.

How do you assess the level of consciousness?

Term and near term babies have periods of sleep and wakefulness. When awake, these babies are visually attentive and respond to external stimuli such as the human voice and other sounds, touch, light and pain. Babies who are sleeping can be aroused into a fully awake state, and those who are crying can be soothed. Motor and feeding behaviors are well organized. They respond to hunger, and exhibit well developed primitive reflexes such as rooting, suck, grasp and Moro. When the palms or soles are "tickled", a withdrawal of the stimulated limb is noted.

When assessing the level of consciousness of a term and near term baby, it is important to note the presence or absence of all or some of the described behaviors. For example, babies with encephalopathy may appear to be alert or hyperalert, but on closer inspection are deficient in many of the other behaviors expected in normal wakefulness.

Assessment of brainstem reflexes:

Examination of functions mediated by cranial nerves is an important part of the neurological examination of the newborn, as the brainstem is an important site of injury in acute neonatal encephalopathy. The essential reflexes to assess are,

- sucking – the presence of strong and rhythmic sucking is normal from 36 to 38 weeks gestation and is tested using a gloved finger inserted into the baby's mouth
- gag reflex – the presence of a strong gag reflex is normal and is tested by touching the baby's throat with a gloved finger or catheter
- tongue fasciculation – the presence of quivering movements along the lateral tongue margins is abnormal
- pupillary reflex to light – normal reaction is present from 28 to 30 weeks gestation
- corneal reflex – the eyelids should close when the cornea is gently touched by the tip of a cotton swab
- oculocephalic – the eyes should deviate in the opposite direction when the head is turned from one side to the other in a baby lying supine (doll's eyes reflex).

The baby continues to breathe regularly at 54/minute. Heart rate remains at 160 bpm, the pulse is easy to palpate over the femoral arteries, and the blood pressure is normal.

She is noted to be mostly sleeping and to have only short periods of wakefulness after stimulation. When examined awake, she does not visually connect with the examiner's face or track a coloured object. She is not attentive when being talked to, but responds by withdrawing the leg when her sole is tickled using a cotton swab. Rooting is absent, and sucking, grasp and Moro are weak.

The anterior fontanel is flat. The pupils are equal and reactive to light. The corneal, oculocephalic and gag reflexes are present; tongue fasciculation is not present.

There are no abnormal movements. Deep tendon reflexes are present and of normal intensity in the upper and lower extremities.

You decide to place a call to your pediatric colleague to determine if further investigations are warranted.

You call the lab and learn that the cord arterial pH was 6.98, with an arterial base deficit of 18 mmol/L. The baby's capillary glucose is 3.5 mmol/L (63 mg/dL).

The baby met none of the alerting signs of the Resuscitation, Respiratory or Cardiovascular Sequences. Therefore, there is no need to consider interventions at this time to treat the metabolic acidosis indicated by the base deficit of 18. With adequate cardiorespiratory function, it is anticipated that the metabolic acidosis will gradually resolve on its own.

Causes of abnormal tone include:

- neonatal encephalopathy
- sepsis
- hypoglycemia
- intracranial hemorrhage
- drugs/anesthesia
- chromosomal abnormality
- congenital CNS disorders
- inborn errors of metabolism
- hypermagnesemia due to maternal administration of magnesium sulfate
- spinal cord injury

In acute conditions such as neonatal encephalopathy, a baby's tone may be normal, increased or decreased at birth; however, the baby may later become hypotonic and develop other neurologic manifestations, including seizures. In other conditions, such as Trisomy 21 or neuromuscular disorders, the baby is hypotonic at birth and this does not change over time.

> Based on the historical findings of poor variability and late decelerations on the fetal heart rate tracing which triggered the urgent Cesarean section, the finding of a placental abruption, the baby's condition at birth and cord blood gas results, and the current physical findings, your working diagnosis is neonatal encephalopathy resulting from perinatal asphyxia.

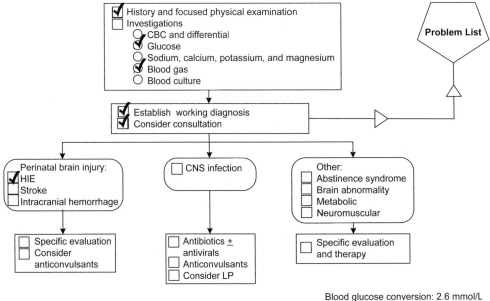

Blood glucose conversion: 2.6 mmol/L is equivalent to 47 mg/dL

What is neonatal encephalopathy?

Neonatal encephalopathy is a condition defined and described for term and near-term babies. Neonatal encephalopathy describes a constellation of abnormal clinical findings which may evolve over hours or days. These findings include a combination of abnormal consciousness, tone, reflexes, feeding, respiration, and/or seizures. Hypoxic-ischemic encephalopathy (HIE) is a common cause of neonatal encephalopathy; less common causes include CNS infections, inborn errors of metabolism and intracranial hemorrhage.

Neonatal encephalopathy may or may not result in permanent neurologic impairment. However, cerebral palsy subsequent to an intrapartum hypoxic-ischemic injury only develops in babies who present with neonatal encephalopathy.

Important considerations in the management of neonatal encephalopathy

Babies with neonatal encephalopathy require:
- Careful observation to ensure that ventilation and oxygenation are within the normal range
  - assisted ventilation may be required
  - there is no therapeutic role for hyperoxia
  - hypocarbia and alkalosis must be avoided
- Assessments for clinical signs of poor perfusion, low pulse pressure or low blood pressure (Cardiovascular Sequence) and maintainance of adequate circulation
  - an echocardiogram and ECG may be helpful in babies with signs of poor circulation
  - volume expanders or inotropes may be required
- Most babies with neonatal encephalopathy are initially oliguric or anuric (Fluid & Glucose Management Sequence)
  - restrict initial fluid intake to 2 to 3 mL/kg/hour (approximately 50 to 75 mL/kg/day) of D10%W
  - monitor blood glucose every 2 to 4 hours until stable: restricted fluid intake may not meet glucose requirements
  - monitor serum sodium every 12 hours: excessive fluid intake will lead to hyponatremia (serum Na < 135 mmol/L)
- Maintenance of body temperature within the normal range
  - hyperthermia must be avoided
  - ongoing studies are trying to determine if therapeutic hypothermia of babies with hypoxic ischemic encephalopathy is efficacious and safe.

Having formulated a working diagnosis and management plan, you exit the Neurology Sequence and continue with the Fluid & Glucose Management Sequence as identified in the Problem List.

One of the questions raised as you completed the Primary Survey was whether this baby with alerting signs on the Neurology Sequence should be fed.

How do you determine if this baby should be orally fed?

A baby should not be fed unless the level of consciousness is normal, the airway protective reflexes (gag and cough) are present, and the suck-swallow mechanism is mature. The suck-swallow mechanism is noted by examining for the presence of rooting, and coordinated sucking and swallowing. This coordination is rarely in place before 32 to 34 weeks gestation.

Babies with neonatal encephalopathy and those suspected of having had a hypoxic-ischemic event should not be fed for 24 to 48 hours as they may have sustained bowel ischemia.

Your pediatric colleague returns your call. She agrees with your working diagnosis of neonatal encephalopathy and with your management plan. She suggests that this baby should remain in the observation nursery so her progress can be followed more closely. She agrees with your decision to withhold feedings for now.

Neurology Case # 2 – A 6 hour-old baby with seizures

Continued from Case #1

The baby is now 6 hours old.

An intravenous with D10%W at 3 mL/kg/hour is infusing. She is lying quietly in her incubator, breathing easily, and is pink in room air. You take a blood pressure and auscultate her heart and lungs. Her heart rate is 120 bpm and regular. Blood glucose has remained > 3.3 mmol/L (> 60 mg/dL) on regular monitoring.

As you remove the blood pressure cuff, the baby's arm begins to twitch rhythmically. You observe her movements carefully. There are rhythmic movements of all extremities that do not stop when the extremities are held. At the same time, her eyes deviate to the left, and she has a glazed look.

You decide the baby is having a seizure.

You determine the baby shows none of the Alerting Signs for immediate resuscitation.

You perform a Primary Survey.

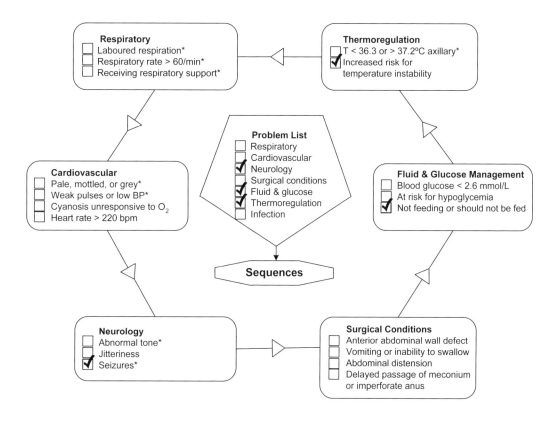

You enter the Neurology Sequence and complete the Core Steps.

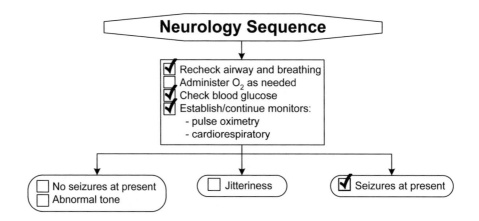

The SpO_2 is 92% on room air, the airway is clear and there are no abnormalities on auscultation of the chest. The blood glucose done at the bedside using a glucose meter is 3.9 mmol/L (70 mg/dL).

Clinical assessment of seizures

Seizures that occur in newborns can be categorized in one of four types:

1. **Subtle** (30% of time)
- horizontal tonic deviation of the eyes with or without jerking movements
- repetitive blinking of the eyelids or staring episodes
- chewing, lip smacking or drooling
- bicycling and purposeless movements
- apnea
- sudden tachycardia at rest, or increase in blood pressure or decrease in SpO_2
- posturing of a limb

2. **Clonic** (25% of time)
- rhythmic, slow movements (1 to 3 jerks/second) involving the face and/or the upper and/or lower extremities on one side of the body (therefore called focal)
  - the baby is usually conscious during focal seizures
- coarse, jerking movements of one or two limbs that migrate to the contralateral part of the body (therefore called multifocal) in a non-orderly fashion
  - when movements generalize to involve both sides of the body, loss of consciousness usually occurs.

3. **Tonic** (20% of time)
- sustained, rigid posturing of a limb or asymmetric posturing of the trunk or neck (focal) with or without tonic eye deviation
- premature babies may develop generalized tonic seizures that include flexion or extension of the neck, trunk and upper extremities and extension of the lower extremities (similar to decorticate or decerebrate posturing), with or without autonomic phenomena

4. **Myoclonic** (25% of time)
- rapid contractions of flexor muscles in one limb (focal), several parts of the body (multifocal) or the whole body (generalized)
  - in "benign sleep myoclonus", which usually disappears by 6 months of age with no sequelae, any of the three forms can be present

I. **Based on the information collected so far, how would you describe the seizures this baby is having?**

_____ **and** _____

You organize the care of this baby on the basis that seizures are present and the blood glucose is in the normal range.

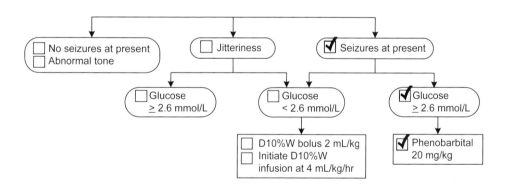

As this baby is not hypoglycemic, the physician orders phenobarbital 20 mg/kg intravenously over 10 to 15 minutes.

The total loading dose of phenobarbital is approximately 40 mg/kg. The second half-loading dose is usually necessary to achieve seizure control and mid-high therapeutic drug levels. Addition of a second anticonvulsant, usually phenytoin, may be necessary when seizures are refractory.

 Anticonvulsants: Phenobarbital & phenytoin

II.   **Calculate the half-loading dose of phenobarbital for this 3500 gram baby.**

> You prepare to administer the phenobarbital and start documenting the seizure activity of this baby.

What should you note when documenting seizure activity?

Time	At what time did the seizure occur?
Duration	How long did the seizure last?
State	Was the baby awake or asleep?
Site& spread	Where did the seizure originate (e.g., arm, leg, or face)? Did the seizure spread to other parts of the body? If so, where?
Suppression	Were the movements suppressed by grasping the extremity or if the baby is wakened?
Eye movements	Were there accompanying eye movements such as horizontal deviation of the eyes, jerking or staring?
Mouth movements	Was there lip-smacking, chewing, tongue movements or drooling?
Level of consciousness	Was the baby or awake or asleep? Did the baby, <ul><li>respond to visual and auditory stimuli?</li><li>rouse from sleep with tactile stimulation?</li><li>cry periodically while awake?</li></ul>
Autonomic changes	Were there changes in heart rate and blood pressure before, during or after the seizure?

Other signs	Was there a change in the baby's color?
	Were there signs of regurgitation or choking?
	Did the baby have difficulty breathing?
	Did the baby have apnea?

> You do a focused neurological examination and note the baby is lethargic and hypotonic. The deep tendon reflexes are increased, and 3 to 4 beats of myoclonus can be elicited in the ankle joints. The Moro reflex is incomplete. Sucking is weak. The gag reflex is present. The pupils are small but reactive to light. The corneal and oculocephalic reflexes are present. Respiration is regular and airway secretions minimal.

What are the common causes of seizures in a newborn?

1. hypoxic ischemic encephalopathy
2. intracranial hemorrhage
3. metabolic disturbances
4. CNS infection (meningitis/encephalitis)
5. underlying brain abnormality
6. neonatal abstinence syndrome

The age of the baby is a clue to the cause of the seizures.

Age	Cause
At birth	• acute drug withdrawal caused by naloxone administration to the baby of a narcotic-using mother • local anesthetic injected into fetal scalp during pudendal block
Day 1	• HIE seizures usually present at 6 to 18 hours of age, worsening over the next 24 to 48 hours • hypoglycemia • metabolic abnormalities such as hypocalcemia • trauma, including subdural hemorrhage
Day 2 to 3	• neonatal abstinence syndrome • meningitis • metabolic disturbances
Day 3 to 7	• cerebral infarct • hypocalcemia • underlying brain abnormality • meningitis/encephalitis • subarachnoid hemorrhage
Day 7	• neonatal abstinence syndrome due to methadone withdrawal • meningitis/encephalitis

1. Hypoxic ischemic encephalopathy

Most babies who are exposed to a perinatal hypoxic ischemic event are asymptomatic and have a normal neurological examination in the postnatal period. These babies have a normal long term outcome. Other babies develop a form of neonatal encephalopathy called hypoxic-ischemic encephalopathy (HIE).

The signs and symptoms of HIE develop in the early postnatal period, but vary depending on the severity of the insult as well as on when the insult occurred. Not all babies with HIE develop long-term sequelae.

HIE occurs when oxygen levels and/or blood supply are inadequate to meet the needs of the baby's organs. As a result, the affected organs develop hypoxemia, lactic acidosis, and cellular injury and death. The insult to the brain is global resulting in a fairly symmetric distribution of dysfunction and injury, as seen on clinical examination and neuroradiological examination. The pattern and duration of the insult determines which areas of the brain are most affected, i.e., the areas of highest energy requirement (basal ganglia and brain stem) when the insult is very acute and global, or areas with the most fragile blood supply (watershed regions of the cortex and subcortex), when the insult is partial but prolonged.

Babies who have suffered a significant perinatal hypoxic ischemic event[1,2] are identified by the presence of:
1. Apgar score 0 to 3 for $\geq$ 5 minutes.
2. Neonatal encephalopathy (hypotonia, seizures, coma).
3. Evidence of multi-organ system dysfunction in the immediate neonatal period.
4. Umbilical cord arterial pH < 7.0.
5. Umbilical cord arterial base deficit $\geq$ 16 mmol/L.
6. Early imaging study showing evidence of acute, non-focal cerebral abnormality.

Because of the global nature of the hypoxic ischemic insult, other organs are usually affected. HIE is most commonly accompanied by evidence of kidney, heart, liver, and bowel dysfunction.
- Kidney damage is recognized by decreased urine output, microscopic hematuria, elevation of serum creatinine and low serum sodium.
- Signs of cardiac injury include poor contractility, low blood pressure, reduced peripheral perfusion, and occasionally, overt heart failure and arrhythmias.
- Hepatic injury manifests as elevation of liver enzymes.

[1] The Task Force on Neonatal Encephalopathy and Cerebral Palsy. Neonatal encephalopathy and cerebral palsy: Defining the pathogenesis and pathophysiology. The American College of Obstetricians and Gynecologists and American Academy of Pediatrics, Washington DC, 2003.
[2] Society of Obstetricians and Gynecologists of Canada. Policy Statement from the Task Force on Cerebral Palsy and Fetal Asphyxia. SOGC CPG FHS in Labour No. 112, March 2002.

- Bowel injury may manifest itself as ileus or necrotizing enterocolitis.
- In some cases there may be clotting abnormalities.

Clinical assessment of severity in HIE

	Mild	Moderate	Severe
Consciousness	"hyperalertness"	lethargy	stupor/coma
Tone	normal/increased	decreased	flaccid
Tendon reflex	increased	increased	depressed
Moro	exaggerated	incomplete	absent
Seizures	absent	present	difficult to control
Breathing	regular	variable	apnea
Suck reflex	present	weak	absent
Gag reflex	present	present	absent

Adapted from Sarnat HB et al: Neonatal encephalopathy following fetal distresss: A clinical and encephalographic study. Arch Neurol 33:695,1976.

The clinical signs of HIE evolve over the first several hours and days after birth. Some babies present with moderate to severe HIE shortly after birth; others may start with minimal signs or signs of mild HIE and then develop signs of moderate or severe HIE, usually over a period of 24 to 48 hours and after the onset of seizures.

For example, a baby with severe HIE may progress over the first three days with the following clinical signs:

Birth to 12 hours
- depressed LOC
- irregular respirations
- intact pupillary response
- hypotonia
- seizures

12 to 24 hours
- decreasing LOC
- apneic spells
- weakness
- increased seizure activity

24 to 72 hours
- stupor or coma
- respiratory arrest
- brainstem disturbances
- seizures absent or present (EEG only or clinical)

> 72 hours
- stupor diminishes
- disturbed suck, swallow, gag
- hypotonia more common than hypertonia
- weakness

Long term neurodevelopmental sequelae of HIE

Not all babies with HIE develop long-term sequelae.

Possible long-term sequelae of HIE include spastic quadriplegia (a form of cerebral palsy) with or without a movement disorder, seizures, cognitive impairment, sensorineural deficits and feeding difficulty.

Almost all babies with mild HIE have a normal outcome, and almost all babies with severe HIE either die or develop long-term sequelae. Death is uncommon in babies with moderate HIE, but long term sequelae develop in approximately 20 to 30%. Seizures which are persistent or difficult to control, a prolonged abnormal neurological examination beyond a week of age or at the time of discharge, inability to feed requiring prolonged gavage feeding are also indicative of risk for long-term sequelae.

Neuroimaging, such as CT or MRI scanning, are useful assessment tools with diagnostic and prognostic value.

2. Intracranial Hemorrhage

Subarachnoid hemorrhage usually occurs in the absence of hypoxic insult or trauma.
- Small subarachnoid hemorrhages are common, present with minimal symptoms, and usually have a good prognosis.
- If seizures occur, they often do so on the second or third postnatal day, and the baby appears well between seizures.

Periventricular (PVH) or intraventricular (IVH) hemorrhage originates in the germinal matrix, a fragile loosely-supported capillary network in the external wall of the lateral ventricles. PVH/IVH is more common in sick, ventilated preterm babies, but may also be found in otherwise healthy preterm babies; it is uncommon in term babies.
- Babies with PVH/IVH are usually asymptomatic.
- In severe cases, PVH/IVH may be accompanied by subtle seizures, decerebrate posturing, and/or generalized tonic seizures.

Subdural hemorrhage may be associated with head trauma (for example, as a result of a difficult delivery). It is a space-occupying lesion that may exert pressure on brain tissue, sometimes causing focal seizures.

Intracranial bleeding may be due to other causes, for example, allo-immune thrombocytopenia.

3. Metabolic Disturbances

Hypoglycemia, hypocalcemia, hypomagnesemia, hyponatremia, and hypernatremia can lead to generalized seizure activity. Of these, hypoglycemia may be associated with long term neurodevelopmental abnormalities.

Inborn errors of metabolism are rare. Early diagnosis and prompt management are of critical importance.

4. CNS Infection

Bacterial (meningitis) or non-bacterial (encephalitis) intracranial infections can result in altered level of consciousness, abnormal tone, and seizures.
- Tests, including blood culture, (± lumbar puncture), white cell and differential count, and platelet count may be needed to rule out sepsis.
- Antibiotics should be started pending test results.

If viral or bacterial meningitis is suspected, a lumbar puncture is necessary to confirm this diagnosis. Performing a lumbar puncture may be beyond the scope of practice of some clinicians. When bacterial meningitis is suspected, obtaining cerebral spinal fluid (CSF) for analysis is less of a priority than initiating antibiotic treatment. Before performing a lumbar puncture, it is important to determine if there are contraindications to this procedure present, such as thrombocytopenia.

5. Underlying Brain Abnormalities

These involve conditions that result in abnormalities of brain growth and anatomy. Causes include single gene, chromosomal or other genetic abnormalities, and exposure in utero to chemical or infectious agents.

6. Neonatal Abstinence Syndrome

Drug withdrawal from opiates such as heroin or methadone, benzodiazepines, and alcohol can result in neonatal seizures.
- Naloxone should not be given to a baby whose mother has a history of long-term narcotic use as this may result in severe seizure activity.

The working diagnosis remains hypoxic ischemic encephalopathy. The presence of seizures indicate the baby now has to be considered as having moderate HIE.

The physician consults with the specialist at the referral center, relating the events of the past several hours. Together, it is decided that the baby should be transported to the referral facility for further evaluation, which will likely include specialized neuroimaging.

The physician tells the parents their baby has started having seizure activity and phenobarbital has been initiated. The parents ask, "How can we tell if our baby will be OK?"

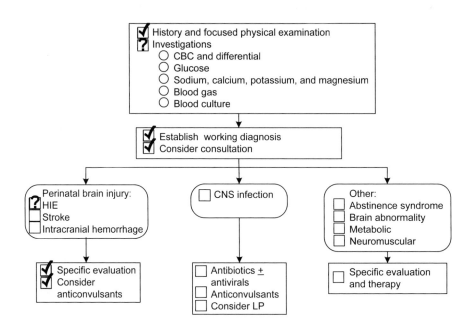

III.   What would you say to the parents when they ask you if their baby "will be OK"?

_____

_____

_____

_____

What is usually included in the further evaluation of a newborn with neonatal seizures or abnormal neurologic findings?

- clinical documentation of seizures and neurologic events
- radiological evaluation, including cranial ultrasound, computerized tomography (CT scan), and magnetic resonance imaging (MRI)
- electroencephalogram (EEG)
- laboratory evaluation, including liver enzymes, urea and creatinine, and urinalysis
- toxicology screen
- metabolic work-up
- lumbar puncture to rule out meningitis

> The transport team arrives. As part of the nursing handover, a copy of the seizure log below is given to the transport team.

Seizure log:

Time/ duration	Suppress by holding	Origin/ spread	Eye/mouth movements	LOC	Autonomic changes	Other signs
09:00 h 20 sec	No	Arm, then all extremities	Eyes deviated to left	Normal crying, auditory and visual responses when not seizing	No	No

Neurology Case # 3 – Baby born to a substance-using mother

As the pediatric resident on call, you are asked to see a 14-hour old baby boy who the nurse reports as jittery and irritable. On arrival to the observation area in the nursery, you find, from the birth record, that he was born at 39 weeks gestation to a 21-year-old primagravida and weighed 3000 grams. The mother had no antenatal care. The nurse is rocking the baby, trying to console him because he has been crying constantly.

You determine the baby shows none of the Resuscitation Signs.

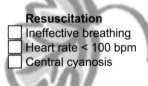

Resuscitation
- [ ] Ineffective breathing
- [ ] Heart rate < 100 bpm
- [ ] Central cyanosis

You carry the baby to the examination table, turn on the over-bed warmer, and complete the Primary Survey. He is lying with flexed arms, sucking his fists vigorously. His legs are tremulous, but the movements cease when you grasp his feet. Vital signs are stable and within normal limits. He has been bottle fed four times since birth, as his mother has declined to breastfeed. The nurses have noticed his suck is not well coordinated.

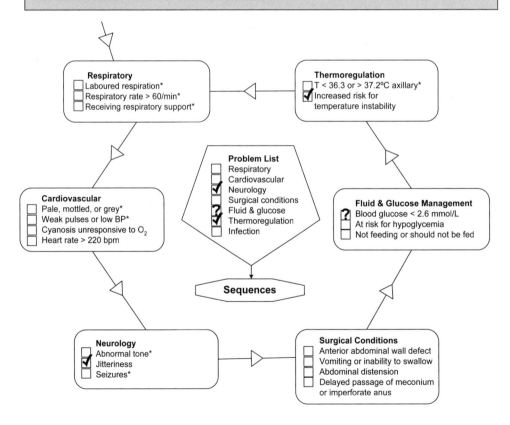

Respiratory
- [ ] Laboured respiration*
- [ ] Respiratory rate > 60/min*
- [ ] Receiving respiratory support*

Thermoregulation
- [ ] T < 36.3 or > 37.2°C axillary*
- [x] Increased risk for temperature instability

Cardiovascular
- [ ] Pale, mottled, or grey*
- [ ] Weak pulses or low BP*
- [ ] Cyanosis unresponsive to O₂
- [ ] Heart rate > 220 bpm

Problem List
- [ ] Respiratory
- [ ] Cardiovascular
- [x] Neurology
- [ ] Surgical conditions
- [?] Fluid & glucose
- [x] Thermoregulation
- [ ] Infection

Fluid & Glucose Management
- [?] Blood glucose < 2.6 mmol/L
- [ ] At risk for hypoglycemia
- [ ] Not feeding or should not be fed

Sequences

Neurology
- [ ] Abnormal tone*
- [x] Jitteriness
- [ ] Seizures*

Surgical Conditions
- [ ] Anterior abdominal wall defect
- [ ] Vomiting or inability to swallow
- [ ] Abdominal distension
- [ ] Delayed passage of meconium or imperforate anus

I.   Is the baby having seizures?

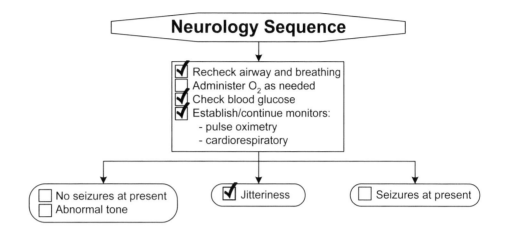

Causes of jitteriness include:

1. **Hypoglycemia**
    Discussed in the Fluid & Glucose Management Chapter

2. **Hypocalcemia**
    Low serum calcium (ionized calcium ≤1.0 mmol/L or total serum calcium ≤ 2.25 mmol/L or 9 mg/dL) may be a result of poor intake, induced alkalosis, prematurity, or metabolic disorders.

3. **Neonatal abstinence syndrome**
    Opioids (heroin, methadone, morphine and related drugs), CNS stimulants (cocaine, amphetamines), CNS depressants (alcohol, sedatives), and hallucinogens used during pregnancy have been demonstrated to cause neonatal abstinence syndrome, also called drug withdrawal, in the baby.

4. **CNS irritability**
    May be due to underlying brain abnormality, neonatal encephalopathy, or CNS stimulants.

The baby has no respiratory distress and SpO$_2$ is 93% on room air. No oxygen is required. The glucose meter reads 4.5 mmol/L (81 mg/dL). Because the baby is jittery but normoglycemic, you proceed directly to Next Steps.

The mother says she used heroin during her pregnancy, including on the day of delivery. She has no co-existing medical conditions. She came to hospital fully dilated and delivered quickly. Membranes ruptured at the time of delivery. No paternal history is available. The baby was vigorous at birth. Apgar scores were 8 at 1 minute and 9 at 5 minutes.

On examination, the baby is irritable and yawns and sneezes frequently. He has a shrill cry and is difficult to console. Tone is increased and he startles easily. There are no other positive physical findings. You order a CBC and differential, but feel that no other blood work is indicated at this time, because your working diagnosis is neonatal abstinence syndrome. You place a call to the attending pediatrician to review your findings and plan the baby's Specific Management.

A positive and supportive relationship between health care providers and the mother is an essential component of management. Inquiring about drug use, as with prescription medications, should be part of routine care and not reserved for those occasions when drug use is suspected. Enquiry should be made in a sensitive way, and in a health care context.

When there is a history of drug use, further information should be obtained to determine the type of drug(s) used, the timing with respect to pregnancy and delivery, and the frequency and route(s) of administration. The need for screening for infectious agents prevalent in populations using intravenous drugs should be explained. If indicated, treatment protocols for the prevention and treatment of perinatal transmission of infectious agents, such as hepatitis B or HIV, should be implemented.

Toxicology studies of mothers and babies have limited therapeutic value as treatment decisions are based on the severity of symptoms. Other concerns regarding their use include,

- false negative results, particularly if a drug was not used shortly prior to birth or if a sample is not obtained shortly after birth,
- false positive results, possible due to interactions with other medications or foods
- the potential use of the results outside of a health care context.

Toxicology studies in mothers or babies require informed consent. It is controversial whether newborn toxicology testing should be performed under the general consent for care - this practice is not recommended.

Neonatal abstinence syndrome (NAS)

The clinical presentation of NAS varies with the substance being used by the mother, the quantity, frequency, duration of intrauterine exposure, and when the drug was last used prior to delivery.

The substance may be therapeutic (for example, morphine for chronic pain) or illicit.

For both heroin and methadone, the newborn appears physically and behaviourally normal at birth. Withdrawal from methadone tends to appear later than withdrawal from heroin because of methadone's long half-life.

Signs and symptoms found in babies with NAS include:

W wakefulness
I irritability, increased tone, increased Moro reflex
T tremulousness (jittery), temperature instability, tachypnea
H hyperactivity, high-pitched cry, hiccoughs, hypersensitivity to sound, hyperreflexia
D diarrhea (explosive), diaphoresis, disorganized suck
R runny nose, regurgitation, respiratory distress, rub marks
A apnea, autonomic dysfunction (change in heart rate and respiratory rate)
W weight loss
A alkalosis (respiratory)
L lacrimation (tearing of eyes) and lethargy
S snuffles, sneezing, seizures,

Babies suspected or known to be at risk for or to have neonatal abstinence syndrome should be,
- loosely swaddled
- handled gently
- placed in a quiet and dimly lit environment
- fed frequently to ensure adequate fluid and calorie intake
- observed for seizures.

The baby's temperature must be monitored to avoid hyperthermia.

Observation and subsequent management of babies with NAS is best achieved using an objective/semi-objective tool. The most commonly used tools are based on the 21-symptom Neonatal Abstinence Scoring (NAS) system developed by Finnegan. Even though the neonatal abstinence score was designed for opiate withdrawal, it is commonly used for monitoring of babies with other intrauterine drug exposures.
- All symptoms exhibited during the entire scoring interval are included.
- Babies are not awakened to elicit reflexes and specified behaviors.
- If awakened for scoring, no score is given for diminished sleep after feeding.
- If crying, babies should be calmed before assessment.
- A score is assigned for prolonged crying, even though it may not be high-pitched in quality.

Sample Neonatal Abstinence Score

System	Signs and Symptoms	Score	Time						Comments
	excessive high pitched cry	2							
	continuous high pitched cry	3							
	sleeps < 1 hour after feeding	3							
	sleeps < 2 hour after feeding	2							
	sleeps < 3 hour after feeding	1							
	hyperactive Moro reflex	2							
	markedly hyperactive Moro reflex	3							
CNS	tremors disturbed	2							
	mild tremors undisturbed	3							
	moderate-severe tremors undisturbed	4							
	increased muscle tone	2							
	excoriation (specify area)	1							
	myoclonic jerks	3							
	generalized convulsions	5							
	sweating	1							
Metabolic	fever 37.2 to 38.3°C	1							
	fever > 38.4°C	2							
	frequent yawning > 4 x /interval	1							
	mottling	1							
Vasomotor	nasal stuffiness	1							
	frequent sneezing > 4 x /interval	1							
	nasal flaring	2							
Respiratory	respiratory rate > 60/minute	1							
	respiratory rate > 60/minute + retractions	2							
	excessive sucking	1							
	poor feeding	1							
GI	regurgitation	2							
	projectile vomiting	3							
	loose stools	2							
	watery stools	3							
Total score									
Scorer's initials									

Adapted from Finnegan L et al., Neonatal Abstinence Syndrome: Assessment and Management. Addictive Diseases 1975; 2:141-158.

- The initial score, at around 2 hours of age, reflects baseline behavior. Subsequent scores are performed at 4 hour intervals.
- If a score is ≥ 8, the frequency of scoring is increased to every 2 hours until 24 hours from the last score of 8.
- A higher score implies a more severe abstinence syndrome.
- If scores consistently remain under 8 until 48 hours of age, observation continued every 8 hours for 5 to 7 days may detect late withdrawal.
- Pharmacotherapy may be titrated using the scoring system. Response to treatment is inferred from a lowered score.
- Babies < 32 weeks gestation may not demonstrate typical withdrawal symptoms, and the decision to evaluate by abstinence scoring should be done on an individual basis.

Pharmacologic intervention is usually considered after ruling out other medical conditions in babies with a total abstinence score > 8 on 3 consecutive scoring periods or whose average score is > 8. These babies usually have,
- inconsolable, continuous crying
- persistent tremors or jitteriness when undisturbed.

In babies known or suspected of opioid withdrawal, the drug of choice is oral morphine, starting with 0.1mg/kg every 6 hours or 0.05 mg/kg every 3 hours. The dose is then titrated up or down with the abstinence score. Some babies may require treatment up to 4 weeks.

Naloxone (Narcan) should not be given to a baby whose mother has been using opioids as this may result in acute withdrawal symptoms.

You leave orders for the baby to be nursed in a quiet environment with low lighting, and increase the feeding frequency to every 2 to 3 hours.

You order morphine 0.1 mg/kg PO every 6 hours to treat his current episode of inconsolable irritability. Neonatal abstinence scoring is continued to assist in titrating the morphine dosing.

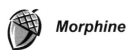 ***Morphine***

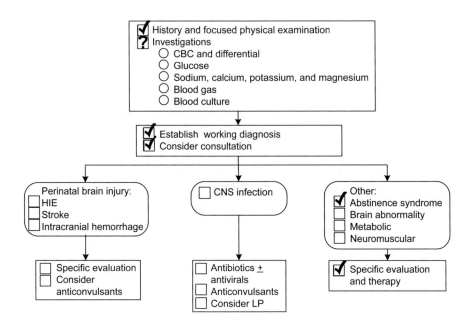

Answers to the questions in Chapter 5

Case #1 – The floppy baby

I.   What four key pieces of information have you obtained so far that may assist you in obtaining a focused history to arrive at a working diagnosis?

Late decelerations and minimal variability

Apgar scores of 1 at 1 minute and 3 at 5 minutes

Requirement for bag and mask ventilation for several minutes

Persistent hypotonia

Case #2 – 12-hour-old baby with a seizure

I.   Based on the information collected so far, how would you describe the seizures that this baby is having?

Clonic multifocal   **and**   subtle

II.   Calculate the half-loading dose of phenobarbital for this 3500 gram baby.

20 mg/kg x 3.5 kg = 70 mg phenobarbital

III.   What would you say to the parents when they ask you if their baby "will be OK"?

We cannot answer the question immediately with certainty.

Not all babies with seizures/encephalopathy develop long term sequelae.
Further tests and observation of his condition in hospital will assist in determining the degree of CNS injury and his level of risk for long term sequelae.

Long term outcome will only be certain as we observe development over time.

Case #3 – Baby born to a substance-using mother

I.   Is the baby having seizures?

No. The baby is not having seizures because the movements stop when the extremities are held.

Bibliography

Finnegan L, Connaughton J, Kron R, Emich J. Neonatal abstinence syndrome: Assessment and management. Addictive Diseases 1975; 2:141-158.

Gomella TL, Cunningham MD, Eyal FG, Zenk KE. Neonatology: Management, Procedures, On-Call Problems, Diseases, and Drugs. 4th Edition. Stamford Conn: McGraw-Hill/Appleton & Lange, 1999.

Mizhari EM. Neonatal seizures and neonatal epileptic syndromes. Neurol Clinics 2001; 19(2):427-63.

Neonatal drug withdrawal. American Academy of Pediatrics Committee on Drugs. Pediatrics 1998; 101(6):1079-88.

Society of Obstetricians and Gynecologists of Canada. Policy Statement from the Task Force on Cerebral Palsy and Fetal Asphyxia. SOGC CPG FHS in Labour No. 112, March 2002.

The Task Force on Neonatal Encephalopathy and Cerebral Palsy. Neonatal encephalopathy and cerebral palsy: Defining the pathogenesis and pathophysiology. Washington DC: The American College of Obstetricians and Gynecologists and American Academy of Pediatrics, 2003.

Volpe JJ. Neurology of the Newborn. 4th Edition. Philadelphia: WB Saunders Company, 2001.

Young TE, Mangum B. Neofax 2003. 16th Ed. Raleigh NC: Acorn Publishing Inc, 2003.

Chapter 6
Surgical Conditions

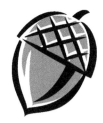

Objectives

Upon completion of this section, you will be able to:
1. Provide immediate management for babies born with an anterior abdominal wall defect.
2. Identify and provide immediate management for babies with gastrointestinal obstruction.
3. Apply the Surgical Conditions Sequence.
4. Stabilize and prepare a baby for surgical care.
5. Recognize when to exit to the other ACoRN Sequences.

Key Concepts

1. Babies with major surgical conditions represent a special category of babies requiring stabilization. These babies require specialized coordinated medical and surgical care in a regional facility.
2. Early recognition, preferably in utero, improves quality of care and outcomes.
3. Medical stabilization precedes surgery in all babies presenting with major surgical conditions.
4. The optimal timing of surgical intervention varies based on the type of condition and degree of medical stabilization. In most cases surgical intervention can be delayed until optimal medical stabilization is achieved.

Skills

*   Bowel bag application

Introduction

Surgical conditions that will be covered in this chapter are those associated with anterior abdominal wall lesions or obstruction of the gastrointestinal tract. Surgical conditions of the respiratory and cardiovascular system have been discussed in the respective chapters. Other surgical conditions will not be covered in this edition of ACoRN.

Many babies with major surgical conditions are diagnosed prenatally. When this is the case, medical and surgical care is facilitated,

- a more thorough prenatal diagnosis may identify or exclude associated conditions, and causes (such as chromosomal anomalies)
- medical and surgical information and counseling can be made available to the parents, facilitating decision making at and after birth
- the type of facility that will be needed to care for the baby can be anticipated, and prenatal transfer considered
- the family may be able to visit the physical space in which their baby will be cared for, and meet members of the medical and surgical team
- if needed, the timing of birth may be pre-determined.

However, babies with major surgical conditions may present at any time in any facility. Subsequent care and outcomes are optimized by,

- prompt recognition
- stabilization of the medical condition
- optimal pre-surgical care
- early transport to an appropriate facility.

Alerting Signs

A baby who demonstrates one or more of the following Alerting Signs enters the Surgical Conditions Sequence:

Surgical conditions
☐ Anterior abdominal wall defect
☐ Vomiting or inability to swallow
☐ Abdominal distension
☐ Delayed passage of meconium or imperforate anus

Anterior abdominal wall defect

In these conditions, internal organs are either exposed to the environment or covered by a membrane which may be intact or ruptured.

These include,
- gastroschisis
- omphalocele
- less common conditions, such as extrophy of the bladder or cloaca.

Vomiting or inability to swallow

Babies with obstruction of the intestinal tract proximal to the junction between the jejunum and ileum usually present with vomiting.

Vomiting due to obstruction of the gastrointestinal tract can be clear or bilious depending on whether the obstruction is located proximal or distal to the point where the bile duct enters the duodenum.

Clear vomiting may be of functional (non-surgical) origin. Surgical causes of clear vomiting include some cases of duodenal atresia, stenosis or duodenal web, when the obstruction is proximal to the exit of the bile ducts into the duodenum.

Bilious vomiting is likely to be of surgical origin. Causes include,
- most cases of duodenal atresia, stenosis or duodenal web
- malrotation with obstruction
- more distal obstruction
  o may be preceded or accompanied by abdominal distension.

Babies with esophageal atresia/tracheo-esophageal fistula (abbreviated as EA/TEF) present with noisy and labored respiration, and inability to swallow (EA) as opposed to actual vomiting. Babies with isolated TEF present with respiratory distress ± signs of aspiration.

Abdominal distension

Babies with obstruction of the intestinal tract distal to the junction between jejunum and ileum usually present with abdominal distension.

When the abdomen is tender in addition to being distended, it is important to exclude causes of acute abdomen such as necrotizing enterocolitis, intestinal perforation, volvulus and peritonitis.
- It is important to remember that an acute abdomen can present with distributive shock, and may require substantial isotonic fluid replacement to normalize perfusion and blood pressure.

Delayed passage of meconium or imperforate anus

Babies with functional or anatomic obstruction of the distal intestinal tract present with failure or delay in the passage of meconium (> 48 hours of age in term, and > 72 hours of age in preterm babies). Causes include,
- anal atresia with or without a perineal or genitourinary fistula
- meconium ileus
- congenital absence of myoenteric plexus (Hirschprung's disease).

These conditions should be suspected early, preferably before the onset of abdominal distension in order to minimize complications such as colitis due to bacterial overgrowth.

Routine newborn exam should always include inspection of the anus. Note that in anal atresia, meconium can leak from a perineal or genitourinary fistula.

Surgical Conditions Sequence

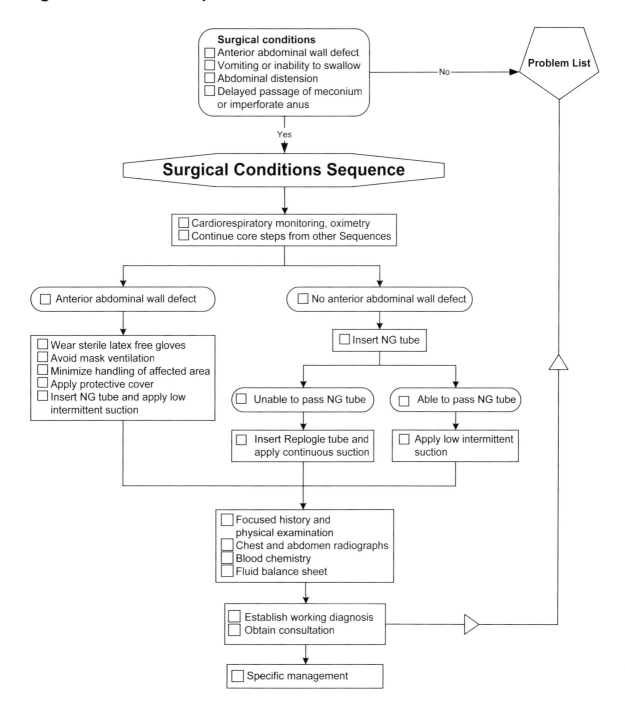

Core Steps

The monitoring activities and interventions that apply to babies in the Surgical Conditions Sequence are to,
- establish cardiorespiratory monitoring and oximetry
- continue the Core Steps from other applicable Sequences.

Organization of Care

The course of action for babies presenting with Surgical Conditions depends on whether,
- the baby presents with an anterior abdominal wall defect or not
- a nasogastric tube can be inserted or not, in babies with signs of gastrointestinal obstruction (vomiting, abdominal distension, delayed passage of meconium or an imperforate anus).

Response

In Surgical Conditions, the response is aimed at optimizing the baby's condition and minimizing complications prior to surgery.

Anterior abdominal wall defect

For babies with anterior abdominal wall defects,
- sterile technique and latex free gloves should be used when handling the exposed areas or bowel, starting in the delivery room
- bag and mask ventilation should be avoided in order to minimize gaseous distension of the gastrointestinal tract
- handling of the affected area should be minimized to prevent secondary damage and infection
- the exposed viscera or area should be covered as soon as possible
  - by placing the baby, up to and including the nipple line, inside a transparent, sterile plastic "bowel bag"
  - to minimize the risk of breakdown, infection, thermal, fluid and electrolyte losses
- the gastrointestinal tract should be decompressed by inserting a nasogastric tube and keeping it to open drainage or low intermittent suction.

A "bowel bag" is preferable over moist gauze dressings. The latter do not allow direct visualization, are rough on the exposed surfaces, absorb fluid from the lesion, and may leave residual particles.

 Bowel bag application

Unable to insert NG tube

Babies in whom a nasogastric tube cannot be inserted should be suspected of having esophageal atresia. Continuous suction is required as these babies cannot swallow their oral secretions. This is best done using a Replogle suction catheter, which is a clear, double lumen tube that allows continuous suction through one lumen and venting to the atmosphere through the other lumen to prevent its end holes from generating a vacuum against the mucosa.

Able to insert NG tube For babies in whom a nasogastric tube can be inserted, the gastrointestinal tract should be decompressed by keeping the tube to open drainage or low intermittent suction.

How do you set up low intermittent suction?

When using a regular gastric tube to decompress the gastrointestinal tract, intermittent suction must be used.
- Intermittent suction has on and off cycles, allowing for safe stomach and gastrointestinal decompression.
- Continuous suction using a regular gastric tube may cause the stomach to collapse leading to direct suctioning of the mucosa, ulceration, hemorrhage or perforation.

Use a regulator that has an intermittent suction setting, with preset on-and-off cycles, and set the initial level of suction within the "low range" (0 to 80 mmHg), starting between 40 to 60 mmHg. The suction level should not exceed 80 mmHg. Intermittent suction only works properly if the collection bottle is positioned 30 cm (12 inches) higher than the level of the stomach. Mucosal damage may result if the collection bottle is lower than the level of the stomach.

Next Steps

The Next Steps are to obtain a focused history, conduct a physical examination, order diagnostic tests, and initiate a fluid balance sheet.

Focused History Essential information to gather during the focused neonatal infection history includes:

Antepartum
- medical, obstetrical and family history
- was a serum "triple screen" done between 16 and 20 weeks gestation
- was a detailed prenatal ultrasound done
- was an amniocentesis done
- was there polyhydramnios
  - time of onset

Intrapartum
- preterm labour
- time of rupture of membranes
- mode of delivery

Neonatal
- need for resuscitation
- management in delivery room
- gestational age: preterm or term

Focused physical examination In addition to the examination conducted during the Primary Survey and other applicable sequences, a focused physical examination for Surgical Conditions includes:

Measurement of vital signs: respiratory rate, heart rate, temperature, blood pressure, current weight compared to birth weight

Observation and examination
- birth weight: small, appropriate or large for gestational age
- skin color for the presence of jaundice
- color of material in nasogastric tube
- signs of dehydration
  - dry mucous membranes
  - excessive weight loss since birth (> 10%)
  - sunken anterior fontanel
- anterior abdominal wall
  - presence/type of defect
  - distension
  - visible bowel loops or peristalsis (sometimes referred to as a "ropey abdomen")
  - redness or other discoloration
  - tenderness
- measurement of abdominal girth
- presence of other anomalies

Diagnostic tests A few simple tests may assist in reaching a working diagnosis, and determine the subsequent course of action:

1. **Chest radiograph**
   - to determine if there are signs of aspiration
   - when a nasogastric tube cannot be inserted and esophageal atresia is suspected, to determine
     - the position of the Replogle or nasogastric tube
     - if a proximal esophageal pouch can be seen
   - to determine if there are abnormalities in heart shape/size, or vertebral abnormalities

2. **Abdominal radiograph** (see examples on pages 6-10 and 6-11)
   In many cases, plain abdominal radiography is able to provide enough information to establish the subsequent course of action,
   - a decubitus radiograph may help identify free air in the peritoneal cavity or air-fluid levels within bowel loops
   - when esophageal atresia is suspected, the radiograph will determine if there is air in the stomach (confirming the presence of a distal fistula)

- in gastrointestinal atresias, to determine/estimate the location of the atresia
  - isolated stomach bubble in pyloric atresia (a rare condition)
  - double bubble in duodenal atresia
  - level of proximal air in more distal atresias
  - presence of distended loops
  - presence of air-fluid levels on a decubitus radiograph
  - presence or absence of air in the rectum
- in meconium peritonitis, to look for calcified amorphous material in the peritoneal cavity
- presence of free air in the peritoneal cavity
- presence of vertebral or sacrococcygeal abnormalities

3. **Blood chemistry**
   - to determine if there are electrolyte abnormalities resulting from excessive water or electrolyte losses by evaporation (abdominal wall defects) or vomiting, suctioning or third spacing (intestinal obstruction)

Fluid balance sheet

Initiate a fluid balance sheet in order to monitor intake and output volumes, including gastric aspirate volume in babies with intestinal obstruction and other losses.

Establish a Working Diagnosis

The evaluation to establish a working diagnosis is aimed at determining the type and level of lesion present, the presence or absence of associated anomalies, and the general condition of the baby.

Consultation and referral to a facility that specializes in the care of babies with surgical conditions should be made as soon as possible.

Specific Management

Specialized diagnostic workup may be needed to diagnose the type and level of lesion present, and the presence or absence of associated anomalies. This may include,

1. **Radiographic study using contrast material**
   - when plain radiographs are inconclusive of type and location of lesion/defect

2. **Rectal suction biopsy**
   - to determine if there are ganglion cells in the rectal/intestinal myoenteric plexus when suspecting Hirschprung's Disease
   - if a suction biopsy is not conclusive, a surgical biopsy may be needed
   - if the biopsy indicates Hirschprung's Disease, additional biopsies are needed to determine the "zone of transition", the most distal segment where ganglion cell can be found

3. **Echocardiography**
   - to rule in or out the presence of associated congenital heart disease

4. **Assessment by a general or subspecialty pediatrician ± medical geneticist ± chromosome analysis**
   - when a genetic syndrome or chromosomal abnormality is suspected to confirm the diagnosis, and provide specialized counseling and support
     - for example, nearly 40% of babies with a duodenal atresia have trisomy 21, and 30% of babies with an omphalocele have a genetic/chromosomal abnormality

Duodenal atresia

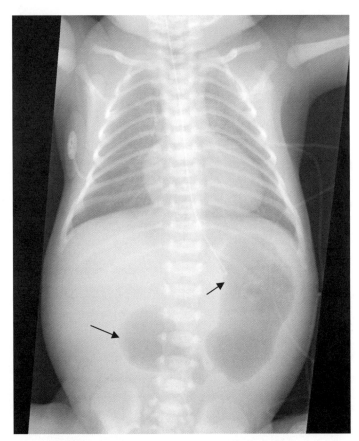

- Abdominal radiograph shows the typical double bubble.
- The longer arrow points at the dilated duodenum, proximal to the atresia. The other larger bubble is the dilated stomach.
- The shorter arrow points at the tip of a gastric tube, which should be advanced into the distended stomach to provide better drainage and decompression.

Ileal atresia

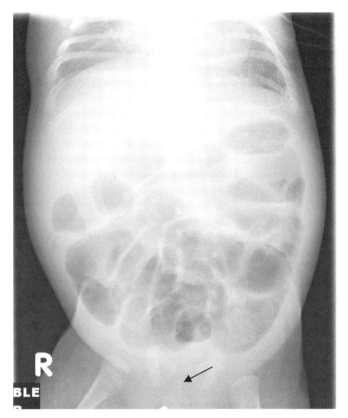

- Abdominal radiograph shows a distended abdomen with multiple distended bowel loops. The arrow is pointing to the absence of air in the rectum.
- Clinically the baby presented with progressive abdominal distension, which was followed by onset of bilious vomiting.

Surgical conditions Case # 1 - Abdominal wall defect

You are called to attend the birth of a 37 week gestation baby. At birth you notice that she has an obvious abdominal wall defect with loops of small bowel extruded. She is breathing regularly and is pink in room air.

You determine that the baby shows none of the Resuscitation Signs, and begin a Primary Survey.

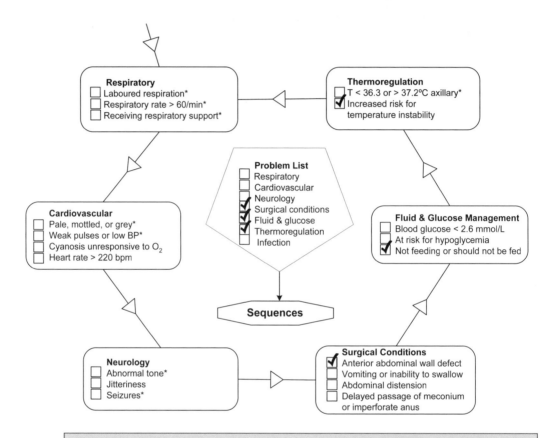

The baby has no Alerting signs corresponding to the Respiratory, Cardiovascular or Neurology Sequences, but the baby meets one of the Alerting Signs for the Surgical Conditions Sequence.

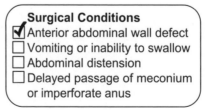

You enter the Surgical Conditions Sequence.

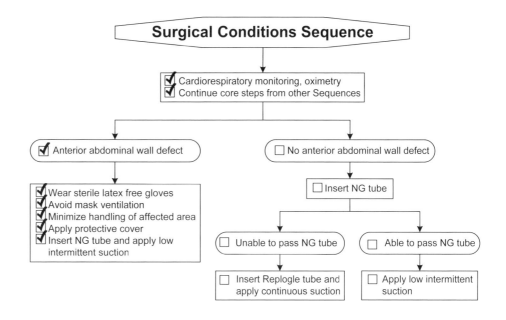

Surgical Conditions Sequence

☑ Cardiorespiratory monitoring, oximetry
☑ Continue core steps from other Sequences

☑ Anterior abdominal wall defect

☐ No anterior abdominal wall defect

☑ Wear sterile latex free gloves
☑ Avoid mask ventilation
☑ Minimize handling of affected area
☑ Apply protective cover
☑ Insert NG tube and apply low intermittent suction

☐ Insert NG tube

☐ Unable to pass NG tube

☐ Able to pass NG tube

☐ Insert Replogle tube and apply continuous suction

☐ Apply low intermittent suction

Cardiorespiratory monitoring and pulse oximetry are initiated.

You ensure the baby has been handled from birth with sterile technique and latex free gloves. The baby is on sterile drapes under a radiant warmer. The nurse administers intramuscular vitamin K, and carefully puts on a bowel bag as a protective cover enclosing the exposed viscera and lower part of the baby. This is secured at the axillary line.

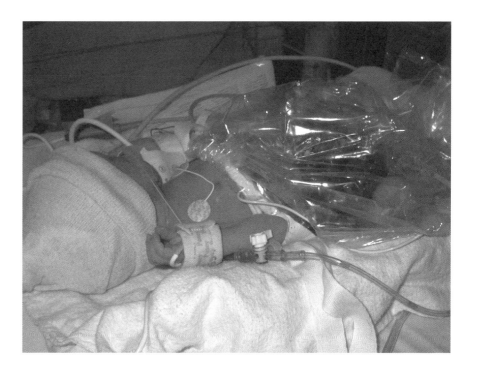

You insert a # 8 Fr orogastric tube, aspirate stomach contents with a syringe. You leave the tube open to air while you set up for low intermittent suction in order to decompress the stomach and prevent further distention of the intestines.

Gastroschisis and omphalocele are the two common defects in the anterior abdominal wall.

Gastroschisis A small opening exists in the abdominal wall, just to the right of where the umbilical cord attaches. The umbilical cord is not involved, and is normal in contents, shape and length. The small intestine and sometimes other organs (stomach, large bowel, spleen) escape through the defect, uncovered by a peritoneal membrane. The intestine is usually anatomically normal, but may contain atresias or be of reduced length. The exposed intestine often appears thick and matted.

Coexisting anomalies are unusual in babies with gastroschisis. The risk for gastroschisis is elevated in mothers who are younger than 25 years, especially if younger than 20 years. Other antenatal risk factors include,
- poor prenatal care/low socioeconomic status
- smoking
- medications such as cycloxygenase inhibitors, for example aspirin and ibuprofen, and decongestants
- occupational or hobby exposure to solvents
- "recreational" drug use of amphetamine-related drugs or cocaine.

Most of the substances listed above are vasoactive, supporting the hypothesis that gastroschisis may be due to a fetal vascular accident.

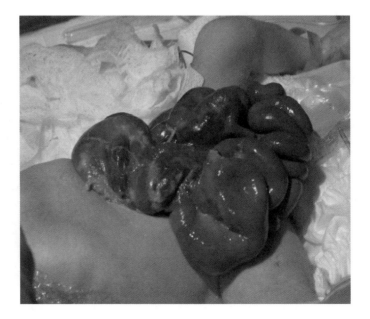

Omphalocele An opening exists at the base of the umbilical cord through which abdominal contents herniate. The defect is covered by a transparent peritoneal membrane and its contents can be seen. The umbilical cord arises from within the affected area. In most cases of omphalocele only the small intestine is visible, however, when the omphalocele is large (also called "giant omphalocele") the liver and other organs may be visible. A giant omphalocele (pictured below) is particularly difficult to repair as there may not be enough space in the abdominal cavity to replace the herniated abdominal contents.

It is important to determine if the membrane covering the omphalocele is intact or ruptured at the time of birth, admission to the nursery and subsequent observations.

There is a high frequency (30 to 40%) of associated conditions and chromosomal abnormalities in babies with omphalocele. These include congenital heart disease, congenital diaphragmatic hernia, intestinal atresia or volvulus, imperforate anus, other anterior wall defects such as extrophy of the bladder or cloaca, spina bifida, and chromosomal abnormalities such as trisomy 13 and 18. Babies with Beckwith-Wiedemann syndrome have omphalocele, hypoglycemia due to high insulin levels, are large for gestational age, and may have other anomalies.

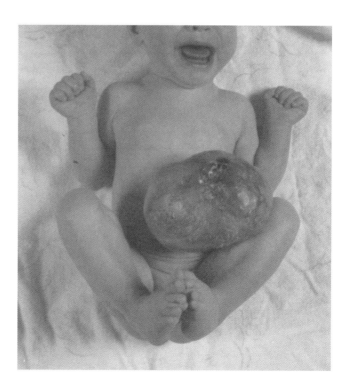

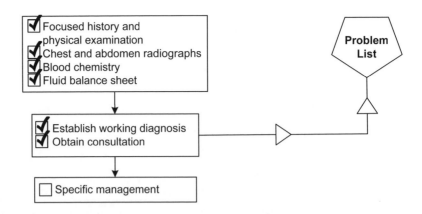

You obtain a focused history and learn that the mother is 17 years old and had minimal prenatal care.

The internal viscera visible in the bowel bag include several loops of small intestine, which look pink and well perfused.

The focused physical examination is otherwise unremarkable and does not suggest dysmorphic features or other anomalies.

A chest and abdominal radiographs are done. These are normal.

Blood chemistry is not done at this time as the baby was just born.

A fluid balance sheet is started.

Your working diagnosis is gastroschisis with no obvious associated anomalies. However, further specialized assessment is needed.

You call your regional center for consultation and request transport.

Having formulated a working diagnosis, you exit the Surgical Conditions Sequence and continue with the Fluid & Glucose Management Sequence and the Thermoregulation Sequence.

Babies with abdominal wall defects are at special risk for,
- hypothermia
- excessive fluid losses and electrolyte imbalance
- infection
- cardiorespiratory instability.

What is the surgical repair for abdominal wall defects?

Gastroschisis should be repaired as early as possible to prevent infection and to preserve gut viability. The treatment modalities vary depending on the size of the defect and the ability to reduce the exposed viscera into the abdomen. The main modalities are primary repair and staged repair using a silo.

The urgency to repair an omphalocele depends on whether the sac is ruptured or not. The timing of the surgery also depends on the dimension of the defect, the size of the baby, and the presence or absence of other anomalies. A silo may be necessary for large defects.

The baby is transferred to the regional centre.

The exposed bowel is reduced and a primary repair is performed.

Post-operatively, she requires mechanical ventilation for 3 days, close observation of intra-abdominal pressure and careful adjustment of fluid and electrolyte to maintain hemodynamic stability.

She will receive parenteral nutrition. It is anticipated that oral feeds will not be started for 2 to 3 weeks, and the baby will be slow to achieve full feeds.

Surgical conditions Case # 2: Inability to pass a nasogastric tube

You are called to examine a 3 hour old, term baby who was initiating breastfeeding when he started coughing and struggling, had an apneic episode and was noted to have colostrum returning through his nose.

The mother tells you that her baby has been drooling and mucousy since birth, and that she had wiped his mouth with a soft cloth several times. She had put her baby to breast in the delivery room, and that had been well tolerated. However, the breastfeeding attempt at 1 hour of age also resulted in coughing and struggling and was abandoned.

The baby is now breathing regularly and is pink in room air, but his respiration is noisy. You notice that saliva drools from the corners of his mouth. A few rales are heard bilaterally on auscultation of the chest.

You determine that the baby shows none of the Resuscitation Signs, and begin a Primary Survey.

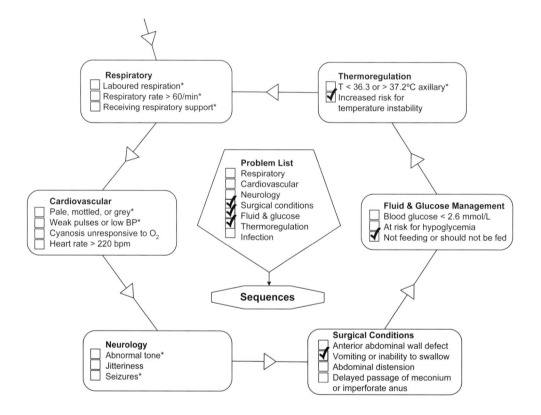

The baby enters the ACoRN Sequences indicated in the Primary Survey.

The baby has no Alerting signs corresponding to the Respiratory, Cardiovascular or Neurology Sequence, but the baby meets one of the Alerting Signs for the Surgical Conditions Sequence. A decision is made to withhold further attempts at feeding, to observe in the nursery under a radiant warmer, and to initiate an intravenous infusion of D10%W.

The airway is patent and the baby continues to breath regularly remaining pink in room air, but his respiration is still noisy. Saliva still drools from the corners of his mouth. A few rales are heard bilaterally on auscultation of the chest.

You enter the Surgical Conditions Sequence.

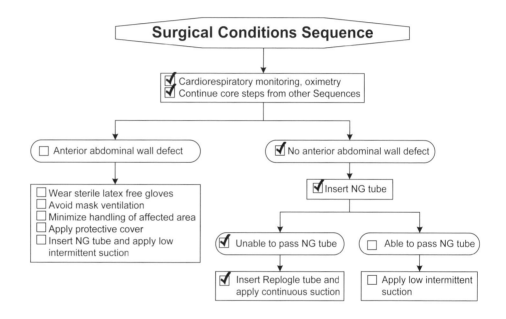

You gently suction the baby's mouth and nose then attempt to pass a nasogastric tube to the stomach. However, you meet resistance at about 10 to 12 cm.

Why do you attempt to insert a nasogastric tube as part of the Surgical Conditions Core Steps?

Babies who present with anterior abdominal wall defects or with suspicion of gastrointestinal tract obstruction, at any level, benefit from the placement of a nasogastric tube to,
- decompress the gastrointestinal tract and decrease vomiting
- rule out esophageal atresia.

> You suction the baby's mouth and nose again, and request a vented Replogle tube be set up and inserted to a distance of 10 cm. You then tell the mother her baby may have an interruption in his esophagus and he will need to be examined more carefully.

How do babies with esophageal atresia present?

Babies with esophageal atresia (EA) typically present with an inability to swallow, drooling and coughing. Nasal returns of saliva and feeds are also commonly seen.

After the first or second breastfeeding attempt, as letdown and milk production begin, the baby increasingly struggles with feeds, choking, coughing and showing milky returns through the nose. At this time there may also be periods of cyanosis and apnea as the baby aspirates milk into his lungs.

Respiratory distress due to aspiration pneumonia may occur in these babies, but this is usually not an early alerting sign.

Anatomic variation in esophageal atresia/tracheo-esophageal fistula.

The figure below shows the five main anatomic variations of EA/TEF.

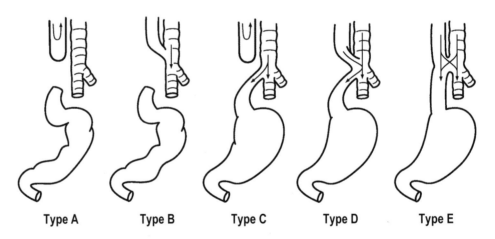

| Type A | Type B | Type C | Type D | Type E |

Type C is the most common anatomic variation of EA/TEF (80% of cases). The proximal esophagus ends in a pouch, preventing swallowing and the insertion of a nasogastric tube beyond 10 to 12 cm. The distal trachea, near the carina, and distal esophagus are connected by a "tracheo-esophageal" fistula. Due to the distal fistula, the stomach bubble is radiographically visible.

Type A, esophageal atresia without fistula (EA), is the second most common anatomic variation. It is also called "pure esophageal atresia", and occurs in approximately 10% of cases. Air does not enter the stomach due to the EA and absence of a distal fistula.

Type E (also known as "H-fistula") is a TEF without EA. An H-fistula is difficult to diagnose, and may present later in the newborn period with coughing and choking during feeds, or in childhood with a history of recurrent pneumonia. It occurs in approximately 5% of cases.

You obtain a focused history and learn the maternal symphysis-fundal height was increased beyond expectation in the last 4 weeks of pregnancy. An ultrasound had been done that showed a mild degree of polyhydramnios. The physical examination does not suggest dysmorphic features. The cardiovascular clinical examination is normal. The anus is patent.

The chest radiograph is shown below.

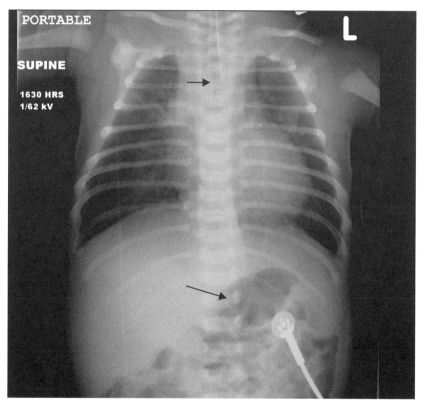

- o The top arrow shows the level at which the tip of the Replogle tube is placed. This is the level of the proximal esophageal pouch.
- o The bottom arrow shows air in the stomach and intestines. This indicates there is a distal tracheo-esophageal fistula.
- o In addition, the lung fields show some infiltrates which are suggestive of congestion / aspiration.
- o The cardiac shadow is of normal size and appearance.
- o There are no vertebral body abnormalities.

Blood chemistry is not done at this time as the baby was just born.

You initiate a fluid balance sheet in order to keep track of the volume aspirated by the Replogle tube and other intake and output volumes.

Your working diagnosis is isolated esophageal atresia with tracheo-esophageal fistula. No other anomalies have been detected, however, further specialized assessment may have to be done.

You call your regional center for consultation and transport.

Having formulated a working diagnosis, you exit the Surgical Conditions Sequence and continue with the Fluid & Glucose Management and Thermoregulation Sequences.

You also proceed to raise the head of the bed to 30 to 40 degrees and institute comfort measures to minimize crying in order to decrease the risk of gastric distension and reflux through the TE fistula.

What is the usual outcome of babies with EA/TEF?

Most babies with EA/TEF type C can have an early primary repair consisting of anastomosis of the esophagus and ligation of the TEF.

However, in many babies with isolated EA, type A, a primary anastomosis in the newborn period may be more difficult and the attempt at repair may be delayed. In these babies, in addition to the usual workup, surgeons are interested in pre-determining the length of the gap between the proximal and distal esophagus.

Post operative complications of EA/TEF repair include anastomotic leaks. In the long term, most babies with EA/TEF have good functional outcomes, but some may develop strictures in the anastomotic area, or have esophageal dysmotility, gastroesophageal reflux, or tracheomalacia.

What other conditions are associated with EA/TEF?

EA/TEF is usually an isolated occurrence, but babies may have associated anomalies such as,
- chromosomal abnormalities, such as trisomy 21, 18 or 13
- other intestinal atresias, such as duodenal atresia
- imperforate anus
- congenital heart disease, such as VSD or tetralogy of Fallot
- vertebral abnormalities
- renal or urinary tract abnormalities
- non-chromosomal syndromes, such as VATER syndrome.

Bibliography

Freeman NV, Burger DM, Griffiths M, Malone PSJ, eds. Surgery of the newborn. Churchill Livingstone, 1994.

Lockridge T, Caldwell AM, Jason P. Neonatal surgical emergencies: Stabilization and management. JOGNN 2002:31(3):328-399.

Chapter 7
Fluid & Glucose Management

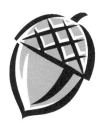

Objectives

Upon completion of this chapter, you will be able to:

1. Identify babies who require fluid and glucose management.
2. Recognize the need for and administration of intravenous fluids.
3. Apply the Fluid and Glucose Management Sequence.
4. Identify contraindications to enteral feeding.
5. Recognize and manage babies with and those at risk for hypoglycemia.
6. Recognize when to exit to the other ACoRN Sequences.

Key Concepts

1. Healthy term babies without risk factors for hypoglycemia should be breastfed on cue and do not require supplemental fluids or investigation of blood glucose levels.
2. Well babies who are at-risk for hypoglycemia require monitoring of blood glucose levels during the period of risk, starting at 2 hours of age after an initial feed.
3. Unwell babies and those who are unable to feed require fluid and glucose management to maintain normal water balance and energy supply.
4. Water and electrolyte balance requires careful attention in babies receiving intravenous fluids.
5. Dehydration, overhydration and hypoglycemia may have serious short- and long-term complications if not appropriately managed.
6. Reliable and accurate measurement of blood glucose, sodium and potassium levels should be available within the hour in all institutions caring for babies.
7. If point-of-care devices are in use, these should be quality controlled.

Skills

- Emergency venous access – Umbilical vein catheterization

Introduction

Term, healthy babies meet their requirements for fluid, glucose and electrolytes through feeding. This is best achieved by breast feeding on cue, and requires no supplementation.

The Fluid and Glucose Management Sequence focuses on the initial intake of water, sodium and glucose in both unwell and at-risk babies.

Fluid requirements

Fluid requirements in an unwell or at-risk baby consists of,
- maintenance fluids
- volume expanders (as required)
- replacement of excessive losses (as required).

Dehydration or hypovolemia occurs when fluid intake does not keep up with losses. Overhydration occurs when fluid intake exceeds losses. Hyponatremia is a sign of overhydration in babies receiving solutions containing a low sodium concentration.

1. **Maintenance fluid**

   Babies require a minimum water intake per day to,
   - replace normal losses from
     - urine and stool
     - evaporation through skin and breathing
   - supply the water accumulated during normal growth (80% of appropriate daily weight gain is water).

   The minimum water requirement in the first days of life is usually 50 to 70 mL/kg/day (2 to 3 mL/kg/hour), but may be as high as 100 mL/kg/day (4 mL/kg/hour) in extremely premature babies cared for under radiant warmers.

   Milk meets a baby's nutritional needs when taken in a quantity $\geq$ 150 mL/kg/day. Fluid intake usually exceeds minimum water requirements, in order to provide adequate caloric intake. This increased volume should not be given to babies on days 1 to 2 of life or to babies with renal dysfunction resulting in decreased urine output as they cannot excrete the excess water.

   Water requirement should be considered separately from volume expanders and replacement for surgical losses. Volume expanders and replacement losses require management with isotonic, sodium containing solutions.

   The following table provides suggested guidelines for oral and intravenous fluid intake to meet *minimum* water requirements. Electrolytes are normally added to intravenous fluid on or after the second day, or once urine output is established and electrolyte status has been assessed.

Postnatal age	Baseline oral intake (if not breastfed on cue)	Baseline intravenous intake (if not feeding)
Day 1	Up to 12 mL/kg every 3 hours	D10%W at 3 mL/kg/hour
Day 2	Up to 12 mL/kg every 3 hours	D10%W at 4 mL/kg/hour
Day 3	Up to 15 mL/kg every 3 hours	D10%W with 20 mmol/L of NaCl at 5 mL/kg/hour
≥ Day 4	Up to 18 to 20 mL/kg every 3 hours	D10%W with 20 mmol/L of NaCl at 6 mL/kg/hour (other electrolytes may be needed)

2. **Volume expansion**

Unwell babies often require volume expansion with isotonic solutions. The solution of choice is 0.9% NaCl (normal saline).

Volume expanders are required to replace lost intravascular volume in situations such as,
- hypovolemia (such as in acute blood loss causing hypovolemic shock)
- abnormal vessel tone (distributive shock)
- "third spacing" or loss into body cavities
- surgical losses

The volume of loss is often difficult to estimate but is best evaluated by the response to repeated boluses of 10 mL/kg of a volume expander given over several minutes.
- The effectiveness of volume replacement is judged clinically by observing an improvement in the baby's condition and vital signs,
  o perfusion
  o heart rate
  o blood pressure.

Volume replacement fluid should be considered separately from maintenance fluid requirements.

3. **Replacement of excessive ongoing losses**

Excessive ongoing losses may occur due to,
- excess evaporative loss from an open lesion
- surgical drainage
- excessive diuresis.

The optimal way to manage excessive ongoing losses is by replacement with an electrolyte solution similar to the loss, usually 0.9% NaCl. Replacement of abnormal ongoing losses should be considered separately from maintenance fluid or volume expansion.

The Fluid and Glucose Management Sequence

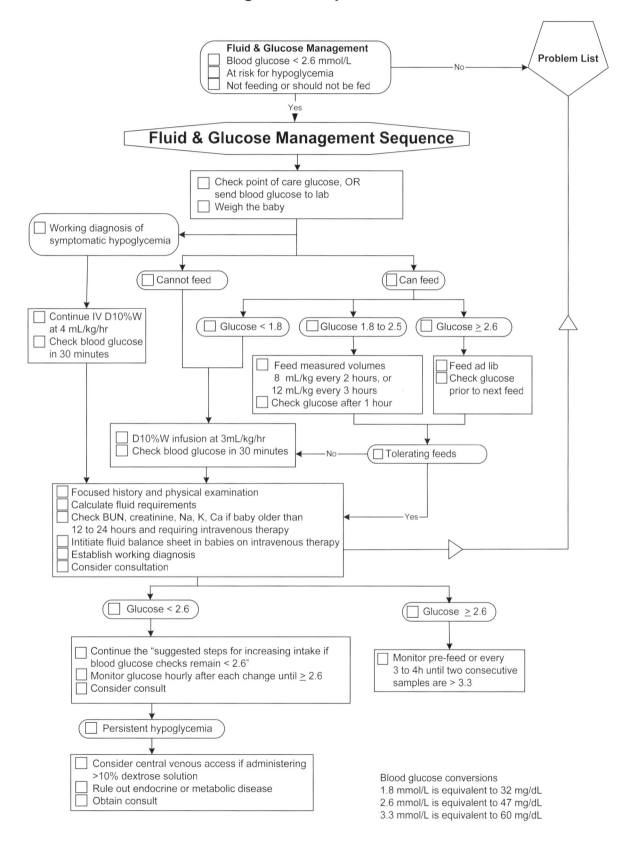

Fluid & Glucose Management
- Blood glucose < 2.6 mmol/L
- At risk for hypoglycemia
- Not feeding or should not be fed

No → **Problem List**

Yes ↓

Fluid & Glucose Management Sequence

- Check point of care glucose, OR send blood glucose to lab
- Weigh the baby

- Working diagnosis of symptomatic hypoglycemia

- Cannot feed
- Can feed

- Glucose < 1.8
- Glucose 1.8 to 2.5
- Glucose ≥ 2.6

Continue IV D10%W at 4 mL/kg/hr
Check blood glucose in 30 minutes

Feed measured volumes
8 mL/kg every 2 hours, or
12 mL/kg every 3 hours
Check glucose after 1 hour

Feed ad lib
Check glucose prior to next feed

D10%W infusion at 3mL/kg/hr
Check blood glucose in 30 minutes ← No — Tolerating feeds

- Focused history and physical examination
- Calculate fluid requirements
- Check BUN, creatinine, Na, K, Ca if baby older than 12 to 24 hours and requiring intravenous therapy
- Intitiate fluid balance sheet in babies on intravenous therapy
- Establish working diagnosis
- Consider consultation

← Yes

- Glucose < 2.6
- Glucose ≥ 2.6

Continue the "suggested steps for increasing intake if blood glucose checks remain < 2.6"
Monitor glucose hourly after each change until ≥ 2.6
Consider consult

Monitor pre-feed or every 3 to 4h until two consecutive samples are > 3.3

- Persistent hypoglycemia

Consider central venous access if administering >10% dextrose solution
Rule out endocrine or metabolic disease
Obtain consult

Blood glucose conversions
1.8 mmol/L is equivalent to 32 mg/dL
2.6 mmol/L is equivalent to 47 mg/dL
3.3 mmol/L is equivalent to 60 mg/dL

Glucose requirements Glucose is the main source of energy for brain cells. An adequate blood glucose concentration is essential because neurological compromise can occur if the brain is deprived of glucose.

At the time of birth, the principal source of blood glucose must shift from the placenta to the baby's own energy stores within minutes. The process of making glucose from energy stores, known as gluconeogenesis, is triggered by the natural fall in blood sugar level that occurs in the first one to two hours after birth.

As a result, the glucose levels of term, healthy babies are lowest at 1 to 2 hours after birth, subsequently reaching adult levels by 24 to 72 hours of age. During this time, term, healthy babies activate metabolic processes referred to as counter regulation, including,

- the ability to make new glucose from internal sources (glycogenolysis and gluconeogenesis)
- direct utilization of alternative fuels as substrates for brain metabolism (lactate, ketones, and fatty acids)
- decreased glucose utilization by the body when availability is limited.

Routine blood glucose monitoring in the term, healthy baby is not indicated in the absence of risk factors, as it may interfere with routine care, bonding, and the establishment of breastfeeding.

When counter regulation is not well developed, such as in preterm babies, or is overwhelmed by stress or medical conditions, clinically significant hypoglycemia can occur.

Babies with hypoglycemia may be asymptomatic or may present with signs such as:

- jitteriness, tremor, seizure, or coma
- irritability, lethargy, or stupor
- hypotonia or limpness
- apnea or cyanotic spells
- poor feeding, having previously fed well
- hypothermia

These signs are non specific as similar signs occur with a variety of other important neonatal conditions, such as neonatal encephalopathy and sepsis. Individualized assessment is important.

Hypoglycemia is more likely to result in long-term neurological complications if it is,

- symptomatic or persistent, or
- occurs in a baby who has other risk factors for adverse outcome, such as preterm or low birth weight babies.

Asymptomatic hypoglycemia may also be associated with adverse outcomes, hence the importance of screening at-risk babies.

Persistent and/or symptomatic hypoglycemia requires investigation and prompt treatment with intravenous dextrose solution.

Alerting Signs   A baby who demonstrates one or more of the following Alerting Signs enters the Fluid & Glucose Management Sequence:

> **Fluid & Glucose Management**
> ☐ Blood glucose < 2.6 mmol/L
> ☐ At risk for hypoglycemia
> ☐ Not feeding or should not be fed

Blood glucose < 2.6 mmol/L (< 47 mg/dL)   Normal blood glucose ranges from 3.3 to 6.0 mmol/L (60 to 108 mg/dl), but may be lower during transition and for the first 24 hours of life.

Healthy, term babies do not require blood glucose screening. The blood glucose levels may be as "low" as 1.8 to 2.0 mmol/L (32 to 36 mg/dL) at 1 to 2 hours of age, increasing to > 2.6 mmol/L (> 47 mg/dL) by 2 hours of age and to normal adult levels (> 3.3 mmol/L or > 60 mg/dL) in the next two days.

Blood glucose < 2.6 mmol/L (< 47 mg/dL) is not acceptable in unwell or at-risk babies. Observational data suggest that persistent (repeated or prolonged) blood glucose levels < 2.6 mmol/L (< 47 mg/dL) may be associated with adverse neurological outcome in at-risk populations. This value, measured in plasma or serum, has been adopted as ACoRN's operational definition of hypoglycemia and requires active management in unwell and at-risk newborns.

Babies with glucose levels of 2.6 to 3.3 mmol/L (47 to 60 mg/dL) require monitoring until two consecutive pre-feed glucose levels are > 3.3 mmol/L (60 mg/dL).

At risk for hypoglycemia   Glucose screening is indicated in newborns at risk for hypoglycemia,
- born to a mother treated with propanolol or oral hypoglycemic agents, or whose mother received glucose infusions during labour
- preterm
- low birth weight (LBW)
- small for gestational age (SGA)
- large for gestational age (LGA)
- infants of diabetic mothers (IDM)
- all babies who meet the ACoRN Alerting signs for the Fluid & Glucose Management Sequence
- unwell babies, such as those with,
  - respiratory distress
  - sepsis
  - perinatal acidemia (pH < 7.0)
  - Apgar score ≤ 3 at 5 minutes
  - babies with non-specific signs/symptoms which could be due to hypoglycemia
  - unable to feed.

Not feeding or should not be fed

Healthy, term babies feed approximately every 3 to 5 hours on the first day of life, and with increasing frequency thereafter until maternal milk supply is established on the 2nd to 4th day of life. A term baby who does not wake, display feeding cues, nor "work" at feeding requires evaluation by an individual experienced in feeding problems, as well as an assessment using the ACoRN primary survey.

Babies who are not feeding or who should not be fed because they are unwell should receive intravenous fluid and glucose. These include babies with,
- ACoRN Respiratory Score ≥ 5 (moderate to severe)
- cardiovascular instability (shock, cyanosis, or tachyarrhythmia)
- seizures and/or abnormal tone
- neonatal encephalopathy, or Apgar ≤ 3 at 5 minutes
- surgical conditions such as gastroschisis, omphalocele, tracheo-esophageal fistula, etc.
- abdominal distention, vomiting, gross blood in the stools (except when it is due to swallowed maternal blood).

In addition to the risk of hypoglycemia, preterm and small for gestational age babies may develop feeding intolerance and are predisposed to necrotizing enterocolitis (NEC), an inflammatory condition of the bowel. For this reason, intravenous fluids should be considered for these babies during the first 24 to 48 hours of life.

Core Steps

The interventions and monitoring activities that apply to all babies who enter the Fluid & Glucose Management Sequence are to,
- check blood glucose level (if not already done)
- weigh the baby.

Determine blood glucose level

An initial blood glucose screen should be obtained on admission in all unwell and symptomatic babies.

In asymptomatic term and near term babies at-risk for hypoglycemia who stay with their mothers and receive early feeds, the glucose screen should be performed at 2 hours of age.

There are two methods of determining blood glucose levels. Each has specific indications and limitations.

1. **Point of care glucose measurement:**
   Blood glucose may be estimated rapidly at the bedside using "point of care" technology.
   - Visual estimation of color change using reagent strips. These should not be used because they are subjective and unreliable for blood glucose levels found in the newborn.
   - Specialized blood glucose meters are simple to operate and provide immediate results, however they do not have internal quality control. Abnormal results (particularly those below 3 mmol/L or 54 mg/dL)

require confirmation with laboratory glucose analysis.
- Direct-reading glucose biosensors with internal quality controls. These methods do not require repeat sampling or verification.

In purchasing point of care devices, one should ensure they are accurate and validated in the low range of plasma glucose (1 to 3 mmol/L or 18 to 54 mg/dL). These devices minimize the need for repeated sampling for laboratory confirmation and unnecessary interventions. Staff should be trained in their use, quality control procedures and limitations.

2. **Laboratory glucose analysis**:
A rapid turn around for laboratory blood glucose results is essential in the management of the at-risk or hypoglycemic baby.

The blood specimen should be chilled, quickly transported (or collected in containers with additives that inhibit glycolysis) and immediately analyzed in order to minimize post-sampling glycolysis. Delays of greater than 15 minutes in processing samples may result in artificially lowered blood levels and unnecessary interventions.

Weigh the baby   Body weight and its variation after birth is a valuable tool in determining both the degree of dehydration and risk factors for hypoglycemia.

Weigh the baby to,
- determine whether the baby is AGA, SGA, or LGA
- assess weight change (loss/gain) from birth or from previously recorded weight
- calculate daily fluid and glucose requirement.

Babies should be weighed naked, using a baby scale with values to the nearest gram. Scales used to weigh babies require routine maintenance and quality assurance procedures.

Organization of Care   Care is first organized on the basis of whether the baby is entering from the Neurology Sequence with a working diagnosis of symptomatic hypoglycemia or not.

For babies without a working diagnosis of symptomatic hypoglycemia, care is organized on the basis of their ability to take enteral (oral or gavage) feeds, and the blood glucose level.
- Babies who are not feeding or should not be fed, including those who fail to tolerate feeds, should be fully managed intravenously.
- Babies who can feed but have critical hypoglycemia – blood glucose < 1.8 mmol/L (< 32 mg/dL) – should be fully managed intravenously initially.
- Babies who can feed but have hypoglycemia with blood glucose between 1.8 and 2.6 mmol/L (32 and 47 mg/dL) should be fed using measured volumes to ensure a predictable intake.
- Babies who can feed and do not have hypoglycemia – blood glucose ≥ 2.6 mmol/L (47 mg/dL) – should be fed ad lib, if mature enough to

do so. Babies managed in this way are usually term or only moderately premature (34 to 35 weeks gestation) with stable vital signs and no gastrointestinal or surgical complications.

Feeding intervals are dependent on the gestational age and volume the baby tolerates

- term babies can generally tolerate 12 ml/kg every 3 hours
- babies 34 to 35 weeks gestation require more frequent feeds of smaller volume, such as 8 ml/kg every 2 hours
- babies < 34 weeks gestation usually require intravenous supplementation.

Response

Babies in this Sequence either need intravenous fluids, measured oral feeds, ad lib oral feeds, or a combination.

Babies requiring intravenous fluids

Babies require an intravenous dextrose infusion if they:

- have a working diagnosis of symptomatic hypoglycemia
- cannot feed or should not be fed
- have critical hypoglycemia – blood glucose < 1.8 mmol/L (< 32 mg/dL)

Almost all babies who require intravenous fluids on the first day of life can be maintained with,

- D10%W at 3 ml/kg/hour, if asymptomatic
- D10%W at 4 ml/kg/hour, if entering from the Neurology Sequence with a working diagnosis of symptomatic hypoglycemia

After day one of life, D10%W should be initiated at the infusion rate appropriate for age in days.

Babies with symptomatic or critical hypoglycemia require,

- continuous intravenous dextrose infusion, and
- close monitoring of blood glucose in order to
  - make necessary adjustments in glucose intake
  - decide if other interventions are needed in a timely manner.

All babies being treated for hypoglycemia with intravenous fluids require a blood glucose determination 30 minutes after starting the infusion.

Can feed but have asymptomatic hypoglycemia ≥ 1.8 mmol/L (32 mg/dL)

Babies who are ≥ 34 weeks gestation and can feed but have hypoglycemia with blood glucose between 1.8 and 2.6 mmol/L (32 and 47 mg/dL) require early feeding (oral or gavage) using measured volumes to ensure a predictable intake.

- If the baby is being fed every 2 hours, the recommended intake is 8 mL/kg per feed.
- If the baby is being fed every 3 hours, the recommended intake is 12 mL/kg per feed.
- Intravenous dextrose infusion is indicated if early feeding fails to raise the blood sugar to ≥ 2.6 mmol/L (47 mg/dL).

Babies who are < 34 weeks gestation usually require supplemental intravenous fluids as they may not tolerate rapidly increased feeds.

All babies being treated for hypoglycemia with feeds require a blood glucose determination 1 hour after administering the feed.

Can feed and do not have hypoglycemia

Babies who can feed ad lib (term and near-term) and do not have hypoglycemia, should be fed ad lib (usually every 3 to 4 hours). They require blood glucose determination prior to feeds until blood glucose is stable in the normal range (> 3.3 mmol/L or 60 mg/dL).

Next Steps

The Next Steps are to obtain a focused history, conduct a physical examination, calculate daily fluid and electrolyte requirements, order diagnostic tests, and establish a working diagnosis.

Focused history

Important information to gather during the focused fluid and glucose management history includes:

Antepartum
- maternal diabetes
- maternal infection

Intrapartum
- excessive maternal glucose infusion during labour (> 100 mL/hour of D10%W)
- non-reassuring fetal heart rate

Neonatal
- cord pH < 7.0
- need for resuscitation at birth
- Apgar score ≤ 3 at 5 minutes
- prematurity
- need for intensive or transitional care
- birth weight and classification as AGA, SGA, or LGA, using growth charts
- difficulty with feeding or inability to feed
- suspected or proven infection
- seizures, jitteriness, irritability, or lethargy
- number of wet diapers/day
- passage of meconium

Physical examination   A focused fluid and glucose management physical examination includes:

Observation:
- current weight compared to birth weight and any previously documented weight
- skin colour for jaundice or plethoric appearance
- surgical conditions or congenital anomalies
- respiratory effort

Measurement of vital signs: temperature, respiratory rate, heart rate, and blood pressure.

Examination:
- signs of dehydration – dry mucosa, and/or poor skin turgor, sunken fontanel
- neurological status – level of alertness, jitteriness, irritability, or seizures
- signs of circulatory instability
- feeding readiness (ability and intensity of suck-swallow and level of energy)
- the abdomen for presence of distention, tenderness, and bowel sounds

Calculate fluid requirements   Use the Maintenance Fluids table on page 7-4 of the Introduction section. Add ongoing losses if significant (> 10 mL/kg/day), and replace prior losses.

Surgical conditions:

As with medical conditions where feeding is contraindicated, surgical conditions require a combination of maintenance fluids according to age, volume expanders (as required), and replacement of losses.
- Most surgical losses include electrolytes and should initially be replaced using isotonic, sodium-containing fluids. Certain losses have typical patterns and should be replaced accordingly,
- Babies with abdominal wall defects may lose 5 to 10 ml/kg/hour during the preoperative and immediate post-operative period, requiring replacement with 0.9% NaCl.
- A perforated bowel may result in hypovolemia due to third spacing, requiring initial volume expansion followed by replacement of ongoing losses of 5 to 10 ml/kg/hour.
- Nasogastric aspirate exceeding 10 ml/kg/day should be replaced with equal quantities of 0.9% NaCl with added potassium chloride 2 mmol per 100 ml.

Diagnostic tests Diagnostic tests included in the Fluid and Glucose Management work-up are:

- Blood chemistry (BUN, creatinine, sodium, potassium, calcium) in babies older than 12 to 24 hours of life who require intravenous therapy to identify the imbalances that may accompany dehydration (typically, hypernatremia) and overhydration (typically hyponatremia).
  - Hypocalcemia may be seen early in newborns, especially in premature and asphyxiated babies, and infants of diabetic mothers.

Initiate fluid balance sheet A fluid balance sheet should be kept on a per-shift and cumulative basis. Record the following categories:

Intake (volume and composition)	Output (volume)
Volume of all fluids given as maintenance, nutrition and with medications	Urine output
Replacement fluids	All measurable abnormal losses (such as gastric or other surgical drainage)

The table below outlines glucose monitoring guidelines to ensure normal values are achieved after treatment is initiated:

Blood glucose level	Monitoring guideline
< 2.6 mmol/L (< 47 mg/dL)	One hour after enteral feed and prior to the next feed, or 30 minutes after an IV bolus or starting an IV infusion.
2.6 to 3.3 mmol/L (47 to 60 mg/dL)	Prior to feeds; or every 4 to 6 hours if on an IV infusion
> 3.3 mmol/L (> 60 mg/dL)	Every 2nd to 3rd feed or every 6 to 8 hours if on an IV infusion. Transition to enteral feeds: discontinue monitoring after two consecutive glucose levels > 3.3 mmol/L (> 60 mg/dL).

Establish a Working Diagnosis

If hypoglycemia resolves with glucose administered as recommended, it is unlikely the problem is due to increased glucose utilization or decreased counter-regulation associated with endocrine or metabolic disorders.

Hypocalcemia and other electrolyte, nutritional, or metabolic needs are addressed after the initial stabilization is complete, and therefore are not part of ACoRN unless they manifest as one of the ACoRN Alerting Signs such as seizures.

Consider consultation

Babies whose hypoglycemia fails to correct with initial management may require specialized assessment and management.

Specific Management

The focus of Specific Management is to achieve and maintain a blood glucose ≥ 2.6 mmol/L (> 47 mg/dL).

In babies with normal metabolic needs, the glucose requirement is usually 4 to 6 mg/kg/minute. This glucose requirement is met by,
- 4 mL/kg/hour of milk (given as boluses of 12 mL/kg every 3 hours)
- 3 mL/kg/hour of D10%W (5 mg/kg/minute of glucose)
- a combination of enteral and IV intake.

Glucose requirements are higher in infants born to diabetic mothers (6 to 8 mg/kg/minute), and in babies with endocrine or metabolic disorders (> 8 mg/kg/minute).

Babies who have received enteral or intravenous fluids at the recommended rate for day 1 of life and have a blood glucose ≥ 2.6 mmol/L (> 47 mg/dL) are "normoglycemic". Their blood glucose must be monitored every 3 to 4 hours until the blood glucose is ≥ 3.3 mmol/L (> 60 mg/dL) in two consecutive samples.

If the blood glucose remains < 2.6 mmol/L (47 mg/dL), increase the amount of glucose being administered in a stepwise fashion:
- Ensure volume of enteral intake by converting from ad lib to measured feeds
- Increase the volume of measured feeds beyond baseline.
- Convert to full intravenous dextrose if,
  - enteral intake is not tolerated
  - blood glucose < 2.6 mmol/L (< 47 mg/dL) one hour after the measured feed
  - blood glucose < 1.8 mmol/L (< 32 mg/dL).
- Increase intravenous dextrose rate.
- Increase intravenous dextrose concentration.

Suggested steps for increasing glucose intake if blood glucose checks remain < 2.6 mmol/L (< 47 mg/dL)

Steps	Enterally fed	IV dextrose infusion
Baseline	Breastfeed on cue, or Feed every 2 to 3 hours	D10%W, 3 mL/kg/hour (= 5 mg/kg/minute of glucose)
Step 1	Feed measured volume 8 mL/kg every 2 hours or 12 mL/kg every 3 hours, or Start IV dextrose infusion at baseline	D10%W, 4 mL/kg/hour (= 6.7 mg/kg/minute of glucose)
Step 2	Go to IV dextrose infusion step 1, and proceed from there	D12.5%W, 4 to 5 mL/kg/hour (= 8.3 to 10.4 mg/kg/minute of glucose) Obtain consultation and investigations Consider central access Consider glucagon or other pharmacological intervention

D12.5%W is the highest dextrose concentration that can be administered via peripheral intravenous access. Dextrose solutions > 12.5% irritate the lining of peripheral veins and should be given centrally (for example, an umbilical venous catheter).

In babies with persistent hypoglycemia (requiring glucose intake of > 8 mg/kg/minute), it is necessary to consider a diagnosis of endocrine or metabolic disorder. Investigation and consultation are indicated. Pharmacological intervention (glucagon, hydrocortisone, somatostatin, or diazoxide) may be required. This level of care is beyond the scope of ACoRN, and consultation is recommended.

Retrospective analysis is the key to diagnosis of endocrine and metabolic conditions. During the time when the baby is hypoglycemic, a blood sample should be drawn for later analysis of insulin, glucose, ketones, glucagon, cortisol, and growth hormone, at a specialized laboratory.

After a stable blood glucose level > 2.6 mmol/L (> 47 mg/dL) is established for 12 hours, it is reasonable to start weaning the intravenous dextrose while increasing the oral feeds.

Fluid & Glucose Management Case # 1 – Infant of a diabetic mother

A baby girl is born at 37 weeks gestation in your community hospital. The mother has juvenile-onset diabetes and has been insulin-dependent for 10 years. Her blood glucose was reasonably well controlled in pregnancy until 3 weeks ago. This is her first baby. There was no need for resuscitation at birth.

The baby weighs 4000 grams. She appears "chubby" and plethoric, but is alert and responsive.

Her behaviour is normal for a healthy newborn. She is bundled and given to the mother to put to the breast as early as possible.

You identify this baby as "at risk" (IDM and LGA) and proceed with the ACoRN Primary Survey.

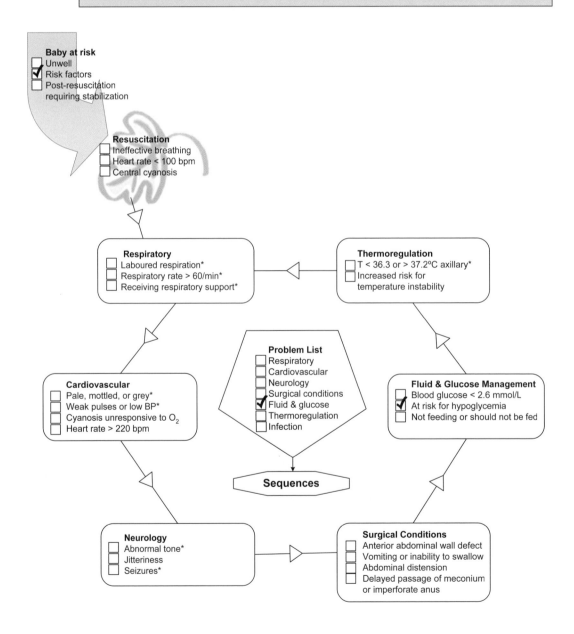

The only area of concern on the Problem List is Fluid & Glucose Management. You enter the Fluid & Glucose Management Sequence and carry out the Core Steps.

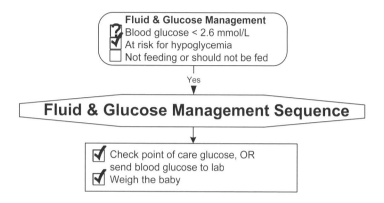

I. At what age do you initially do a blood glucose screen in a well, term baby who is breastfeeding but is at risk for hypoglycemia?

_____

Glucose Screening   Symptomatic and unwell babies require immediate glucose testing.

In asymptomatic at-risk babies, blood glucose screening should be performed at 2 hours of age and every 3 to 6 hours after this, in keeping with frequency of feeding.

Testing may be discontinued,
- after 12 hours of age in LGA babies and IDMs if blood glucose levels remain ≥ 2.6 mmol/L (47 mg/dL),
- after 36 hours of age in SGA babies and preterm babies if feeding has been established and blood glucose levels remain ≥ 2.6 mmol/L (47 mg/dL).

The baby has been suckling well.

The result of the blood glucose screen done at 2 hours of age by glucose meter is 2.0 mmol/L (36 mg/dL).

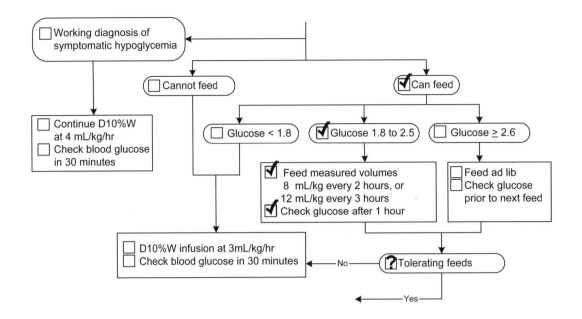

Your care of this baby is now Organized on the basis that this baby can feed, and the blood glucose is 1.8 to 2.5 mmol/L at two hours of age despite breastfeeding ad lib.

Because babies in the first two hours of life may only be consuming a few mL of colostrum, and this baby is hypoglycemic at two hours of age despite ad lib breast feeding since birth, the Response is to administer measured feeds of 12 mL/kg every three hours and to check blood glucose one hour after the feed is completed.

You explain to the mother that because her baby's blood glucose is low despite breastfeeding, it is necessary to start feeding measured amounts until the blood glucose is stable.

You initiate supplementation while encouraging the mother to continue breastfeeding and to pump to establish her milk supply.

You decide to check the blood glucose 1 hour after administering the measured feed.

II.   Calculate the amount of measured feeds for this baby.

_____

_____

Feeding intervals are dependent on the gestational age and volume the baby tolerates.

- Babies who are term usually tolerate a 12 mL/kg feed and can be fed every three hours.
- Babies who are premature (34 to 36 weeks gestation) may require more frequent feeds of smaller volumes.
- Babies who are < 34 weeks gestation, are unlikely to tolerate the whole amount of feeds and will likely require early intravenous supplementation.

Despite this being a term baby you may decide to start with smaller feeds (for example, 8 mL/kg every 2 hours), and gradually increase to 12 mL/kg every 3 hours as the volume is tolerated.

> The baby tolerates the 50 mL feed well so you decide the next feed will be in three hours.
>
> You proceed to Next Steps.

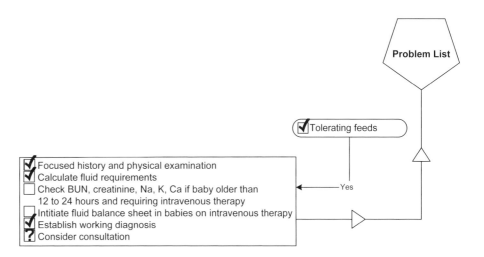

> You are aware of the mother's history, as she has been a patient in your practice for several years. You complete the remainder of the baby's physical examination which reveals a moderately enlarged liver but no other positive findings.

III. **What is the fluid requirement of a baby in the first 24 hours? Are you meeting or exceeding that fluid requirement?**

_____

_____

IV.   What determines the range of fluid requirement/tolerance?

_____

_____

> Because the baby is only 2 hours old, you do not check a BUN, creatinine or electrolytes at this time.

It may be necessary to check electrolytes at 12 to 24 hours of age if the blood glucose remains low, < 2.6 mmol/L (47 mg/dL) or borderline, 2.6 to 3.3 mmol/L (47 to 60 mg/dL), and the baby requires fluid intake over the recommended daily requirements in order to maximize glucose intake.

V.   What is your working diagnosis?

_____

Infants of diabetic mothers (IDMs)   Infants of diabetic mothers (IDMs) may have transient hyperinsulinism, which presents in the first couple of hours of life and usually resolves in 3 to 7 days.

Blood glucose levels decline more abruptly in the IDM than in normal babies, with the lowest point occurring at 1 to 2 hours of age. Hypoglycemia is not likely to have its onset beyond 24 hours after birth.

If macrosomic (large for gestational age), IDMs are at even greater risk of becoming hypoglycemic.

Large for gestational age (LGA) babies   LGA babies (> 90th percentile) have a reported incidence of hypoglycemia of approximately 8%. Hypoglycemia is not likely to have its onset beyond 8 hours after birth.

In both the IDM and LGA baby, if the initial blood glucose is low, the baby should receive measured feeds. If a pre-feed glucose drawn at > 3 hours of age is normal, it is unlikely that supplements will be required and the baby may be treated as a healthy baby.

You exit the Fluid & Glucose Management Sequence and return to the Problem List. As there are no other problems in the Problem List you continue to observe the baby's progress and address the Specific Management of your working diagnosis.

One hour after the measured feed, the blood glucose by glucose meter was 2.8 mmol/L (50 mg/dL). The blood glucose two hours later, just before the next feed is due, is 1.8 mmol/L (33 mg/dL).

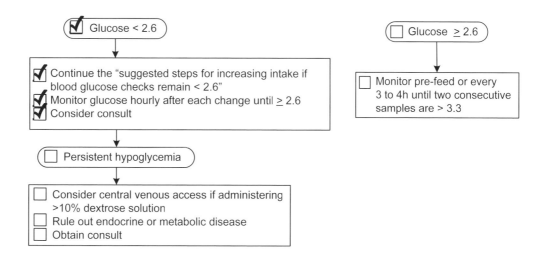

Remember the suggested steps for increasing intake if blood glucose checks remain < 2.6 mmol/L (47 mg/dL)?

Steps	Enterally fed	IV dextrose infusion
Baseline	Breastfeed on cue, or Feed every 2 to 3 hours	D10%W, 3 mL/kg/hour (= 5 mg/kg/minute of glucose)
Step 1	Feed measured volume 8 mL/kg every 2 hours or 12 mL/kg every 3 hours, or Start IV dextrose infusion at baseline	D10%W, 4 mL/kg/hour (= 6.7 mg/kg/minute of glucose)
Step 2	Go to IV dextrose infusion step 1, and proceed from there	D12.5%W, 4 to 5 mL/kg/hour (= 8.3 to 10.4 mg/kg/minute of glucose) Obtain consultation and investigations Consider central access Consider glucagon or other pharmacological intervention

> You have been feeding measured amounts of milk, 12 mL/kg every 3 hours, which is the maximum amount likely to be tolerated.
>
> According to the Table you must now initiate a D10%W intravenous infusion at 4 mL/kg/hour.
>
> You order a blood glucose level hourly after each change.
>
> You plan to proceed stepwise, using the Table as a guide, if the blood glucose remains < 2.6 mmol/L (47 mg/dL).

If fluid administration exceeds the daily requirements for day 1 of life, a consultation for specialized care should be obtained. This may include an endocrine diagnostic workup.

If a dextrose concentration > 12.5% is required, central venous access should be established. A securely sutured, umbilical venous catheter in a low position (2 to 3 cm below skin level) is adequate for short-term central access.

 Emergency venous access: Umbilical vein catheterization

Intravenous or enteral feeding? Due to its content of fat and protein, milk (67 to 70 kcal/100 mL) contains 50 to 70% more energy than dextrose solutions. However, fat and protein only become a source of additional energy when counter-regulation is present.

When hypoglycemia persists despite full enteral feeds, counter-regulation can be assumed to be depressed and that blood glucose is dependent on the intake of simple carbohydrates such as dextrose. Blood glucose will be more stable with an intravenous infusion of D10%W or D12.5%W, which contains 1½ to twice as much carbohydrate as milk.

The table below compares the amount of glucose provided by milk and intravenous dextrose.

Content per 100 mL volume	Early breast milk (mature milk)	Term formula	D10%W	D12.5%W
Energy (kcal)	67 (70)	68	40	50
Protein (g)	2.4 (1.3)	1.4	--	--
Carbohydrate (g)	6.1 (7.0)	7.2	10.0	12.5
Fat (g)	3.8 (3.9)	3.7	--	--

Once the blood glucose becomes stable, feeds should be reintroduced gradually. As counter-regulation is re-established, fat and protein become additional energy sources.

> You initiate a D10%W infusion at 16 ml/hour (4mL/kg/hour).
>
> One hour later, the blood glucose increases to 2.7 mmol/L (48 mg/dL). When repeated three hours later, the blood glucose is 3.3 mmol/L (60 mg/dL). The baby remains asymptomatic.
>
> You gradually reintroduce oral feeding and are able to decrease the intravenous dextrose solution over the next 12 hours.

Fluid & Glucose Management Case # 2 – A baby with symptomatic hypoglycemia

As the family practice resident on call, you are asked to see a 4 hour old baby boy who the nurse reports as jittery and irritable. On arrival to the observation area in the nursery, you are told the baby was born at 40 weeks gestation to a 21-year-old primigravida and weighed 2300 grams. The nurse noticed the baby was jittery as she was helping the mother with breastfeeding.

The baby is pink and breathing, and the heart rate is 140 bpm. You determine that the baby shows none of the Resuscitation Signs.

Resuscitation
- [ ] Ineffective breathing
- [ ] Heart rate < 100 bpm
- [ ] Central cyanosis

You proceed to perform a Primary Survey and develop an ACoRN Problem List.

The baby has no respiratory distress, a respiratory rate of 48/minute, is pink and well perfused. He looks small for gestational age with "skinny" extremities and little subcutaneous tissue. He is alert, active, and seems hungry. He is jittery, and irritable. His legs are tremulous, but the movements cease when you grasp his feet.

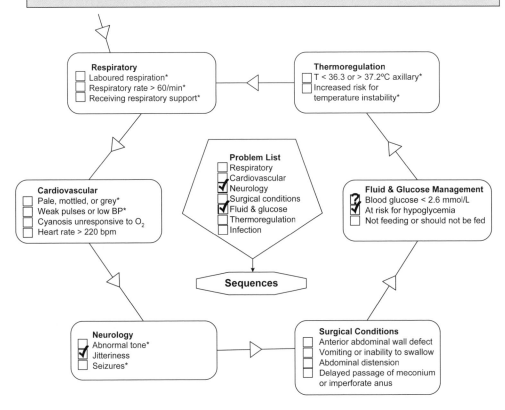

Respiratory
- [ ] Laboured respiration*
- [ ] Respiratory rate > 60/min*
- [ ] Receiving respiratory support*

Thermoregulation
- [ ] T < 36.3 or > 37.2°C axillary*
- [ ] Increased risk for temperature instability*

Problem List
- [ ] Respiratory
- [ ] Cardiovascular
- [x] Neurology
- [ ] Surgical conditions
- [x] Fluid & glucose
- [ ] Thermoregulation
- [ ] Infection

Cardiovascular
- [ ] Pale, mottled, or grey*
- [ ] Weak pulses or low BP*
- [ ] Cyanosis unresponsive to O_2
- [ ] Heart rate > 220 bpm

Fluid & Glucose Management
- [?] Blood glucose < 2.6 mmol/L
- [x] At risk for hypoglycemia
- [ ] Not feeding or should not be fed

Sequences

Neurology
- [x] Abnormal tone*
- [x] Jitteriness
- [ ] Seizures*

Surgical Conditions
- [ ] Anterior abdominal wall defect
- [ ] Vomiting or inability to swallow
- [ ] Abdominal distension
- [ ] Delayed passage of meconium or imperforate anus

You enter the Neurology Sequence and perform the Core Steps.

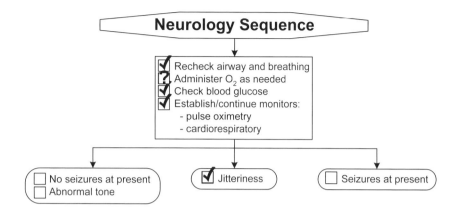

The airway is patent, and breathing is regular. Oxygen is not needed because the pulse oximetry reads 93% on room air.

The Core Steps in the Neurology Sequence include a blood glucose determination, which the nurse performs at the bedside using a glucose meter.

The blood glucose result is immediately available: 1.0 mmol/L (18 mg/dL).

What are the possible causes of jitteriness in this baby?

The most common causes of jitteriness are,
- hypoglycemia
- hypocalcemia
- drug withdrawal
- neonatal encephalopathy.

This baby has jitteriness and hypoglycemia. He should be considered to have symptomatic hypoglycemia until proven otherwise, and managed accordingly.

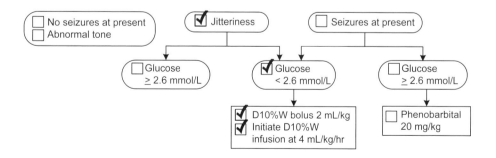

> You administer a minibolus of 2 mL/kg of D10%W and initiate a D10%W infusion at 4 mL/kg/hour.

The administration of a bolus of D10%W for symptomatic hypoglycemia is controversial,

- it may reduce the time to normalization of the blood glucose level
- it may stimulate insulin secretion and suppress glucagon secretion, resulting in rebound hypoglycemia
- it remains in circulation for only 20 minutes.

The key to the management of a critically hypoglycemic baby is to,

- start a D10%W infusion at 4 mL/kg/hour, and
- monitor blood glucose every 30 minutes until ≥ 2.6 mmol/L.

> The history and physical examination indicate the mother had gestational hypertension and decreased amniotic fluid in the week prior to birth.
>
> Labour was induced and lasted 19 hours. Apgar scores were 8 and 9, at 1 and 5 minutes. The baby was active and eager to feed at birth; he has been exclusively breastfeeding. Mother asked that no blood work be done on the baby.
>
> The baby is small for gestational age (birth weight < 10th percentile, and length and head circumference 25th percentile), with thin extremities and little subcutaneous tissue.
>
> He is alert, active and seems hungry, but is irritable and jittery. He has been sucking vigorously at the breast but mother has not heard any swallowing. She does not feel there is much milk being produced yet.
>
> You hold the baby's arms and legs and they stop shaking.
>
> You plan to repeat a blood glucose 30 minutes after initiation of the D10%W infusion.

I.   **What is your working diagnosis?**

_____

_____

You exit the Neurology Sequence and enter the next Sequence in your Problem List: Fluid & Glucose Management.

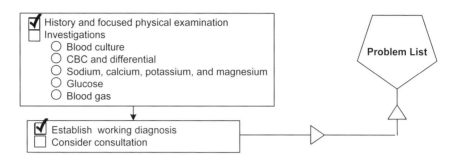

II. When should the initial blood glucose be obtained in babies at-risk for hypoglycemia, who are well and feeding by breast or bottle?

In addition, the blood glucose would have been monitored before every feed until the baby had established oral feeding and had two consecutive samples > 3.3 mmol/L (> 60 mg/dL).

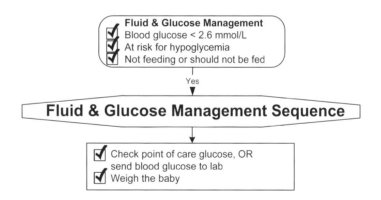

This baby is now in the Fluid & Glucose Management Sequence because of the symptomatic hypoglycemia. He is being fully managed using intravenous dextrose. He remains at risk for hypoglycemia.

You obtain a blood glucose by glucose meter and send a simultaneous sample to the laboratory. The baby had been previously weighed.

The blood glucose by glucose meter is 2.8 mmol/L (50 mg/dL).

The baby is less irritable and no longer jittery.

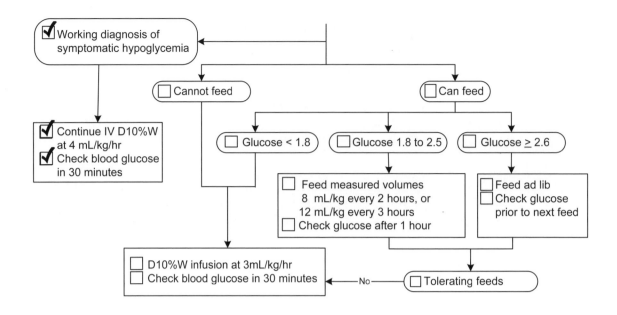

The baby has a working diagnosis of symptomatic hypoglycemia but his blood glucose is > 2.6 mmol/L (> 47 mg/dL).

- You do not increase the dextrose infusion at this time as it is already infusing at 4 mL/hour.
- You must check a blood glucose level in 30 minutes.

You proceed to Next Steps.

☑ Focused history and physical examination
☑ Calculate fluid requirements
☐ Check BUN, creatinine, Na, K, Ca if baby older than
   12 to 24 hours and requiring intravenous therapy
☑ Intitiate fluid balance sheet in babies on intravenous therapy
☑ Establish working diagnosis
☑ Consider consultation

No additional focused history is available at this time.

You calculate that the baby is currently receiving approximately 70 mL/kg/day of fluids.

You decide you will not check a BUN, creatinine or electrolytes until 24 hours of age, unless you need to increase the daily fluid intake over the upper range of recommended daily requirement of 100 mL/kg/day in order to maximize glucose intake.

You initiate a fluid balance sheet.

Your working diagnosis remains symptomatic hypoglycemia in a baby with intrauterine growth restriction, but you note that the baby is no longer symptomatic or hypoglycemic.

You decide to obtain a specialist consultation.

You exit the Fluid & Glucose Management Sequence and return to the Problem List.

As there are no other problems in the Problem List you continue to observe the baby's progress and address the Specific Management of your working diagnosis.

Thirty minutes later the blood glucose is 2.2 mmol/L (40 mg/dL).

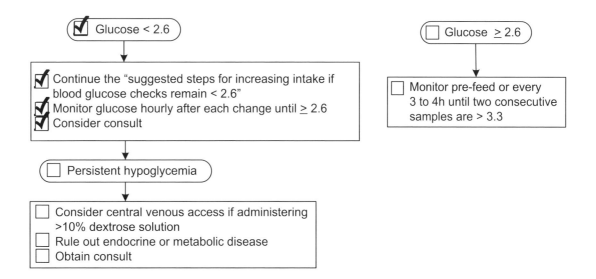

III. **What is the next step for increasing glucose intake?**

_____

IV. **What other steps would you consider in addition to increasing glucose intake?**

_____

_____

_____

> The blood glucose increases to 3.3 mmol/L (60 mg/dL) 30 minutes after increasing the concentration to D12.5%W infusion.
>
> You decide to observe the blood glucose level over the following several hours, and to gradually reintroduce feeds if it remains > 3.3 mmol/L.
>
> The mother reinitiates breastfeeding the following day and you are able to decrease the intravenous dextrose concentration to D10%W. As feeding increases, you gradually decrease the IV infusion rate. The baby establishes full oral feeds and maintains blood glucose > 3.3 mmol/L (60 mg/dL) by 48 hours of age.

Answers to the questions in Chapter 7

Case # 1:

I.   At what age do you initially do a blood glucose screen in a well, term baby who is breastfeeding but is at risk for hypoglycemia?

At 2 hours of age

II.   How do you calculate the amount of measured feeds for this baby?

Every 3 hours: Wt (kg) x 12 mL/kg = 4 x 12 ~ 50 mL

Every 2 hours (if 50 mL is not tolerated): Wt (kg) x 8 mL/kg = 4 x 8 ~ 30 mL

III.   What is the fluid requirement of a baby in the first 24 hours? Are you meeting or exceeding that fluid requirement?

The fluid requirement of a baby receiving enteral feeds, in the first 24 hours of life, is 50 to 100 mL/kg/day.

You are currently giving 96 mL/kg/day of enteral feeds, which is within these limits.

IV.   What determines the range of fluid requirement/tolerance?

The ability or inability to excrete extra water by increasing urine output

The presence or absence of increased insensible or measurable losses

V.   What is your working diagnosis?

LGA baby of a diabetic mother with hypoglycemia

Case # 2:

I.   What is your working diagnosis?

Symptomatic hypoglycemia in a baby with intrauterine growth restriction

Possibly insufficient milk intake

II. **When should the initial blood glucose be obtained in babies at-risk for hypoglycemia, who are well and feeding by breast or bottle?**

At 2 hours of age

III. **What is the next step for increasing glucose intake?**

Change the infusion to D12.5%W (still at a rate of 4 mL/kg/hr).

IV. **What other steps would you consider in addition to increasing glucose intake?**

Obtain central venous access

Seek urgent specialist consultation

Rule out metabolic / endocrine disease

Bibliography

Cornblath M, Hawdon JM, Williams AF, Aynsley-Green A, Ward-Platt MP, Schwarts R, Kalhan SC. Controversies regarding definition of neonatal hypoglycemia: suggested operational thresholds. Pediatrics 2000 May;105(5):1141-5.

Cornblath M, Ichord R. Hypoglycemia in the neonate. Semin Perinatol 2000 Apr;24(2):136-49.

Hawdon JM, Ward Platt MP, Aynsley-Green A. Prevention and management of neonatal hypoglycemia. Arch Dis Child Fetal Neonatal Red 1994 Jan;70(1):F60-4; discussion F65.

Hypoglycaemia of the Newborn, Review of the Literature. World Health Organization, Geneva. 1997. http://www.who.int/child-adolescent-health/New_Publications/NUTRITION/hypoclyc.htm

Kalhan SC, Parimi PS. Disorders of Carbohydrate Metabolism. In: Fanaroff AA and Martin RJ. Neonatal-Perinatal Medicine, Diseases of the Fetus and Infant, 7th Edition, Volume Two, Mosby Inc 2002, St. Louis, Missouri.

Mehta A. Prevention and management of neonatal hypoglycemia. Arch Dis Child Fetal Neonatal Red 1994 Jan;70(1):F54-9; discussion F59-60.

Stenninger E, Flink R, Eriksson B and Sahlen C. Long term neurological dysfunction and neonatal hypoglycemia after diabetic pregnancy. Arch Dis Child Fetal Neonatal Ed 1998;79:F174-9.

Chapter 8
Thermoregulation

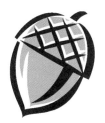

Objectives

Upon completion of this chapter, you should be able to:
1. Apply the Thermoregulation Sequence.
2. Identify the risk factors for and causes of temperature instability.
3. Recognize and manage hypothermia and hyperthermia.
4. Understand the importance of a thermally controlled environment.
5. Recognize when to exit to the other ACoRN Sequences.

Key Concepts

1. All newborns are at risk for temperature instability.
2. Babies at increased risk for hypothermia include those who are preterm, small for gestational age, low birth weight (LBW ≤ 2000 grams), very low birth weight (VLBW ≤ 1500 grams), and unwell.
3. A thermally controlled environment is one in which a baby uses the least energy, oxygen, and calories to maintain a normal temperature.
4. Severe cold stress may impede resuscitation and stabilization efforts.
5. Hyperthermia may increase morbidity and mortality.

Introduction

Maintaining temperature within the normal range by providing warmth and minimizing heat loss is an important component of newborn care, especially for preterm babies.

Without prompt attention, body temperature falls rapidly (by 0.2° to 1° C per minute). Caloric expenditure and oxygen consumption increase to compensate for heat loss, resulting in the depletion of energy stores (brown fat and glycogen) within hours.

Appropriate support of body and environmental temperature to prevent hypothermia,
- prevents depletion of valuable energy stores
- may prevent hypoglycemia, metabolic acidosis, and pulmonary hypertension.

Appropriate support of body and environmental temperature to prevent hyperthermia may reduce the extent of organ injury in asphyxiated babies.

Recent information suggests that intrapartum and neonatal hyperthermia may have detrimental effects on all newborns, such as an increased incidence of seizures.

The optimal temperature at which term babies, with or without clinical signs of asphyxia, should be stabilized is presently unknown.
- As with all other interventions, temperature support should be administered and monitored carefully.
- Until further information is available, the accepted approach is to avoid both hyper- and hypothermia.

Alerting Signs

A baby who demonstrates one or more of the following Alerting Signs enters the Thermoregulation Sequence:

> **Thermoregulation**
> ☐ T < 36.3 or > 37.2ºC axillary*
> ☐ Increased risk for temperature instability

Axillary temperature < 36.3° C or > 37.2° C

There is a lack of evidence on what constitutes the "normal" temperature range for a baby. For the purposes of this text, hypothermia is defined as < 36.3° C axillary and hyperthermia as > 37.2° C axillary. Consensus is that axillary temperature should be maintained between 36.3 and 37.2° C (inclusive) and skin temperature between 36.5 and 37.0° C.

Increased risk for temperature instability

All babies are at risk for temperature instability because their ability to regulate body temperature has not yet fully developed. Babies have a surface-area to body-mass ratio that is four times that of an adult, yet their ability to increase heat production is only one third that of an adult. Temperature is especially labile during the transition from intrauterine to the extrauterine environment. Although mild variations from normal are common, wider variations can be detrimental.

Babies who are at increased risk for hypothermia include,
- those who are not dried
- those who are not cared for in a warm, draft-free environment
- preterm babies, who have greater surface area in relation to body weight than term babies and can lack both the white fat needed for insulation and the brown fat needed for heat production
- small for gestational age babies, who have the same risk factors as preterm babies plus a higher metabolic rate
- sick babies, because they use extra oxygen and energy to maintain normal body functions
- babies with congenital anomalies involving open lesions or exposed organs.

Hyperthermia is usually iatrogenic (for example, caused by overheating of the environment) and preventable. Other causes of hyperthermia include dehydration, infection, increased maternal temperature affecting the fetal temperature, administration of PGE_1, and central nervous system disorders.

Body temperature must be considered in the context of the baby's age, weight, birth history and present surroundings. For instance,
- if a baby has an elevated temperature in the immediate newborn period or first 24 hours of age following a normal labor and birth, the cause is likely to be external to the baby (for example, over-heating by a radiant warmer)
- if a baby's temperature remains elevated after controlling for environmental factors or if a previously normothermic baby presents with new onset hyperthermia, a cause of fever, such as sepsis, should be considered.

Body temperature should also be considered in the context of the baby's appearance. For instance,
- a term baby who is externally overheated will implement thermoregulatory mechanisms that increase heat loss, and will appear flushed (vasodilated), while
- a term baby developing a fever may look pale, mottled and have cold, acrocyanotic extremities (vasoconstricted).

The Thermoregulation Sequence

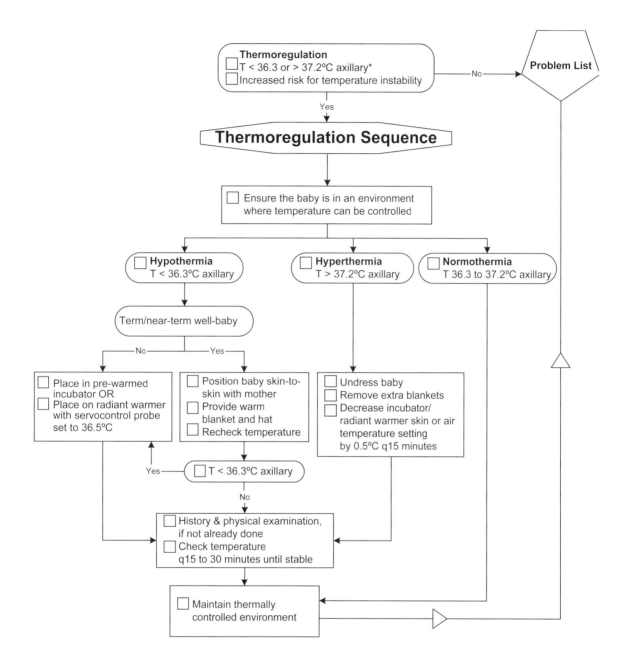

Core Steps

There is only one Core Step in the Thermoregulation Sequence, "Ensure the baby is in an environment where temperature can be controlled". This includes,

- maintaining the temperature of the birthing room between 22 to 25°C to facilitate temperature stability during the transitional period after birth
- using an incubator or radiant warmer if the baby is unwell or requires observation.

Organization of Care

The ability to distinguish between hypothermia, hyperthermia and normothermia depends on accurate temperature readings. There are several sites where temperature can be measured; the axilla is the safest and most convenient route. Temperature measured per axilla is comparable to rectal temperature in both term and preterm babies, if proper technique is used.

Technique for taking an axillary temperature:
1. Ensure the area under the arm is dry.
2. Place the tip of an electronic thermometer into the mid-armpit and fold the baby's arm snugly against his/her body.
3. Hold this position until the electronic thermometer reading is completed.

Rectal temperatures are not recommended because,
- the act of inserting a thermometer into the rectum may induce rectal or sigmoid trauma
- a rectal temperature, usually taken at a depth of 1 cm, is not a better estimate of core temperature than an axillary temperature
  - electronic thermometer probes cannot be safely inserted deep enough (5 cm) to measure core body temperature.

Glass mercury thermometers are not recommended due to concerns regarding potential trauma and mercury exposure from breakage. Tympanic thermometers are not currently recommended for use in children under two years of age due to concerns about accuracy.

Taking the temperature at a central and peripheral site simultaneously (for example, the axilla or abdomen and the sole of the foot), allows identification of relative changes between central and peripheral locations. A change in peripheral temperature precedes a change in central temperature, as peripheral temperatures are subject to variation in perfusion. A drop in peripheral skin temperature may be an early sign of hypothermia, hypovolemia or shock.

Response

There are many ways to restore normothermia to a warm or cool baby. The choice depends on gestational age, whether the baby is sick or well, and how widely the temperature has diverged from normal.

- Term or near term well babies can be effectively rewarmed by positioning them skin-to-skin with their mothers; other babies should be rewarmed in incubators or under radiant warmers.
  - It is not known if rewarming of cool babies should be done rapidly or slowly
- Cooling of hyperthermic babies to achieve normothermia is usually achieved by undressing them, removing extra blankets and decreasing the incubator or radiant warmer temperature.
  - All overheated babies should be cooled.
  - It is likely that cooling babies who are hyperthermic for other reasons is also beneficial.

Next Steps

The frequency with which temperature should be rechecked depends on how widely the baby's temperature has diverged from normal, the stability of the baby's condition, and the mechanism(s) being used to warm or cool the baby.

A complete history and physical examination are indicated if they have not already been completed in a previous ACoRN sequence.

In addition, a focused thermoregulation history includes:

Antepartum
- maternal health during pregnancy

Intrapartum
- maternal infection, fever, and antibiotic administration
- delivery method and complications

Neonatal
- need for resuscitation
- signs of temperature instability
- ambient room temperature

Essential components of the physical examination include:

Observation
- temperature trend since birth
- color (mottling, acrocyanosis)
- room temperature
- servocontrol setting on the radiant warmer or on the skin probe attached to the baby in an incubator, or the air temperature setting in any incubator being used in a non-servocontrol mode

Measurement of vital signs: current axillary temperature, respiratory rate, heart rate, blood pressure, and pulse oximetry

Examination
- a comparison of limb and body skin temperature by touch (e.g. cool extremities, decreased perfusion)

There are no diagnostic tests specific to the Thermoregulation Sequence because this Sequence is concerned with maintaining body temperature within normal range. However, certain underlying medical conditions (for example, sepsis) may affect temperature. The diagnosis and laboratory evaluation of these conditions is dealt with in the other Sequences.

Specific Management

As an ideal, all babies should be cared for in a neutral thermal environment, which is defined as that environment in which a baby uses the least energy, oxygen, and calories to maintain a normal body temperature.

In practical terms, the aim is to provide a controlled thermal environment that maintains the baby's skin temperature at 36.3 to 37.2°C. Babies of different sizes and ages require different amounts of external heat to accomplish this.

For unwell and at-risk babies, an incubator or a radiant warmer not only provide a controlled thermal environment, but also allow close visual observation, and in the case of the radiant warmer, frequent access for procedures.

Incubators

Incubators are heated by circulating warm air inside (convection). They provide a controlled thermal environment despite temperature fluctuations due to uneven room temperature, external radiant heating, phototherapy lights, etc.

Incubators operate in two modes: air temperature control or servocontrol.

Air temperature mode
Air temperature mode heats the air inside the incubator to a chosen temperature. A variety of thermal environment charts have been published to guide the selection of incubator temperature settings, according to the baby's weight and age, with the aim of maintaining a normal body temperature while minimizing energy expenditure.

These charts were developed decades ago. Since then, equipment and care practices have changed substantially (for example, using double-walled incubators, nesting babies, and covering incubators).

The information contained in the charts should be used as an initial guide only as it may not be accurate for current care practices.

Choosing the initial incubator temperature in the first 12 hours of age

Birth weight (grams)	Air temperature setting °C (double wall, humidified incubator)
< 750	39.5 (37.5)
750 to 1000	39.0 (37.0)
1000 to 1200	37.5
1200 to 1500	36.5
1500 to 2000	35.5
> 2000	34

Adapted from: Jaimovich DG, Vidyasagar D. Handbook Pediatric and Neonatal Transport Medicine (2d Edition). Philadelphia: Hanley & Belfus, Inc. 2002, p. 483

Servocontrol Mode

In servocontrol mode, the heating element turns on and off in response to the baby's skin temperature, according to the reading from the servocontrol probe. The servocontrol probe temperature is set at 36.5°C.

Tape the skin temperature probe tip flat on the right upper quadrant of the abdomen, for servocontrol or for simply monitoring the skin temperature.

Humidity

Humidity is important for preterm and particularly very-low-birthweight babies to decrease evaporative heat and water loss. Preterm babies should receive humidity at levels $\geq 70\%$.

- Newer incubators use servocontrolled humidification systems with filters and sterile distilled water to ensure clean air enters the incubator.
- In older incubators, which lack built-in humidification system, providing humidity via a water reservoir increases the risk for infection.
- Follow the manufacturer's instructions and hospital infection control guidelines for care of an incubator humidification system.

Caution!

1. Do not block the air circulation inside the incubator.
2. If the baby's temperature is $> 37.2°$ C and the incubator air temperature has been decreased to its lowest setting, do not turn off the incubator in an attempt to cool the baby or the incubator further. Air flow ceases when the incubator is turned off. Instead, transfer the baby to a radiant warmer or place in a cot.

Radiant warmer

Radiant warmers use infrared heat as the radiant heat source.

Radiant warmers function in two modes: manual and servocontrol (automatic).

- In manual mode, the warmer will continue to heat unless turned off. It is not effective for maintaining a controlled thermal environment since the baby can easily be overheated in this mode. For these reasons, it is recommended servocontrol mode be used for all babies.
- In servocontrol mode, the warmer turns on and off in response to the baby's skin temperature, according to the reading from the servocontrol probe. This decreases the risk for hypo- or hyperthermia.

All babies under a radiant warmer should have the skin temperature probe attached and functioning to avoid overheating and associated complications.

- Set the skin probe temperature to 36.5°C.
- A reflective cover over the temperature probe is necessary to prevent overheating of the probe, which reduces heater output.
- Set high and low temperature alarms 0.5°C above and below pre-set temperature.

Radiant heat to the baby can be blocked by blankets and sterile drapes, plastic shields, equipment, and the hands and heads of care providers. Drafts around the radiant warmer increase the risk of convective heat loss.

Insensible water loss is greater under radiant warmers. Strategies to ensure temperature stability for VLBW babies include covering the radiant warmer bed with plastic wrap when the side panels are up, and supplying warmed and humidified air under the plastic wrap. Removal of these coverings can lead to wide fluctuations in temperature.

After initial resuscitation and stabilization, consider moving the baby to an incubator (or the warmer converted to an incubator like some new models) to ensure adequate thermoregulation, rest, and prevention of insensible water loss.

Thermoregulation Case # 1 - The cold, outborn baby

A baby boy is born in a car on a chilly winter night, and arrives at the rural nursing station when he is approximately 15 minutes of age. You are working alone. As the father passes you the baby wrapped in his sweater, he tells you the baby was born three weeks early.

You place the baby on the examination table and remove the wet clothing. No meconium is noted while you are drying him.

The baby is breathing spontaneously, has a heart rate of 130 bpm, and is peripherally cyanosed. He appears sleepy.

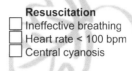

Resuscitation
- [ ] Ineffective breathing
- [ ] Heart rate < 100 bpm
- [ ] Central cyanosis

You determine the baby shows none of the Resuscitation Signs and begin the Primary Survey.

The baby appears small for 37 weeks gestation. He is breathing easily with no signs of respiratory distress. As you easily palpate the brachial and femoral pulses, you notice his limbs are cool to touch and he has acrocyanosis. The heart rate is 120 bpm. Though the baby appears sleepy, his tone is normal. The axillary temperature is 35.5°C. You wrap the baby's heel in a warm towel in preparation for a blood glucose determination. You also note the baby has not fed yet.

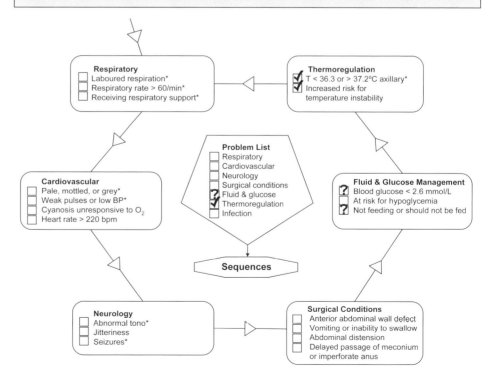

The glucose meter indicates that the blood glucose is within the normal range. You observe that the baby is eager to feed. You decide there are no contraindications to feeding the baby.

According to the order of occurrence in the Problem List, you enter the Thermoregulation Sequence and perform the Core Steps by ensuring that the baby is in an environment where the temperature can be controlled.

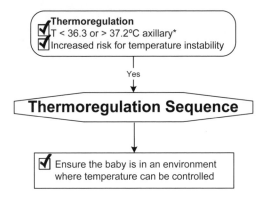

Thermoregulation
☑ T < 36.3 or > 37.2°C axillary*
☑ Increased risk for temperature instability

Yes

Thermoregulation Sequence

☑ Ensure the baby is in an environment where temperature can be controlled

You turn up the thermostat in the room while covering the baby with a warm blanket. The mother is conscious and anxious about her baby. A quick check reassures you the mother is stable.

Body temperature should be interpreted in conjunction with the environmental conditions, age and size of a baby.

I.   **What features of this baby's presentation put him at risk for hypothermia?**

_____

_____

When is a baby said to be cold stressed?

A baby is said to be cold stressed when the body becomes hypermetabolic in an attempt to regulate its temperature. A cold stressed baby may consume twice as much oxygen as a baby who is not hypermetabolic. However, clinicians do not have the tools to determine when a baby is cold stressed, hypermetabolic or consuming oxygen at an accelerated rate.

- Babies with normal temperatures may be experiencing cold stress and be hypermetabolic.
- Conversely, babies being rewarmed may no longer be hypermetabolic even if the body temperature is still below the normal range.

What clinical signs and complications might you see in a baby with cold stress?

Cold stressed babies may show clinical signs such as,
- vasocontriction
- tachypnea
- tachycardia
- fussiness.

Cold stressed babies may also develop complications such as,
- metabolic acidosis
- transient hyperglycemia
- hypoglycemia
- respiratory distress
- apnea
- hypoxemia
- shock
- clotting disorders
- death.

There are four mechanisms of heat loss.

1. Conduction – involves heat transfer from contact between the baby and a cold surface.

2. Evaporation – involves the loss of moisture (for example, amniotic fluid or water) from a warm surface such as the skin or respiratory mucosa. It can be responsible for 25% of heat loss in premature babies due to their increased skin permeability.

3. Convection – involves heat loss due to air currents such as drafts in the environment, or drafts created by movement of people or equipment.

4. Radiation – involves heat transfer from the skin to the surrounding, cooler environment.

Strategies for preventing heat loss should take into consideration the four mechanisms of heat loss.

Heat loss mechanism	Strategy
Conduction	• Pre-warm the radiant warmer or incubator. • Cover cold weigh scales or x-ray plate with a warm blanket. • Change wet for dry bedding and diapers as soon as possible.
Evaporation	• Dry the baby. • Cover abdominal wall and other exposed "open" lesions such as gastroschisis (see Chapter 6). • Warm and humidify oxygen/air supplied to the incubator or ventilator circuit. • Delay bathing until temperature is normal and stable.
Convection	• Maintain air temperature at approximately 22 to 25° C. • Protect the baby from drafts created by air vents, windows, doors, or fans. • Build a "nest" around the baby (see Chapter 11). • Close incubator portholes. • Raise the sides on the radiant warmer.
Radiation	• Maintain the baby in a flexed position. • Place warm blankets under the baby, especially if the radiant warmer is not preheated. • Apply a pre-warmed hat. • Avoid blocking the heat source in a radiant warmer. • Use a servocontrol temperature probe on radiant warmer (not manual setting). • Use a double walled incubator if possible or add a transparent shield over the baby in a single-walled incubator. • Avoid blocking air flow within the incubator. • Cover the incubator for transport.

Can babies warm themselves?

In order to warm themselves, babies must have the ability to generate heat by,
- burning brown fat and release the energy produced as heat instead of storing it as ATP
- converting glycogen into glucose which may lead initially to hyperglycemia and be followed by hypoglycemia (when glycogen stores are depleted)
- generating heat by becoming hyperactive and irritable, even if they do not generally shiver.

The closer to term the gestational age, the higher the ability a baby has to produce endogenous heat to warm itself.

- By 32 weeks' gestation, babies can produce heat and are able to sense and respond to changes in their thermal environment but have difficulty regulating or overcoming heat loss
- Extremely low birth weight babies (< 1000 grams) have limited brown fat stores and glycogen reserves, and cannot warm themselves.

When warming a baby, the goal is to ensure that the temperature steadily increases. An oscillating body temperature is more likely to trigger a hypermetabolic response.

Simple interventions for warming a mildly hypothermic (35.0°C to 36.3°C) term or near term baby who is stable.

There are multiple strategies to warming a term or near term baby (> 2000 grams) who is able to generate endogenous heat:

- Bundle the baby in a pre-warmed blanket
- Apply a warm hat to decrease heat loss from the head.
- Increase the ambient room temperature to approximately 22 to 25° C
- Apply exogenous heat by placing the baby,
  - inside an incubator or under a radiant warmer
  - skin-to-skin with its mother to enhance conductive heat transfer from mother to baby.

Skin-to-skin care Skin-to-skin care is a means of providing warmth to term and stable low birth weight babies.

The baby is placed in an upright position between the mother's breasts, and both mother and baby are covered with a blanket.

The lowest weight and gestational age for using this approach is unknown.

Caution! Heating pads, hot water bottles, surgical gloves filled with warm water, and chemical or gel warming packs carry an extreme risk of skin burns and are therefore not recommended.

The nursing station does not have a radiant warmer, but it does have an older-style, single-walled incubator. You plug it in to warm it up.

In the meantime, the baby is placed skin-to-skin with the mother. The head of the mother's stretcher is raised. You place a warm hat on the baby, position him upright between his mother's breasts, and cover mother and baby with a warm blanket.

Over the next 20 minutes, you have the opportunity to talk with the parents and provide the mother with personal care while continuing to monitor her baby. The mother tells you the baby was born three weeks early. There are no maternal risk factors for sepsis.

The physical examination reveals a term newborn with a birth weight of 2400 grams. He appears to have intrauterine growth restriction but is otherwise healthy.

You apply a pulse oximeter and confirm that the oxygen saturation is over 95% in room air.

The blood glucose is 4.0 mmol/L (72 mg/dL) by glucose meter.

You check the baby's temperature every 15 to 30 minutes until stable.

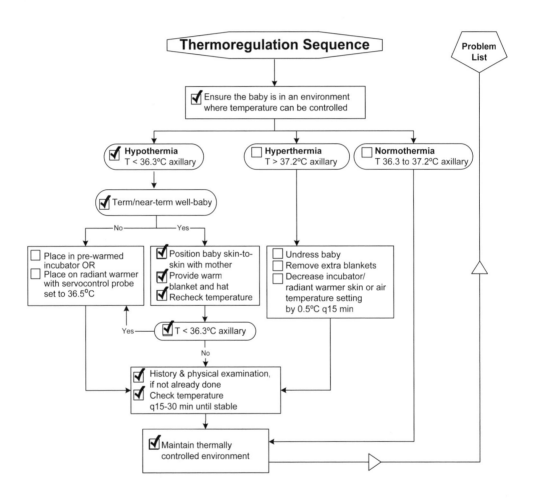

Thirty minutes later, the baby's temperature is 36.3° C axillary. Because the baby's temperature is increasing, you decide to leave the baby skin-to-skin with his mother rather than placing him in an incubator.

Use of external sources of heat for warming a baby

An external source of heat should be used when babies cannot warm themselves with heat conservation measures alone,

- ≤ 32 weeks
- < 2000 grams
- moderately (32.0 to 34.9°C) or severely (< 32.0°C) hypothermic, or
- when simple measures are insufficient

Warming a hypothermic baby using an incubator requires close attention to,

- the type of incubator (single- or double-walled)
- air temperature settings
- provision of humidity
- the baby's weight, gestational age and postnatal age
- the presence of congenital anomalies with open lesions or exposed organs.

Premature babies have high evaporative losses. Adjustments in incubator air temperature alone are insufficient for managing body temperature and the addition of humidity is essential. Adding > 60% humidity to the environment reduces evaporative heat loss.

To warm a baby, the incubator air temperature should be set at 1 to 1.5°C higher than the body temperature, or at 36°C. If the baby's temperature fails to increase, the incubator air temperature may be increased first to 37°C and then to 38°C, and the humidity level to 70%. Attempt to identify sources of ongoing heat loss (usually radiant or convective), and sources that might block exogenous heat from reaching a baby who is producing very little endogenous heat, such as blankets or shields.

The most common complication during rewarming of a baby is apnea. This requires the baby be closely monitored.

Once the baby's axillary temperature reaches the normal range, the incubator is gradually switched back to the recommended air temperature setting for age and weight.

Having completed the Primary Survey, generated a Problem List, and applied the relevant Sequences, you determine there is one Alerting Signs for Infection derived from the ACoRN Alerting Signs with *.

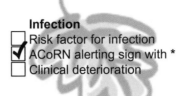

Infection
- [ ] Risk factor for infection
- [x] ACoRN alerting sign with *
- [ ] Clinical deterioration

You exit the Thermoregulation Sequence and enter the Infection Sequence. However, you suspect the reason for the baby's hypothermia is due to being born in a cold environment rather than an infection.

You decide to observe the baby closely and monitor his vital signs every 4 hours.

Thirty minutes later, the baby's temperature is 36.7° C axillary.

You recheck the baby's temperature every 30 minutes. At 2 hours of age, the baby is active and alert. His axillary temperature remains 36.8ºC.

He is showing signs that he is ready to initiate feeding at the breast.

Thermoregulation Case # 2 – A baby with hyperthermia

A baby girl was born vaginally at 40 weeks to a healthy mother. Membranes ruptured at the time of delivery and the amniotic fluid was clear. There was a tight nuchal cord, and she required 1 minute of bag-and-mask ventilation at birth.

It is now 20 minutes after delivery, and the baby remains on a radiant warmer without the servocontrol probe attached. The heater is set to manual.

She is breathing spontaneously but is irritable. Her heart rate is 180 bpm, respiratory rate 60/minute, and skin colour red and flushed. Her temperature is 38.5ºC axillary. Her pulses are bounding.

This baby meets no criteria for immediate resuscitation.

You proceed with an ACoRN Primary Survey.

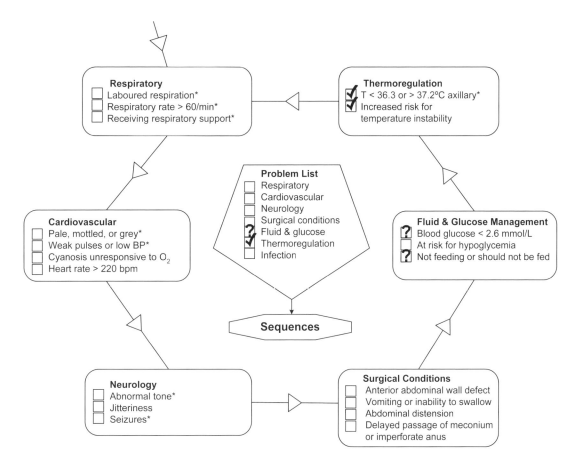

Respiratory
- [ ] Laboured respiration*
- [ ] Respiratory rate > 60/min*
- [ ] Receiving respiratory support*

Thermoregulation
- [✓] T < 36.3 or > 37.2ºC axillary*
- [✓] Increased risk for temperature instability

Cardiovascular
- [ ] Pale, mottled, or grey*
- [ ] Weak pulses or low BP*
- [ ] Cyanosis unresponsive to O₂
- [ ] Heart rate > 220 bpm

Problem List
- [ ] Respiratory
- [ ] Cardiovascular
- [ ] Neurology
- [ ] Surgical conditions
- [?] Fluid & glucose
- [✓] Thermoregulation
- [ ] Infection

Fluid & Glucose Management
- [?] Blood glucose < 2.6 mmol/L
- [ ] At risk for hypoglycemia
- [?] Not feeding or should not be fed

Neurology
- [ ] Abnormal tone*
- [ ] Jitteriness
- [ ] Seizures*

Surgical Conditions
- [ ] Anterior abdominal wall defect
- [ ] Vomiting or inability to swallow
- [ ] Abdominal distension
- [ ] Delayed passage of meconium or imperforate anus

Sequences

In order to complete the Primary Survey, you wrap the baby's heel in a warm towel in preparation for a blood glucose determination. You also note that the baby has not fed yet.

The baby exhibits two Alerting Signs for the Thermoregulation Sequence.

You enter the Thermoregulation Sequence.

Why do you think this baby is hyperthermic?

The source of the hyperthermia (extrinsic or intrinsic to the baby) and its timing relative to birth determines the approach to its management.

Hyperthermia in a newborn is often related to some aspect of the environment (extrinsic). Therefore, attention is first directed to identifying and removing potential causes of overheating before making a judgment about whether the elevated temperature is a fever.

If there are risk factors for sepsis or the baby's condition has changed in the absence of environmental influences, then attention turns to intrinsic causes of hyperthermia (fever) such as sepsis.

Tracking the trend between incubator air and skin temperatures helps differentiate between fever and environmental overheating.

Factors that may result in extrinsic hyperthermia include,
- failure to monitor the temperature of the incubator or the radiant warmer heat output
- malfunction, detachment or failure to use a servocontrol skin probe
- over-dressing for the environmental conditions
- direct sunlight on an incubator (creates a greenhouse effect)
- phototherapy lights
- out-of-hospital incidents such as leaving a baby in an automobile with the windows closed on a hot day.

What features of this baby's presentation suggest that hyperthermia is due to overheating?

Clinical features may help to distinguish whether the elevated temperature is caused by overheating or an increase in heat production.

An overheated baby may display heat-losing mechanisms, such as vasodilatation (resulting in a flushed appearance with warm hands and feet), an extended posture, tachypnea, and, in the full term baby, sweating. On the other hand, the febrile baby increases endogenous heat production during the phase of rising temperature. The baby is vasoconstricted, resulting in pale, mottled skin, and cool hands and feet.

Irritability, tachycardia and bounding pulses may be found in either situation.

If heat stress is severe, the baby may also exhibit apnea, shock, and/or convulsions. The increased metabolic rate and evaporative water loss will ultimately lead to dehydration if the hyperthermia goes untreated.

Controlling the environment to cool the baby

In a bassinet,
- unwrap the baby and remove his/her hat
- move the bassinet out of direct sunlight.

Under a radiant warmer,
- ensure the servocontrol setting is selected
- ensure the heat probe is attached to the radiant warmer, and that it is functioning
- ensure the heat probe is attached over the upper right quadrant of the abdomen, and that the probe has a reflective cover
- ensure the baby is not lying on the probe
- sponge the baby with tepid water to increase evaporative losses if temperature exceeds 41°C.

In an incubator,
- move the incubator or close the window blinds to decrease the potential greenhouse like effect which may be caused by direct sunlight
- decrease the pre-set skin temperature or incubator air temperature by 0.5 to 1.0°C every 15 minutes until the temperature is corrected
- decrease the humidity if air temperature adjustments do not resolve the problem
- never turn off the incubator to decrease the temperature as this will also turn off the airflow inside.

Caution! Servocontrol may mask a fever by lowering heater output in response to increasing skin temperature. A decrease in heat output from a radiant warmer in a previously stable baby may indicate fever.

You attach the servocontrol probe to the right upper quadrant of the baby's abdomen and set the skin temperature servocontrol to 36.5°C but the radiant warmer alarms.

You consider your alternatives to managing the baby's hyperthermia:
- turn the radiant warmer off and risk forgetting to turn it back on; or
- setting the servocontrol probe to the lowest possible setting without putting the radiant warmer to an alarm mode and risk forgetting to decrease the setting as the baby's temperature falls.

You elect to increase the temperature setting of the servocontrol probe to 37.8°C where the alarm condition is corrected (most servocontrol systems alarm if the set temperature is ± 1.5°C different than the baby's temperature), and to check the baby's temperature every 15 minutes.

The focused physical examination reveals a baby that appears flushed, well perfused, and has a capillary refill of 2 seconds. Her hands and feet feel warm, and she is active and responsive. The blood glucose by glucose meter is 6 mmol/L (108 mg/dL).

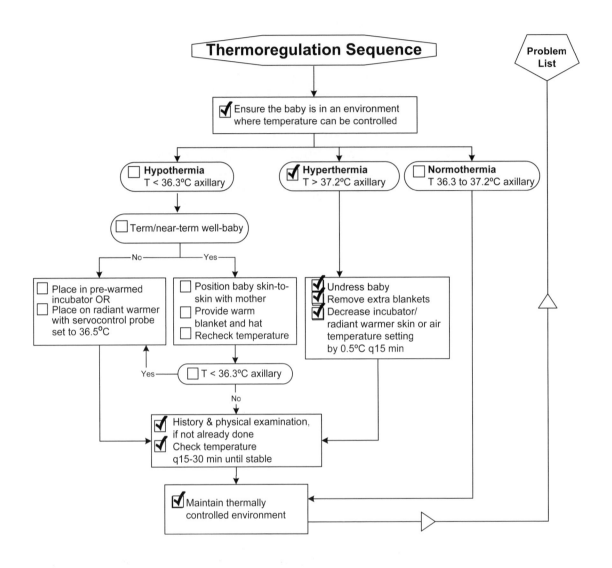

Thermoregulation Sequence

Problem List

☑ Ensure the baby is in an environment where temperature can be controlled

☐ **Hypothermia** T < 36.3°C axillary

☑ **Hyperthermia** T > 37.2°C axillary

☐ **Normothermia** T 36.3 to 37.2°C axillary

☐ Term/near-term well-baby

No / Yes

☐ Place in pre-warmed incubator OR
☐ Place on radiant warmer with servocontrol probe set to 36.5°C

☐ Position baby skin-to-skin with mother
☐ Provide warm blanket and hat
☐ Recheck temperature

☑ Undress baby
☑ Remove extra blankets
☑ Decrease incubator/ radiant warmer skin or air temperature setting by 0.5°C q15 min

Yes ← ☐ T < 36.3°C axillary

No

☑ History & physical examination, if not already done
☑ Check temperature q15-30 min until stable

☑ Maintain thermally controlled environment

Having completed the Primary Survey, generated a Problem List and applied the Thermoregulation Sequence, you determine there is one Alerting Sign for Infection derived from the ACoRN alerting signs with *.

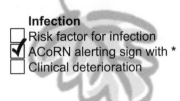

Infection
☐ Risk factor for infection
☑ ACoRN alerting sign with *
☐ Clinical deterioration

You exit the Thermoregulation Sequence and enter the Infection Sequence.

You already know this mother was healthy during her pregnancy and labour, and that the membranes ruptured at birth. There are no other risk factors for infection from your focused history and physical examination. The baby was being nursed under a radiant warmer that was not servocontrolled.

After 15 minutes, the baby's temperature has decreased to 37.7ºC axillary, the heart rate is 156 bpm, and the respiratory rate is 56 breaths/minute.

You continue to reduce the probe setting until it reaches 36.5ºC and continue to monitor the baby's temperature response for another 15 minutes.

The baby's temperature normalizes 20 minutes later.

Answers to the questions in Chapter 8

Case # 1: The cold, outborn baby

I. **What features of this baby's presentation put him at risk for hypothermia?**

Not initially cared for in a warm environment (i.e. born in a car on a chilly winter night)

Not dried at birth (i.e. wrapped in father's sweater which was wet on arrival at the hospital)

Bibliography

Bailey F, Rose P. Temperature measurement in the preterm infant: A Bailey F, Rose P. Temperature measurement in the preterm infant: A literature review. J Neonat Nurs 2000:6(1):28-32.

Health Canada. Family-Centred Maternity and Newborn Care: National Guidelines, Minister of Public Works and Government Services, Ottawa, 2000.

Jaimovich DG, Vidyasagar D. Handbook of Pediatric and Neonatal Transport Medicine (2nd edition). Philadelphia: Hanley & Belfus, Inc. 2002.

Laptook AR, Corbett RJT. The effects of temperature on hypoxic ischemic brain injury. Clinics of Perinatology 2002; 29: 623-649.

LeBlanc Michael H. The Physical Environment. In: Avroy E. Fanaroff and Richard J. Martin (Eds). Neonatal Perinatal Medicine: Diseases of the fetus and Infant (7th ed). St. Louis, Missouri: Mosby, 2002, p. 512-529.

National Association of Neonatal Nurses. Neonatal Thermoregulation Guidelines for Practice. Petaluma, CA, 1997.

Rockwern S. Neonatal thermoregulation. In C. Kenner, J. Wright Lott & A Applewhite Flandermeyer (eds), Comprehensive neonatal nursing: A physiologic perspective (2nd ed). Philadelphia, PA: Saunders, 1998, p. 207-219.

Sinclair JC. Servocontrol for maintaining abdominal skin temperature at 36°C in low birth weight infants (Cochrane Review). In: The Cochrane Library, Issue 3, 2003. Oxford: Update Software.

Woods Blake W, Murray J. Heat balance. In G. Merenstein and S. Gardner (Eds). Handbook of Neonatal Intensive Care (5th ed). St. Louis, Missouri: Mosby, 2002, p. 102-116.

Chapter 9
Infection

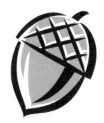

Objectives

Upon completion of this section, you will be able to:
1. Identify the risk factors for perinatal infections.
2. Recognize the early signs of infection.
3. Apply the Infection Sequence.
4. Perform appropriate diagnostic evaluation.
5. Initiate antibiotic treatment and provide supportive care.

Key Concepts

1. Signs and symptoms of sepsis in the neonate are non-specific.
2. The presence of sepsis should be suspected in babies with recognized risk factors for infection, the presence of certain Alerting Signs identified in the ACoRN Primary Survey, or evidence of clinical deterioration.
3. Whenever sepsis is clinically suspected, blood cultures should be obtained and antibiotics initiated without delay.
4. If a lumbar puncture is likely to delay the initiation of antibiotic therapy, it may be done later.

Skills

- Interpretation of complete blood count (CBC) and differential white cell count.
- Antibiotics (dose calculation, frequency of administration, route of administration)

Introduction

Newborns have poor cellular and humoral defense mechanisms, predisposing them to infections. Sick newborns have multiple portals of entry for organisms such as immature skin, breakage in skin barrier at time of IV insertion, placement of central lines or an endotracheal tube.

Sepsis is defined as a condition where there is clinical evidence of an infection and signs that the baby is systemically unwell (as might be detected by the ACoRN Primary Survey and Alerting Signs). Early signs of sepsis in babies may be non-specific and difficult to diagnose. Babies who need resuscitation at birth may already have an underlying infection.

Babies have poor ability to localize infection so rapid dissemination and deterioration is common unless prompt treatment with appropriate antibiotics is given.

Sepsis is most commonly bacterial, and occasionally fungal or viral. Hence, the majority of this chapter is directed towards the early detection and treatment of serious bacterial infections. Where considered relevant, other types of infection are discussed.

In babies suspected to have sepsis, it is important,
- to start antibiotics as soon as appropriate cultures have been taken
- not to delay antibiotics while waiting for results of ancillary tests.

Alerting Signs

A baby who demonstrates one or more of the following alerting signs enters the Infection Sequence:

Infection
- ☐ Risk factor for infection
- ☐ ACoRN alerting sign with *
- ☐ Clinical deterioration

Risk factors for infection

Risk factors for infection may be identified in the antenatal period, during labor or after birth and are listed under the Focused History for Infection.

Alerting signs marked with an asterisk (*)

- from the respiratory chapter,
  - labored respiration
  - respiratory rate > 60/minute
  - receiving assisted ventilation
- from the cardiovascular chapter,
  - pale, mottled, or grey
  - weak pulses or low BP
- from the neurology chapter,
  - abnormal tone
  - seizures

- from the thermoregulation chapter,
  - T < 36.3 or > 37.2° C axillary

Term babies with mild respiratory distress lasting < 4 hours require ongoing observation but do not require entry to the Infection Sequence unless they meet other criteria for entry.

Clinical deterioration Clinical deterioration in a previously well baby or worsening condition in a previously unwell baby requires entry into the Infection Sequence.

Core Steps

In addition to the steps/interventions already undertaken in the relevant Sequences, the Infection Core Steps indicate the need to continue
- performing the ACoRN Primary Survey at regular intervals until stable
- updating the Problem List
- applying the Sequences that remain relevant.

Organization of Care

The course of action for babies who enter the Infection Sequence depends on whether,
- the baby is well or unwell
- the baby is term or preterm
- the mother has signs or symptoms of infection.

Response

Well babies who are term and whose mother has no signs or symptoms of infection generally do not need a blood culture or antibiotics. These babies should be observed for 24 to 48 hours to ensure they remain healthy.

In babies who are unwell, pre-term or whose mothers have signs or symptoms of infection,
- obtain blood cultures
- establish venous access and
- initiate antibiotic therapy.

The choice of initial antibiotic therapy depends on the suspected organisms and is based on the,
- age of baby (early onset/late onset neonatal sepsis)
- the presence or absence of a focus of infection.

First line antibiotics in sepsis occurring in the first three days of life are ampicillin and gentamicin. If meningitis is suspected, cefotaxime should be added.

Similarly, for community acquired infections in the first month of life, ampicillin and gentamicin are appropriate, adding cefotaxime if meningitis is suspected or cannot be ruled out.

Nosocomial (hospital acquired) infections arising after 3 days of age require adjustment of coverage using local microbiological information. In this case one might consider cloxacillin or vancomycin in combination with gentamicin or cefotaxime.

The Infection Sequence

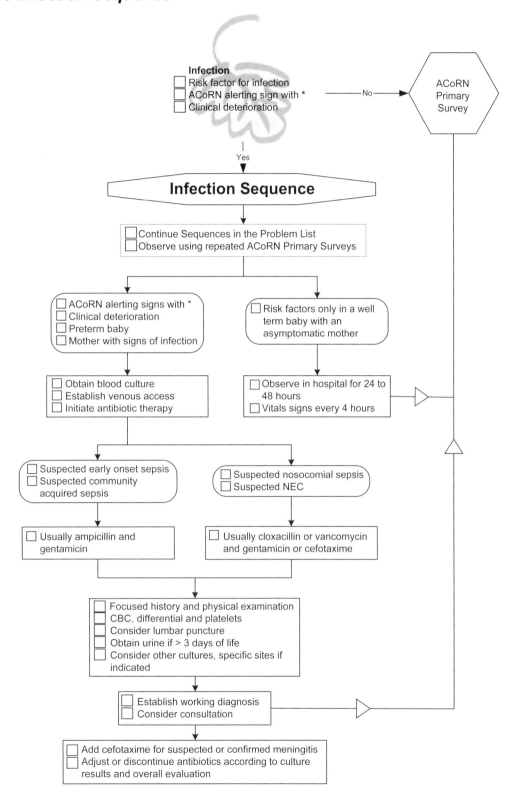

Infection
- [ ] Risk factor for infection
- [ ] ACoRN alerting sign with *
- [ ] Clinical deterioration

→ No → ACoRN Primary Survey

Yes

Infection Sequence

- [ ] Continue Sequences in the Problem List
- [ ] Observe using repeated ACoRN Primary Surveys

- [ ] ACoRN alerting signs with *
- [ ] Clinical deterioration
- [ ] Preterm baby
- [ ] Mother with signs of infection

- [ ] Risk factors only in a well term baby with an asymptomatic mother

- [ ] Obtain blood culture
- [ ] Establish venous access
- [ ] Initiate antibiotic therapy

- [ ] Observe in hospital for 24 to 48 hours
- [ ] Vitals signs every 4 hours

- [ ] Suspected early onset sepsis
- [ ] Suspected community acquired sepsis

- [ ] Suspected nosocomial sepsis
- [ ] Suspected NEC

- [ ] Usually ampicillin and gentamicin

- [ ] Usually cloxacillin or vancomycin and gentamicin or cefotaxime

- [ ] Focused history and physical examination
- [ ] CBC, differential and platelets
- [ ] Consider lumbar puncture
- [ ] Obtain urine if > 3 days of life
- [ ] Consider other cultures, specific sites if indicated

- [ ] Establish working diagnosis
- [ ] Consider consultation

- [ ] Add cefotaxime for suspected or confirmed meningitis
- [ ] Adjust or discontinue antibiotics according to culture results and overall evaluation

Antibiotics (dose calculation, frequency of administration, route of administration)

Next Steps

The Next Steps are to obtain a focused history, conduct a physical examination, and order diagnostic tests.

Focused history

Essential information to gather during the focused neonatal infection history includes:

Antepartum
- maternal infection
- history of a previous baby with Group B Streptococcus (GBS) infection or unexplained stillbirth at term
- rupture of membranes at < 37 weeks gestation
- positive maternal GBS screen or GBS bacteriuria during current pregnancy

Intrapartum
- preterm labor
- rupture of membranes > 18 hours
- maternal temperature ≥ 38°C orally
- choriamnionitis suspected on clinical examination
- suspected or proven maternal bacterial infection from other sources (urine, blood)
- risk of mother-to-baby transmission of viral infections in the perinatal period (for example, active genital herpes, hepatitis B and HIV)

Neonatal
- need for resuscitation
- prematurity/low birth weight
- nosocomial or community-acquired infection

Babies being admitted for or receiving prolonged intensive care are at increased risk of infection.

Focused physical examination

In addition to the examination conducted during the Primary Survey and applicable sequences, a focused physical examination for Infection includes:

Measurement of vital signs: respiratory rate, heart rate, temperature, and blood pressure.

Observation and examination
- sources of infection (skin breakdown, wounds)
- localized infection (abscess, pneumonia, necrotizing enterocolitis, meningitis).

Diagnostic tests

In addition to the blood culture done during Response, a sepsis work-up should include,

- complete blood count with white cell differential and platelet count
- urine culture (by catheter or suprapubic aspiration) in babies > than three days old
  - urinary tract infection is a common cause of sepsis in the first month after birth.

In all babies who are unwell in whom infection is suspected, it should be decided which microbiological samples are required in addition to a blood culture and urine culture,

- lumbar puncture (LP)
  - meningitis is a serious complication of sepsis and is difficult to diagnose without a lumbar puncture
  - lumbar puncture should be considered in any baby with alerting signs in the neurologic system or with a positive blood culture
  - a positive cerebrospinal fluid (CSF) culture guides choice of antibiotics, duration of therapy and follow-up
  - lumbar puncture can be deferred in babies who have respiratory or cardiovascular instability and considered again when the baby is stable or if the blood culture comes back positive
  - only a clinician trained and experienced in lumbar puncture should do this procedure
- cultures from other sites or viral cultures should be considered when clinically indicated, such as,
  - wound drainage
  - stool culture.

Consider other investigations that may not have been addressed in the ACoRN Primary Survey, such as abdominal radiograph if necrotizing enterocolitis (NEC) is suspected

Establish a Working Diagnosis

The evaluation to establish a working diagnosis should aim at determining whether sepsis is disseminated or is localized to an organ or tissue (pneumonia, meningitis, urinary tract, gastrointestinal tract).

Babies with infections may become unstable or develop complications rapidly. Early consultation should be considered.

Specific Management

When an initial working diagnosis of sepsis (disseminated infection without a clear focus) is made, it is often sufficient to administer initial antibiotics until the results of the blood cultures are known.

When the focus of infection is known, antibiotics can be modified to optimize treatment. For example:

- In suspected or confirmed meningitis it is important to use antibiotics with optimal penetration into the CSF. Cefotaxime is usually added pending culture reports.

- In NEC it is important to use antibiotics with good penetration to the intestinal tissues and lumen, and with adequate coverage for intestinal bacteria

Consultation may be appropriate at this time.

Specific management includes,
- reviewing the result of blood cultures and antibiotic sensitivity
- adjusting antibiotic choice, dosing, therapeutic drug monitoring, as required
- determining duration of antibiotic therapy
- considering other diagnostic or therapeutic interventions such as,
  - need and timing of surgical intervention in NEC
  - abscess drainage.

Provide supportive therapy according to needs identified on the Primary Survey, and management of complications (such as coagulopathy).

Neonatal Infection Case # 1 – Baby with respiratory distress and prolonged rupture of membranes

> You are called to examine a baby boy with respiratory distress. He was born by spontaneous vaginal delivery at 37 weeks gestation. Membranes had been ruptured for 19 hours and mother had developed a fever and signs of chorioamnionitis. Mild tachypnea was present at birth, and he was admitted to the nursery for closer observation. Over the next 30 minutes his respirations became increasingly labored.

I. Looking at the Primary Survey below, describe the findings in this baby

_____   _____

_____   _____

_____   _____

_____

Baby at risk
☑ Unwell
☐ Risk factors
☐ Post-resuscitation requiring stabilization

Resuscitation
☐ Ineffective breathing
☐ Heart rate < 100 bpm
☐ Central cyanosis

☐ **Support**

Infection
☑ Risk factor for infection
☑ Alerting signs* from ACoRN
☐ Clinical deterioration

Respiratory
☑ Laboured respiration*
☑ Respiratory rate > 60/min*
☐ Receiving respiratory support*

Thermoregulation
☐ T < 36.3 or > 37.2°C axillary*
☑ Increased risk for temperature instability

Cardiovascular
☑ Pale, mottled, or grey*
☑ Weak pulses or low BP*
☐ Cyanosis unresponsive to O_2
☐ Heart rate > 220 bpm

Problem List
☑ Respiratory
☑ Cardiovascular
☐ Neurology
☐ Surgical conditions
☑ Fluid & glucose
☑ Thermoregulation
☑ Infection

Fluid & Glucose Management
☐ Blood glucose < 2.6 mmol/L
☑ At risk for hypoglycemia
☑ Not feeding or should not be fed

Sequences

☐ **Consider transport**

Neurology
☐ Abnormal tone*
☐ Jitteriness
☐ Seizures*

Surgical Conditions
☐ Anterior abdominal wall defect
☐ Vomiting or inability to swallow
☐ Abdominal distension
☐ Delayed passage of meconium or imperforate anus

II. Based on your Problem List, what Sequences will you need to work through?

_____   _____

_____   _____

_____

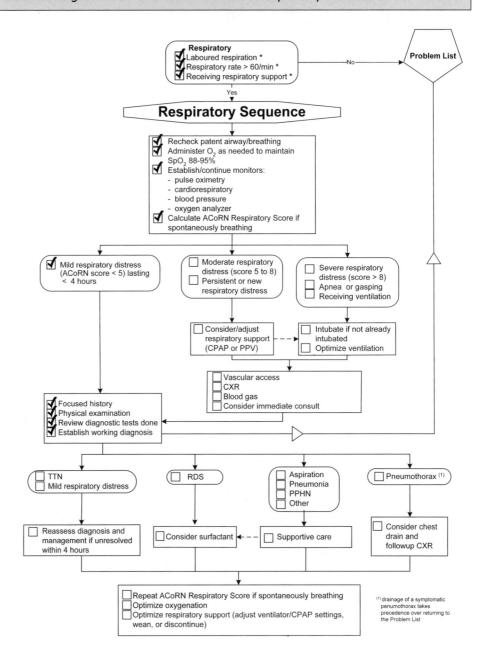

The baby has a respiratory rate of 66/minute, is on 30% oxygen, has mild to moderate retractions, is grunting with stimulation, and breath sounds are easily heard throughout. You calculate the ACoRN Respiratory Score. It is 4.

You complete the Respiratory Sequence and proceed to the Cardiovascular Sequence.

The baby is mottled, and the blood pressure is 45/30 with a mean of 35 mmHg.

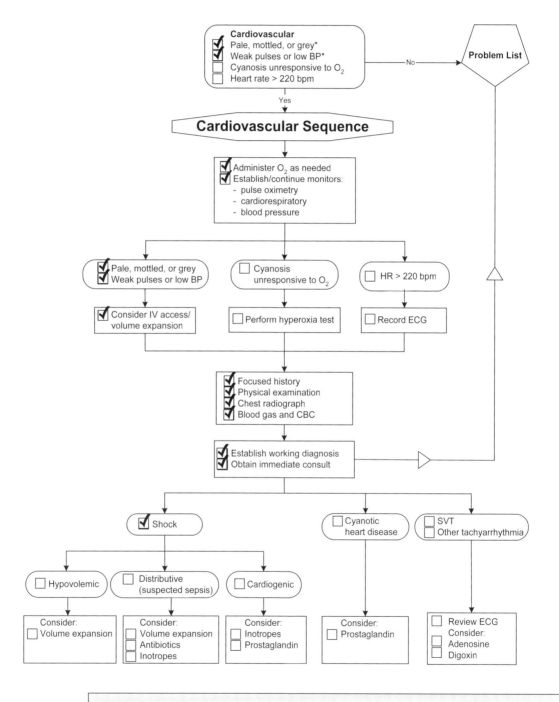

You establish an intravenous line and give 10 mL/kg of 0.9% NaCl for volume expansion. The blood pressure is now 55/35 mmHg but the baby still looks mottled.

III.   Why do you think an immediate consult is necessary?

_____

_____

_____

> You make a decision not to feed the baby. You obtain a point of care glucose and initiate an infusion of D10%W at 3 mL/kg/hour.
>
> There is an increased risk for temperature instability. The baby is under a radiant warmer, an environment where temperature can be controlled.
>
> Having completed the Primary Survey, generated a Problem List and applied the relevant Sequences, you consider the Infection Sequence.
>
> The baby demonstrates two alerting signs for Infection.

Infection
- ☑ Risk factor for infection
- ☑ ACoRN alerting sign with *
- ☐ Clinical deterioration

IV.   What risk factors for infection are present in this baby?

_____   _____

_____

V.   What specific ACoRN alerting signs * from the Primary Survey may indicate Infection in this baby?

_____   _____

_____   _____

In addition to the stabilization steps already undertaken following the relevant Sequences, the Infection Core Steps indicate the need to continue,
- performing the ACoRN Primary Survey at regular intervals until stable
- updating the Problem List
- applying the Sequences that remain relevant.

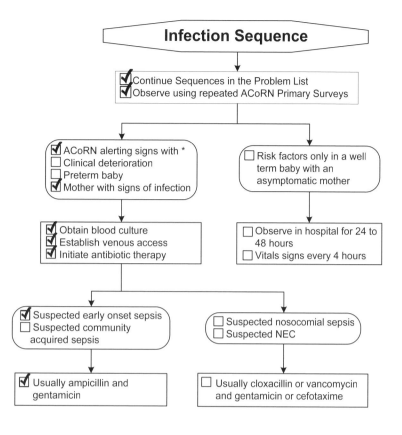

Infection Sequence

☑ Continue Sequences in the Problem List
☑ Observe using repeated ACoRN Primary Surveys

☑ ACoRN alerting signs with *
☐ Clinical deterioration
☐ Preterm baby
☑ Mother with signs of infection

☐ Risk factors only in a well term baby with an asymptomatic mother

☑ Obtain blood culture
☑ Establish venous access
☑ Initiate antibiotic therapy

☐ Observe in hospital for 24 to 48 hours
☐ Vitals signs every 4 hours

☑ Suspected early onset sepsis
☐ Suspected community acquired sepsis

☐ Suspected nosocomial sepsis
☐ Suspected NEC

☑ Usually ampicillin and gentamicin

☐ Usually cloxacillin or vancomycin and gentamicin or cefotaxime

---

The baby is unwell with several ACoRN alerting signs with * and the mother has fever and signs of chorioamnionitis. You obtain a blood culture and initiate antibiotics.

VI.   What antibiotics will you start at this time?

_____   _____

Based on suspected early onset sepsis, you start ampicillin and gentamicin. The objective of giving intravenous antibiotics early in the Infection Sequence is to minimize any delay in implementing specific therapy to treat the infection.

Intravenous antibiotics achieve a more rapid and reliable blood level than intramuscular antibiotics, especially in a baby who is symptomatic and more so in babies with circulatory instability.

If a peripheral IV cannot be started, other forms of intravascular access should be pursued, such as an umbilical venous line.

Significant information is gathered from the antenatal, intrapartum, and neonatal history. The results of her antenatal GBS screen have not been reported. In the second stage of labour, the maternal temperature was 38°C and she received one dose of IV clindamycin (substitute for ampicillin in penicillin-allergic patients) 1 hour prior to birth.

Blood is sent for CBC and differential, Na, K, Ca, and blood culture. A portable chest radiograph shows bilateral "hazy" pulmonary infiltrates. The capillary blood gas reveals a pH of 7.32 and P_{CO_2} of 48 mmHg.

VII. What other investigations would you consider?

On consultation with the neonatologist at the regional centre, you decide to postpone the LP until the respiratory status improves.

VIII. What is the working diagnosis?

What is neonatal sepsis?

Neonatal sepsis generally refers to bacterial infection acquired perinatally or in the first days or weeks of life.

Signs and symptoms Signs and symptoms of sepsis in babies are often non-specific, and vary according to age and how the infection is acquired:
- early onset sepsis (usually in first 72 hours of life) – acquired perinatally or ascended from the birth canal
- late onset sepsis (age > 72 hours) – acquired while in hospital (nosocomial) or in the community.

Early onset sepsis is characterized by respiratory distress, apnea, shock, pneumonia, and meningitis.

Late onset sepsis usually presents with temperature instability, decreased activity, poor feeding, jaundice, etc. Additional signs and symptoms may point to infection in a particular organ system or complications:
- gastrointestinal – abdominal distension, bilious vomiting, blood in stool
- meningitis – seizures, high-pitched cry, bulging fontanel

- pneumonia – cyanosis, grunting
- hematologic – petechiae from low platelet count or disseminated intravascular coagulation.

Common organisms	Early onset sepsis	Late onset sepsis and nosocomial infections

	Gram-positive bacteria
	    Streptococcus agalactiae (GBS)
	    Streptococcus pneumoniae
	    Listeria monocytogenes
	Gram-negative bacteria
	    Escherichia coli (E Coli)
	    Klebsiella pneumoniae
	    Enterobacter spp
	    Proteus spp
	    Salmonella spp
		Gram-positive bacteria
		    Streptococcus agalactiae (GBS)
		    Streptococcus pneumoniae
		
		Gram-negative bacteria
		    E coli
		    Klebsiella pneumoniae
		    Enterobacter spp
		    Proteus spp
		    Others *(Citrobacter , Serratia,*
		        Pseudomonas, Haemophilus,
		        Neisseria)
		
		Nosocomial
		    Staphylococcus aureus
		    Coagulase-negative Staphylococcus
		        (CoNS)
		    Enterococcus spp

GBS is the most common cause of early onset infection and is associated with significant morbidity and mortality. The source is usually the mother. Universal prenatal screening for vaginal and rectal GBS colonization of all pregnant women at 35 to 37 weeks gestation, and administration of intrapartum antibiotic prophylaxis to those who are GBS positive or if in labor at < 37 wks gestation reduces the likelihood of neonatal GBS infection[1].

In the absence of risk factors (rupture of membranes at < 37 weeks or > 18 hours prior to delivery, or fever during labor) the risk of neonatal GBS disease when intrapartum antibiotics are not given is 1 in 200, and when intrapartum antibiotics are given is 1 in 4000.

Since intrapartum antibiotics became commonplace, the overall risk of early onset GBS sepsis has decreased from 1.7 cases per 1,000 live births to 0.4 cases per 1,000 live births. Severe GBS sepsis has become rare.

---

[1] Centre for Disease Control. Prevention of perinatal group B streptococcal disease. August 16, 2002. http:www.cdc.gov/mmwr/preview/mmwrhtml/rr511a1.htm.

Choosing initial antibiotics — Most neonatal units begin with a combination therapy to cover for both gram-positive and gram-negative organisms. The likely causative organisms depend on the age and source/focus of the infection.

	Gram-positive coverage	**Gram-negative coverage**
Suspected sepsis	ampicillin	gentamicin
Suspected meningitis	ampicillin	gentamicin cefotaxime
Suspected nosocomial sepsis	cloxacillin / vancomycin (if multi-resistance suspected)	gentamicin / cefotaxime

Viral and congenital infections

Although infections acquired in the perinatal/neonatal period are mostly bacterial in origin, other less common forms of infection can occur:

Acute viral infections (perinatal) — Amongst the acute viral infections, herpes and varicella disseminate most rapidly and can result in fulminant systemic or central nervous system disease. Diagnosis is difficult and does not depend on the presence of vesicular lesions. Maternal history may be helpful, especially in varicella. If herpes or varicella are suspected, urgent consultation, treatment, and isolation of the baby are necessary.

Congenital infections (in-utero) — Chronic infections acquired in-utero or congenital infections are associated with abnormal physical findings at birth (for example, microcephaly and hepatosplenomegaly). The term "TORCH" is used to describe some of the causative agents:

> **T** = toxoplasmosis
> **O** = other (for example, syphilis or HIV)
> **R** = rubella
> **C** = cytomegalovirus (CMV)
> **H** = herpes

Two hours after antibiotics have been started, the CBC results are reported as follows:

Hemoglobin	140 g/L
Total WBC count	6.0×10^9/L
Total neutrophil count	1.2×10^9/L
Immature neutrophils count (bands)	0.4×10^9/L
Platelets	120×10^9/L

The neutropenia ($< 2 \times 10^9$/L) and high immature-to-total neutrophil ratio of 0.33 (left shift) are supportive of sepsis in this baby.

The WBC and differential count is not a reliable predictor of bacterial sepsis. The decision to treat sepsis in sick babies is a clinical one. When sepsis is suspected, the administration of antibiotics should not be delayed.

 Complete blood count and differential interpretation

You continue to monitor the baby closely by performing the ACoRN Primary Survey at regular intervals. Another bolus of 10 mL/kg of 0.9% NaCl is given and the blood pressure stabilizes.

The baby improves after antibiotic treatment is started. Twelve hours later, the laboratory reports the baby's blood culture and maternal vaginal culture are positive for GBS.

A lumbar puncture is done. The CSF is normal and culture is negative. You continue antibiotics for a total of 7 days.

Answers to the questions in Chapter 9

I. **Based on the Primary Survey below, describe the findings in this baby**

The baby is unwell.

He is at risk for hypoglycemia
He is not feeding or should not be fed.

There are no alerting signs for
immediate resuscitation.

Being a newborn under observation / care, he
is at risk for temperature instability.

He has labored respiration and is
tachypneic.

He has risk factors for infection.
Has ACoRN alerting signs with an * .

His color is pale, mottled or grey.
He needs his BP measured.

II. **Based on your Problem List, what Sequences will you need to work through**

Respiratory

Fluid and glucose

Cardiovascular

Thermoregulation

Infection

III. **Why do you think an immediate consult is necessary?**

Baby has both Respiratory and Cardiovascular instability.

You are considering Shock as a diagnosis. A baby in shock can rapidly deteriorate.

Additional investigations and treatment may be needed.

IV. **What risk factors for infection are present in this baby?**

Rupture of membranes > 18 hours

Suspected chorioamnionitis

Maternal fever

V. **What specific ACoRN alerting signs with * from the Primary Survey may indicate Infection in this baby?**

Labored respiration

Pale, mottled or grey

Respiratory rate > 60 bpm

Weak pulses or low BP

VI. **What antibiotics will you start at this time?**

Ampicilin

Gentamicin

VII. What other investigations would you consider?

You consider a lumbar puncture (LP).

VIII. What is the working diagnosis?

Neonatal sepsis with congenital pneumonia.

Bibliography

American Academy of Pediatrics. Infection control for hospitalized children. In: Pickering LK, ed. *Red Book: 2003 Report of the Committee on Infectious Diseases.* 26th ed. Elk Grove Village, IL: American Academy of Pediatrics; 2003.

Bradley JS, Nelson JD, eds. Nelson's pocket book of pediatric antimicrobial therapy. 15th Ed. Lippincott, Williams and Wilkins, 2002-2003.

Hey E. Neonatal formulary. 4th Ed. BMJ Books, 2003.

Isaacs D, Moxomer ER. Handbook of neonatal infections, a practical guideline. W.B. Saunders, 1999.

Smyth J, McDougal A, Vanderpas E, eds. Neonatal drug dosage guidelines. 4th ed. Vancouver, BC: Children's and Women's Health Centre of British Columbia, 2002.

Young TE, Mangum B. Neofax 2003. 16th Ed. Raleigh NC: Acorn Publishing Inc, 2003.

Chapter 10
Transport

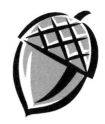

Objectives

Upon completion of this chapter, you should be able to:
1. Recognize some of the factors that influence the decision to transport a sick baby.
2. Describe the information needed by the referral facility at initial contact.
3. Describe the roles of the local facility, the receiving physician, the transport coordinator, and the transport team.
4. Discuss the activities involved in preparing a baby for transport.
5. Recognize the support needs of the family.
6. Describe ways in which the sending facility and the transport team can assist and support each other.

Key Concepts

1. The act of seeking early consultation does not necessarily imply a request for transport.
2. Effective stabilization before transport minimizes morbidity.
3. The earlier the need for more specialized care is identified, the sooner the transport process can be initiated, and the transport team mobilized.
4. Communication with the family is an integral part of the transfer process.

Introduction

The best transport system for a baby is in the uterus. The birth of a sick or at-risk baby can often be anticipated and, provided there is sufficient time, maternal/fetal transport can be arranged to enable delivery at a tertiary care centre. However, some babies with high-risk conditions go unrecognized in the prenatal period or develop rapidly, and some babies are born well but become sick in the hours or days following birth. These babies may need urgent stabilization and transport to a regional facility able to provide a higher level of care, appropriate for the baby's condition. This type of facility will be referred to as the receiving hospital in this Chapter.

Consider the following scenario:

> You are a family physician working in a hospital that averages 75 births per year. Your patient has just delivered a baby girl at 32 weeks gestation. The baby was vigorous at birth, with Apgar scores of 7 at 1 minute and 8 at 5 minutes, but then develops respiratory distress and requires oxygen to remain pink. You complete an ACoRN Primary Survey, generate a Problem List, and progress through the appropriate Sequences.

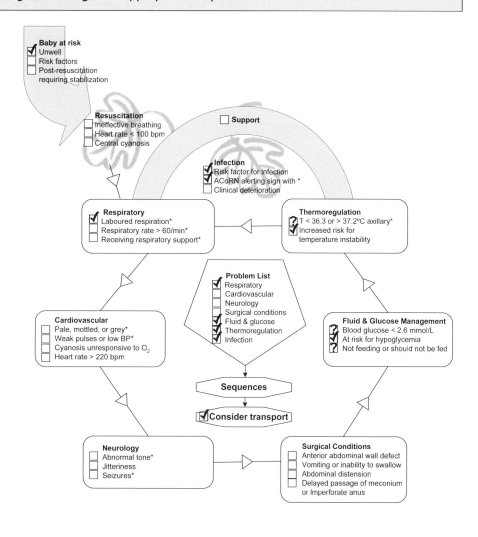

After the initial stabilization, the baby is on a radiant warmer receiving 45% oxygen by oxygen hood to maintain her $SpO_2 > 88\%$. In view of the limited resources in your facility, you decide to consult with your regional hospital regarding transport. In preparation for this consultation, you collect pertinent information about the baby's condition, using your hospital's neonatal pre-transport information sheet.

The neonatologist on call asks you:
- How is the baby breathing?
- What is the oxygen saturation by pulse oximetry?
- If the baby deteriorates, is there someone who can intubate? If so, it would be prudent to alert the person to be available on stand-by.
- What is your estimate of the baby's weight?
- Do you have venous access? If so, where?
- Are you able to draw a blood culture before starting antibiotics?
- Are you able to do a chest x-ray and draw a blood gas?
- How is your health care team coping?
- What are the weather conditions at the airport?

A decision is made to transfer both mother and baby at the same time to the receiving hospital. The neonatologist asks you to remain with the baby at all times, but to limit the amount of handling to the minimum necessary to manage the baby's care as physical handling may worsen her condition. The transport team is available and the airplane can depart within the hour. The estimated arrival time is 2 hours.

The Transport Process

Throughout ACoRN, the importance of early consultation for the purposes of optimizing care has been emphasized. The act of seeking consultation does not necessarily mean you want or need to transport the baby to another facility. However, if the baby's current or anticipated problems cannot be managed at the local facility, the earlier the need for more specialized care is identified, the sooner the transport process can be initiated. Time is critical, especially if there is the potential for the baby's condition to deteriorate.

Making the decision to transport

The decision to transport an unwell or at-risk baby to another facility is based on discussion between the sending facility and the transport-coordinating physician.

A number of factors must be considered,
- the baby's current and changing condition
- the baby's ability to tolerate the inherent risk of transport
- resources (personnel, expertise, equipment, and specialized services) at the sending facility
- regional referral patterns
- mode of transportation required and distance involved
- current or impending weather conditions.

Neonatal Pre-Transport Information Sheet

Date of call: _____ Time of call: _____

Local facility physician's name: _____ Tel number: _____

Consultant physician/
Transport coordinator's name: _____ Tel number: _____

Information about the baby

Name: _____ Diagnosis/reason for consult: _____

Birth date	Time	Sex	Birth wt.	Gestation	Apgar score	Eye prophylaxis? ☐
					1 min: 5 min:	Vitamin K given? ☐

Resuscitation:

Respiration	Compressions	Medications
Spontaneous: Yes ( ) No ( ) Bag ventilation: Yes ( ) No ( ) O_2: Yes ( ) _____% No ( ) Intubated: Time _____ ETT size _____ Suction meconium below cords: Yes ( ) No ( )	Yes ( ) No ( ) Time initiated: Time stopped:	ETT: IV:

Congenital anomalies: _____

Postnatal course: _____

Current status: Heart rate: _____ RR: _____ BP: _____ Perfusion: _____ SaO_2: _____

FiO$_2$: _____ IPPV: _____

Physical exam: _____

Feeding/intravenous: _____

X-rays – results: _____

Laboratory – results: _____

Cord/other blood gases: _____

Information about the mother

Name: _____ Age: ____ G: ___ P: _____ LMP/EDC: _____/_____

Blood group _____ Rh _____ VDRL _____ Rubella _____ HBsAG ____ TB ____ HIV _____

Group B Strep: Pos ( ) Neg ( ) Unknown/not done ( )   Date ____/____/____

Past obstetric history: _____

Labour & delivery

Fetal monitoring: Yes ( ) No ( ) Internal ( ) External ( ) Auscultation ( ) Scalp pH _____

Length of labour: 1st stage _____ 2nd stage _____

AROM ( ) SROM ( ) Date _____ Time _____ Colour _____ Amount _____

Medications: _____ Anesthesia/analgesia: _____

Type of delivery: C. Section ( ) Vaginal ( ) Forceps ( ) Vacuum ( ) Presentation _____

Complications: _____

Date: ____/____/____ Signature and title: _____

Adapted from: PPPESO. Neonatal Transport. Perinatal Nursing Guidelines (3rd Ed). Ottawa, ON: Perinatal Partnership Program of Eastern and Southeastern Ontario, 2001.

An essential role of any transport system is to place babies where they can receive the appropriate level of care.

- The baby and/or mother should be transported to the closest-to-home appropriate hospital unless local capacity has been reached.
- Shortage of resources at the receiving hospital should not result in leaving a baby at a facility unable to meet the mother/baby care needs but requires diversion to an appropriate hospital outside the region.

Initiating contact with the transport coordination centre

Every facility likely to request the services of a neonatal transport team should understand the way in which babies are transported in their region and should have the contact information to access their transport system 24 hours a day, 7 days a week.

A physician, midwife, or delegate at the sending facility, with the authority to make decisions about the baby's care, is responsible for initiating the transport process.

The transport coordination centre is called and communication with the transport-coordinating physician or delegate is initiated.

The sending physician, midwife, or delegate should be prepared to provide,
- the ACoRN Problem List
- a working diagnosis
- management received by the baby
- demographic, antenatal, intrapartum, and neonatal data.

Transport coordination

There are three main aspects to transport coordination,
- clinical coordination
- finding a bed for the baby ± mother
- logistics (mechanics of transport).

The three aspects may be coordinated independently. More commonly, the same personnel perform more than one duty (for example, clinically coordinating the transport plus finding a receiving bed, or organizing the logistics plus finding a receiving bed).

Clinical coordination is provided by a transport-coordinating physician or delegate. It includes,
- provision of medical advice to the practitioner at the sending facility
- ensuring nursing advice on care be available when needed
- medical supervision of the transport team operations
- identification of the receiving facility
- communication with the receiving physician.

The transport-coordinating physician requires information about the mother and baby in order to provide adequate advice to the sending facility and to assist in decision making regarding,
- the need for transport
- the composition of the team to be dispatched
- the mode and urgency of transport
- the level of care needed and the receiving hospital.

The role of logistics coordinators varies from region to region. In general, they organize the mechanics of the transfer and act as liaison with the transport-coordinating physician during the entire process.

Responsibilities of the sending facility

The heath care team at the sending facility plays an integral role in neonatal transfer by,
- providing initial resuscitation, and initial and ongoing stabilization
- identifying the need for consultation and transport
- initiating contact with the transport-coordination centre
- communicating the baby's condition and giving details of the stabilization process
- conveying significant changes in the baby's condition to the transport-coordinating physician
- remaining with the baby to provide ongoing care, and assisting the transport team to optimize pre-transport stabilization until departure from the sending facility.

The sending facility needs to prepare the following material to go with the baby:
- a copy of
  o prenatal, labour and delivery records
  o the mother's chart with all relevant neonatal history
  o the baby's chart
  o laboratory data
- radiographs
  o if the ETT has been repositioned since the last chest film and no new radiographs have been taken, this information should be noted on the last chest radiograph
- clearly labeled specimens if requested, for example
  o the baby's blood cultures (aerobic ± anaerobic)
  o a maternal blood sample
  o a cord blood sample from the placenta, useful mainly for a direct antibody (Coombs') test
- the placenta, wrapped in a sealed plastic bag or placed in a bucket with a lid (no additives or preservatives)
- signed consent forms for transport, admission and care at the receiving hospital, and for transfusion of blood products
- contact information for the baby's parents and family physician.

Responsibilities of the transport-coordinating physician

The transport-coordinating physician is responsible for,
- providing ongoing telephone support to the sending physician, midwife, or delegate and for advising on the baby's medical care pending arrival of the transport team at the sending facility, including
  o further resuscitative interventions
  o the need for additional investigations
  o suggestions for the stabilization process
  o recommendations for starting interim treatment

- communicating with the receiving physician
- providing supervision to the transport team operations
- ensuring that the logistics of transport meet the needs of the baby, and the standards of care requirements and timelines of the region.

These duties begin when initial contact with the sending physician, midwife, or delegate is made, and end when the baby has been transferred to the care of a physician at the receiving hospital.

All communications by the transport-coordinating physician with the sending facility, logistics coordinator, transport team, and receiving physician constitute medical acts that require documentation.

Responsibilities of the receiving physician

A physician at the receiving hospital must accept responsibility for the baby. The receiving physician or delegate is responsible for informing the attending physician at the sending facility and the family of the baby's status once the baby has arrived at the receiving hospital.

Responsibilities of the transport team

The transport team continues and elaborates on the care initiated by the sending facility.

Stabilization in preparation for transport ensures that the baby's condition and management is reviewed and optimized by the team prior to leaving the sending facility.

Safety precautions must be in place to deal with the hostile nature of the transport environment and the fragility of a sick baby. Leaving the sending facility means severing access to hospital staff, equipment, and diagnostic facilities, and taking the baby into a restricted space with limited supplies, lighting and temperature control, high levels of noise and vibration, accelerations and decelerations, and sometimes changes in altitude and atmospheric pressure.

Pre-transport stabilization allows the transport team to be proactive rather than reactive. For example:
- If the baby is not already ventilated, the team may electively intubate and ventilate to ensure support is in place should respiratory function deteriorate during transport.
- If the baby is already ventilated, there needs to be a trial of ventilation using the transport ventilator, so that the settings can be adjusted to mimic the respiratory effects of the local ventilator.
- Any necessary adjustments are guided by a combination of clinical findings, blood gases, and radiographs until the team is satisfied the settings are optimal.
- New vascular access lines may be started and existing access lines re-taped or replaced to ensure that whatever intravenous needs may arise during transport can be met.

The team discusses the scope of stabilization at the sending facility with the transport-coordinating physician, who retains significant responsibility for the medical and administrative acts of the transport team.

The transport team is responsible for updating the sending facility about the team's estimated time of arrival, any unexpected delays in the outward journey, and the safe arrival of the baby at the receiving hospital.

Feedback for staff at the sending facility should always be provided in a supportive way. This is an essential component in establishing and maintaining a collegial and educational environment/network.

Shared responsibilities

The medical responsibility for the baby rests within the sending hospital until the call is placed to the transport-coordinating centre. From that moment forward, until arrival of the transport team, the responsibility for the baby is shared between the sending hospital and the transport system. Upon arrival of the transport team, the primary responsibility for the baby is transferred to the transport team and the transport-coordinating physician but the local physician shares the responsibility until the transport team leaves. The local health care team remains responsible for providing support, space, and equipment as needed. When the baby arrives at the receiving hospital, the receiving physician and facility accept medical responsibility.

Communicating with the Family

Most parents understand when circumstances dictate their sick baby be transported to a facility where the baby will receive a higher level of care. In these situations, every effort should be made to keep the family informed of their baby's status and of the transport arrangements. Family members need time to ask questions, voice their concerns, and express their feelings.

The family should be given every opportunity to be with their baby while preparations for transport are in progress. Providing parents with a digital or rapid-development photograph of their baby can help ease the separation. The photo will likely become a keepsake. Family members should be encouraged to take additional photos or videotape.

It may not always be possible for family members to accompany the baby during transport because of limited space in transport vehicles, but efforts should be made to facilitate this.

The time of separation between parents and baby should be minimized especially when the baby's condition is critical. This may involve facilitating arrangements for early discharge or transfer of the mother.

Provision of appropriate accommodation for parent(s) at the receiving facility should be made by arranging maternal admission, if in-hospital care is still required, or coordinating alternate accommodation if discharged.

If the mother is planning to breastfeed, she should be taught to pump and store her breast milk.

The transport team should meet with the parents prior to departure. It is their responsibility to explain what they will be doing for the baby, to answer the parents' questions, obtain any necessary consents, and provide information about the receiving hospital (contact numbers and names, directions to the neonatal care unit, local accommodation and unit policies, such as breastfeeding and visiting). Personnel from the local hospital should participate in these discussions.

A designated transport team member is responsible for informing the family once the baby arrives at the receiving facility.

Bibliography

Jaimovich DG, Vidyasagar D. Handbook of Pediatric and Neonatal Transport Medicine (2nd ed). Philadelphia, PA: Hanley & Belfus, 2002.

Klaus M, Fanaroff A. Care of the High-risk Neonate. Philadelphia: W.B. Saunders Company. 2001.

Pendray M. Transports. In EMA III – Infant Transport Team Training Program: Transport Resource Manual. New Westminster: Justice Institute of BC, 1997.

Weingarten CT. Nursing interventions: Caring for parents of a newborn transferred to a regional intensive care nursery – A challenge for low risk obstetric specialists. J Perinatol 1988; 8(3):271-275.

Chapter 11
Support

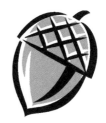

Objectives

Upon completion of this chapter, you should be able to:
1. Describe an approach to care that minimizes physiological stress for newborns.
2. Recognize signs that indicate a baby is stressed.
3. List supportive strategies for babies who demonstrate signs of stress.
4. Discuss the importance of assessing and managing pain in newborns.
5. Describe the types of support families may require throughout the continuum of care.
6. Recognize that newborn stabilization affects members of the health care team differently.
7. Identify opportunities to improve care.

Key Concepts

1. Minimizing extraneous stimulation in the baby's environment may reduce morbidity.
2. Developmentally supportive care should be intrinsic to all phases of newborn care, including stabilization.
3. Newborns experience pain that may have potentially detrimental physiological consequences.
4. Caring for the baby includes caring for the family and the health care team.
5. Case review can help the team recognize what went well and explore opportunities for improvement.

Skills

- Morphine and Fentanyl

Introduction   The importance of resuscitation and stabilization tasks needs to be balanced with provision of supportive care for the baby, family, and health care team. Support should not be considered an "extra", to be attended to once the medical priorities have been addressed. It should be integrated into all aspects of ACoRN, starting at the time of initial contact with the baby and family.

Babies can communicate their tolerance for caregiving activities and their environment through nonverbal cues. Attending to these cues has been shown to reduce morbidity and length of hospital stay. Including the family in this care recognizes the contribution of the family to the wellbeing of the baby. Each family unit is unique and has unique needs for support.

Individuals with various backgrounds, experience, and expertise come together to form a neonatal resuscitation, stabilization and/or transport team. The membership of the "team" may vary, as may the demands placed upon each member by the situation. For the individual and the team to function effectively, support, in the form of training, opportunities to practice, role clarification, and emotional advocacy are essential.

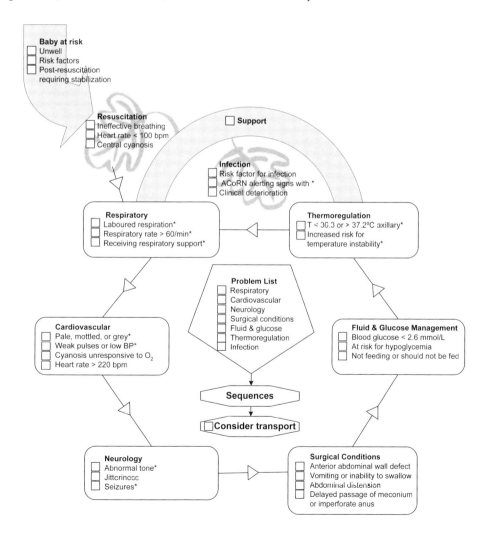

Consider the following scenario:

> You are caring for a 32 week gestation baby who was born 45 minutes ago. During completion of the ACoRN sequences, it becomes evident that he requires transport to your referral facility. The transport team is due to arrive in 90 minutes. The baby is lying on a radiant warmer in the brightly-lit nursery. There are loud voices in the background and the overbed heater alarm is ringing. The doctor is on the ward speaking with the family.
>
> The baby has moderate indrawing, is tachypneic, and requires 40% oxygen to maintain his SpO_2 levels 88 to 95%. His arms and legs are fully extended. There is a blood pressure cuff around his left arm and a pulse oximeter probe on his left foot. As you place a thermometer under his right axilla, he squirms and attempts to bring his left hand to his mouth, but is unsuccessful.
>
> A colleague administers vitamin K intramuscularly and applies erythromycin ointment to his eyes. The baby startles with handling. A capillary blood gas and glucose are drawn via heel poke. The baby cries throughout the procedure. An IV is started after four attempts. The physician returns for an update and you exchange information across the warmer.
>
> The baby now looks exhausted. His respiratory distress is worsening and his oxygen requirements have increased to 55%. His eyes are closed but he startles, flails his arms and legs, grimaces, and cries each time he is handled or hears loud noises. While he is being positioned for a chest film, he stops breathing and becomes bradycardic. You initiate bag-and-mask ventilation. Discussion ensues about whether to intubate.

Supporting the Baby

Babies have limited reserves to deal with sensory overload manifesting responses such as increased heart rate, decreased oxygen saturation, increased need for respiratory support, and disruption of the sleep/wake cycle. Interventions aimed at decreasing the baby's stress response and promoting physiological stability include,

- clustering and pacing care activities
- controlling sensory stimuli
- positioning the baby to mimic the intrauterine experience.

Interventions designed to minimize the negative impact of noise, light, other environmental factors, interventions, and caregiving activities on the baby's physiological and neurobehavioral functioning are collectively referred to as developmentally supportive care.

Stability and stress responses

Babies communicate through their autonomic, motor, and behavioral responses. Responses (cues) should be observed in totality, as it is the pattern of responses that indicate the baby's tolerance (stability or stress) to care activities and the environment.

Acquired observation skills are required to detect more subtle cues indicating distress, such as twitches, color changes, and respiratory pauses. If undetected, they may persist and intensify until they become pronounced enough to trigger cardiorespiratory or pulse oximeter alarms.

	Stability Cues	Stress Cues
Autonomic system	• stable vital signs • good colour • feeding tolerance	• change in quality/rate of respiration • change in heart rate • desaturation • colour change (pale/mottled/dusky) • tremors • gagging/spitting up/hiccoughing
Motor system	• hand to face or mouth • hand or foot clasping • grasping • leg or foot bracing • rooting/sucking • flexed posture	• frowning/facial grimacing • truncal arching • finger splaying/saluting • airplane movement (arms rigidly extended out from body like airplane wings) • flaccidity • averting gaze • sitting on air (lying supine with hips fully flexed knees extended)
Behavioural	• definite sleep state • ability to maintain a quiet alert state • attention to caregiver • attention to stimuli in environment rhythmical robust crying • self quieting/consolability • shiny-eyed alertness • cooing/smiling/looking around	• diffuse sleep or awake states • panicked/worried alertness • glassy-eyed • strained alertness • fussing/crying • staring • looking away • roving eye movements

I.   **Does the baby demonstrate any stability cues?**

II. **Looking back at the case, what stress cues is this baby demonstrating?**

_____

_____

_____

_____

_____

_____

Incorporating developmentally supportive care into neonatal care

1. Reduce noise levels.
   - avoid loud jarring noises (for example, snapping porthole doors shut)
   - avoid unnecessary noise (for example, using the incubator as a writing surface or talking over the incubator)
   - speak in a calm, quiet voice
2. Reduce light exposure.
   - shade the baby's eyes
   - partially cover the incubator and reduce ambient light when not directly involved in providing care
3. Nest the baby to provide motor containment.
   - flex the limbs and contain them close to the trunk
   - surround the baby with rolled towels to contain movement

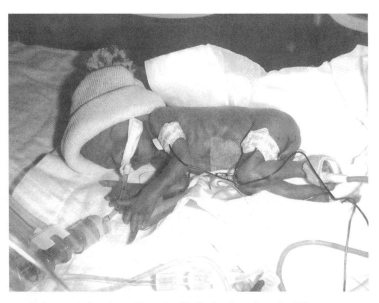

Baby nested and positioned with limbs flexed and midline.

4. Promote self-calming.
   - position the baby to allow hands to touch mouth or face
   - provide a soother
   - handle the baby gently
   - avoid sudden postural changes
   - limit social interactions (for example, talking and/or stroking the baby)
5. Base caregiving on the baby's sleep/wake cycle.
6. Before beginning any caregiving activity, hold your hands still above the baby to allow the baby to sense your presence.
7. Pace caregiving according to the baby's responses.

Care should be individualized. Interventions that work for one baby may not work for another. There will be times when the baby will display stress cues despite developmentally supportive care measures.

In critical situations, it may not be possible to pause if the baby becomes distressed. However, every attempt should be made to provide positional support and comfort during and following procedures. Whenever possible, the baby should be given time to recover from stressful or painful procedures.

Let's revisit the case using principles of developmentally supportive care.

> You are caring for a 32 week gestation baby who was born 45 minutes ago. During completion of the ACoRN sequences, it becomes evident that he requires transport to your referral facility. The transport team is due to arrive in 90 minutes. The baby is lying on a radiant warmer in the brightly lit nursery. There are quiet voices in the background and the overhead heater alarm is silenced promptly. The doctor is speaking with the family at the mother's bedside.
>
> You gently flex the baby's limbs and position a U-shaped nest around him to help contain his arms and legs. He squirms slightly, splays his fingers, and pushes against the sides of the nest with his feet. The boundaries of the nest contain the baby's arms and legs. You place your hands on the baby to settle him and help him maintain a quiet state before beginning your assessment. You talk softly as you pace your care according to the baby's behavioural cues, giving him time to recover when necessary. You decline the offer from another nurse to help admit the baby, preferring to do one intervention at a time to avoid overwhelming him. On arrival of the physician, the two of you move away from the radiant warmer and engage in quiet discussion.
>
> The baby demonstrates moderate respiratory distress and is receiving 40% oxygen. He still requires blood work, an IV, and antibiotics. You provide positional support and comfort during the IV start and blood draw.
>
> The baby's respiratory distress worsens somewhat and his oxygen requirements increase to 45% during the IV start. You position the baby prone and notice that he frequently brings his hands to his mouth, sucking his fingers to comfort himself. You reinforce the nest around him, ensuring he is still able to bring his hands to his mouth if he chooses.

Assessment and management of pain Babies, even those who are extremely preterm, do perceive pain. Pain can result from noxious procedures, surgical interventions, or the baby's underlying medical condition. Untreated pain has been shown to have physiological and behavioural consequences. The response to untreated pain in the very low birth weight preterm baby may be severe enough to contribute to intraventricular hemorrhage.

Babies cannot self-report pain, therefore, historically, pain has been under-recognized and pain management has not been a priority in neonatal care.

Pain should be anticipated, prevented if possible and, when present, assessed and appropriately treated.

Common indicators of pain include,
- physiological signs, such as
  - increased heart rate
  - increased or irregular respiratory rate
  - increased blood pressure
  - decreased oxygen saturation
  - palmar sweating
- behavioral signs such as,
  - strained crying
  - posturing
  - restlessness
  - changes in facial expression such as brow bulging or eye squeezing.

Signs of pain can vary depending on the baby's gestational age and status. Extremely preterm babies may exhibit a less robust behavioral response to pain. Babies who are ventilated, medically paralyzed, or neurologically depressed are difficult to assess.

Which non-pharmacologic strategies minimize a baby's discomfort and/or pain?

Mild discomfort and/or pain can often be managed using non-pharmacologic strategies such as,
- nesting the baby
- providing a soother
- reducing noxious stimulation such as noise and frequent handling.

Moderate to severe pain warrants the use of pharmacologic agents (analgesics) in conjunction with developmentally supportive care measures.

The prophylactic administration of sedatives to reduce stress, and analgesics to reduce pain associated with noxious procedures is prudent.

Morphine and fentanyl are the most commonly used narcotic analgesics (opioids) in neonatal care. Their pharmacological effects can be compared as follows.

	Morphine	Fentanyl
Onset	5 to 10 minutes	3 to 5 minutes
Duration of action	60 to 120 minutes	30 minutes
Cardiovascular stability	variable	yes
Sedation	more sedative effect	less sedative effect
Chest wall rigidity	no	yes, with large doses or rapid administration
Active metabolites	yes	no

Fentanyl is more potent than morphine, by as much as 50 to 100 times. Clinically, a ratio of 10:1 (morphine: fentanyl) is generally used for dose conversion. That is, 10 microgram (mcg) of morphine is equivalent to 1 mcg of fentanyl.

There is limited information in the literature with regard to potential long term effects of analgesic use in newborns.

When analgesics and/or sedatives are administered, it is essential that resuscitation equipment is on hand, appropriate monitoring is in place, and the practitioner has the expertise to evaluate the response to treatment, manage the airway, and deal with complications and side effects.

The particulars of pain assessment and management are outside the scope of ACoRN. If there is no one available locally to provide direction, consultation should be sought from the referral centre.

 Morphine and Fentanyl

Supporting the Family

> The baby's parents arrive in the nursery. They seem nervous and apprehensive. You encourage them to see and touch their son. As you speak with them, you refer to the baby by name, focusing on him as a person. You show them how to touch, support, and comfort him, yet not over-stimulate him.

III. Can you think of other ways to support the family?

_____

_____

_____

Emotional support for the family is an integral part of caring for a baby. No matter how prepared the parents are that their baby may be unwell, seeing their sick baby for the first time, attached to monitors and receiving ventilatory support, may be overwhelming. They may grieve the unexpected loss of their "perfect" baby.

There may not have been an opportunity to see the baby at birth if the baby was quickly removed for initiation of resuscitation and stabilization. As soon and as often as possible, the parents should be allowed to see, touch, and talk to the baby. If possible, they should be encouraged to be present during resuscitation and stabilization. This allows them to observe what is being done for their baby and the level of effort and care involved. It may also help alleviate their fears, and in the event that the baby dies, facilitate the grieving process.

Supporting the family includes asking them what they need or want to help cope with this event. Families need ongoing information about the baby's status, the equipment being used, the procedures being performed, and the plan of care. Information should be provided both in anticipation of the family's needs and in response to their questions, and repeated as often as necessary in different ways to ensure comprehension. The focus should be on the baby rather than the technology. This will also help the family understand that the team sees their baby as an individual.

A parent's response may depend on many factors; for example, the effectiveness of their coping strategies, their ability to concentrate on the information they are receiving, other events occurring in their lives, the nature and availability of family support systems, and whether the baby will be cared for locally or transferred to another community. Most parents understand the need for transport of their sick baby to a facility where a higher level of care is available. In these situations, every effort should be made to keep the family informed of the status of transport arrangements (see Chapter 10).

IV. **Can you think of ways to support the family if they must be separated from their baby who is being transported to the tertiary centre, a 4 hour flight away?**

_____

_____

_____

_____

Supporting the Health Care Team

> This is the first time you have cared for a baby this small. Now that the baby and his mother have left with the transport team, the team members gather to discuss the resuscitation, stabilization, and ongoing care of this baby.

Team members who suddenly find themselves resuscitating or stabilizing a sick baby may experience their own feelings of distress. This is especially true if these situations arise infrequently in their clinical practice. Events can be emotionally charged for staff when,

- the baby's condition acutely deteriorates
- feelings of inadequacy arise during the provision of care
- there is lack of experience in managing this type of case
- personnel and resources are limited
- immediate access to consultants specializing in neonatology is lacking.

Learning from practice

Resuscitation and stabilization are a team effort. Every clinical experience, especially a rare event, provides an opportunity for staff to learn from the situation and each other. Case review can help the team recognize what went well and which areas, if any, need improvement, as well as build self-confidence and self-esteem.

The process should be used as an educational tool or quality improvement activity for proactive problem-solving. Teams should make case review a routine practice so that every case is discussed, not just the difficult ones. Making review a normal part of the learning process helps remove any punitive connotation. All members of the team should participate, as individuals may have disparate ideas and perspectives. Suggestions generated during discussion may stimulate ideas for incorporation into policies and procedures or future training sessions.

Once a baby has been stabilized and/or transported, and the team members have had a chance to relax, the case review might begin with the following questions:

1. How do the team members feel about the case?
2. What went well?
3. Are there things the team or its individual members could have done differently to improve the flow of care and communication?
4. What things might be done differently the next time a similar event presents?
5. What information/knowledge/skills does the team need to review, acquire, and/or practice before caring for a similar baby in the future?
6. Do current policies, procedures, equipment, setups, and supplies need to be updated?
7. Does the team need a professional facilitator to help debrief after a particularly unusual or difficult event?

Using the ACoRN Framework and Sequences to review the clinical experience can provide structure for case review.

Template for case review

Anticipation/preparation Personnel Supplies and equipment	
Communication Between team members Between teams With family members	
Care As per ACoRN framework and sequences	
Recommendations Equipment and supplies Current policies and procedures Communication Staff education/skill maintenance	

Palliative Care

Occasionally, babies will present with conditions that will not improve despite properly performed resuscitation and stabilization. As with individuals at any age, the decision to provide palliative (or comfort care) would be based on the likelihood of either death or survival with unacceptable burden. Palliative care is when you move from active care to save a baby's life, to active care to provide comfort care to the baby, family and health care team as the baby dies.

In these situations, expert opinion on the baby's prognosis will guide parental counseling and decision-making.

When a baby dies

During the difficult time surrounding the death of a baby, the family's and health care team's needs should be supported.

It is helpful for the health care team to demonstrate an open and non-judgmental attitude and a willingness to participate in the bereavement experience with the family. The team should acknowledge that every situation is unique, and that every family has different needs.

Other suggestions to help the team support the family include,

- encouraging the parents to see, touch, and hold their baby if they choose to do so
- offering options such as religious or cultural observances (for example, baptism)
- offering the parents the opportunity to call in their family members/friends or spiritual/religious advisors
- photographing the baby before and after death (some families initially refuse photos but later change their minds, so photos should be taken and kept on file)
- hand/foot prints (some families initially refuse the hand/foot prints but later change their minds, so hand/foot prints should be taken and kept on file)
- encouraging the family to take as much time as they desire with their baby
- dressing the baby in a special outfit
- providing the family with a bereavement kit that includes a variety of resources and reading materials (these can be obtained from some referral centers)
- discuss with parents potential opportunities to donate breastmilk where possible.

Providing end-of-life care for babies and their family can be very intense for members of the health care team. It is important that all members of the team (physicians, nurses and ancillary staff) who interact with the baby and the family receive collegial support. Support can also be obtained more formally from others within the clinical setting, for example: hospice bereavement staff, spiritual care providers, social workers, and employee assistance personnel.

The particulars of perinatal loss are outside the scope of ACoRN. If there is no one available at your centre to provide direction, consultation can be sought from your referral centre.

Answers to the questions in Chapter 10

I.   Does the baby demonstrate any stability cues??

There is no clear evidence of stability cues. Moving his arms and legs may represent the baby's attempt to either seek boundaries or reposition himself midline and flexed.

II.   Looking back at the case, what stress cues is this baby demonstrating?

Respiratory distress with increasing oxygen requirements

Non-flexed posture

Unsuccessful attempt to self-console

Crying in response to handling

Flailing and grimacing in response to loud noises

Apnea and bradycardia in response to positioning for the chest radiograph

III.   Can you think of other ways to support the family?

Provide a comfortable, private area to interact,

Ask whether they would like a visit from other family members, the chaplain or social worker,

Answer their questions and provide information.

IV.   Can you think of ways to support the family if they must be separated from their baby who is being transported to the tertiary centre, a 4-hour flight away?

Have the transport team meet with the parents prior to departure.

If possible, transfer mother with the baby.

Provide parents with a photo of their baby.

If the mother is planning to breastfeed, instruct her how to pump and store her breastmilk.

Bibliography

American Academy of Pediatrics. Committee on Fetus and Newborn. Committee on Drugs. Section on Anesthesiology. Section on Surgery. Canadian Paediatric Society. Fetal and Newborn Committee. Prevention and management of pain and stress in the neonate. Pediatrics 2000; 105(2): 454-61.

Catlin A, Carter B. Creation of a neonatal end-of-life palliative care protocol. Neonatal

Network 2002: 21(4): 37-46.

Coleman M, Solarin K, Smith C. Assessment and management of pain and distress in the neonate. Adv Neonatal Care 2002; 2(3): 123-36.

Finer N, Rich W. Neonatal resuscitation: Toward improved performance. Resuscitation 2002; 53: 47-51.

Health Canada. Family-Centred Maternity and Newborn Care: National Guidelines 2002; Ottawa, ON: Minister of Public Works and Government Services.

McGrath J. Developmentally supportive caregiving and technology in the NICU: Isolation or merger of intervention strategies? J Perinat Neonatal Nurs 2000; 14(3): 78-91.

Puchalski M, Hummel P. The reality of neonatal pain. Adv Neonatal Care 2002; 2(5): 233-46.

Symington A, Pinelli J. Distilling the evidence on developmental care: A systematic review. Adv Neonatal Care 2002: 2(4): 198-201.

Weingarten CT. Nursing interventions: Caring for parents of a newborn transferred to a regional intensive care nursery – A challenge for low risk obstetric specialists. J Perinatol 1988; 8(3): 271-5.

Appendix A
Neonatal Assessment Tool

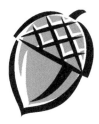

Each unit should have a standardized way in which all babies are assessed. This assessment guide is an optional tool developed to help you complete your physical assessment and documentation. The areas to assess and descriptive terms are meant to be trigger words.

Sequence	Alerting sign	Areas to assess	Descriptive terms
Respiratory	➢ Laboured respirations*[1] ➢ Respiratory rate > 60* ➢ Receiving respiratory support*	• type of airway management • respiratory support • respiratory rate & effort • air entry • breath sounds • chest shape & symmetry • skin colour • pulse oximeter • oxygen requirements • patent nares and choanae • secretions • treatments • medication & effects	• O_2 requirements (%) • nasal prongs, hood, CPAP, ETT • ventilator settings • tachypneic, apneic, gasping • retractions, grunting, nasal flaring • ACoRN Respiratory Score • breath sounds equal bilaterally, presence of 'crackles or wheezes' • symmetry of chest movement, barrel chest, flail chest • presence of cleft palate or micrognathia (small jaw) • pink, pale, plethoric, mottled, grey • chest tube placement, drainage, bubbling of air • response to handling, i.e. increase O_2 requirements • secretions thick, thin, creamy white, clear, blood tinged • surfactant treatment with improvement/no change in breath sounds, chest expansion, SpO_2
Cardiovascular	➢ Pale, mottled, or grey* ➢ Weak pulses or low BP* ➢ Cyanosis unresponsive to O_2 ➢ Heart rate > 220 bpm	• level of arousal • skin colour • central & peripheral perfusion • temperature of extremities • pulses • blood pressure • BP both arms, one leg • heart rate, rhythm & character • point of maximal impulse (PMI) • precordium • monitoring devices • hyperoxia test • blood/volume replacement • medications & effects	• dysmorphic features • active, distressed, listless, lethargic • pink, plethoric, pale, mottled, grey, cyanotic, dusky • capillary refill trunk/extremities, sluggish/brisk • extremities warm, cool • pulses, equal bilaterally, full, bounding, weak, absent, 4-limb comparison • absence/minimal respiratory distress • breath sounds moist, rales • disinterest, fatigue with feed • diaphoretic • brady/tachycardia • location of PMI • presence of murmur (soft, loud), location heard loudest • activity of precordium • edema, pitting • weight gain/loss • type of blood product/volume replacement, response

---

[1] See: Alerting Signs with * (Chapter 1, Chapter 9)

Sequence	Alerting sign	Areas to assess	Descriptive terms
Neurology	➢ Abnormal tone* ➢ Jitteriness ➢ Seizures*	• level of alertness • activity • posture • tone • reflexes • developmental indicators • cry • seizures/abnormal movements • fontanels/sutures • evidence of external injury • treatments • medications & effects • seizure log • neonatal abstinence scoring sheet	• evidence of external injury (such as cephalohematoma, bruising) • awake, asleep, irritable, startles easily • cry high pitched, lusty, quiet • active, lethargic, stupor, hyperalert • flexed, flaccid, hypertonic, hypotonic • fullness/tension of fontanels - soft, flat, full, bulging • sutures approximated, overriding, separated (distance in mm) • suck, swallow, gag • type of movement, jittery, tremulous, twitching, mouthing, bicycling seizure, duration, origin/spread, suppressed by holding, eye/mouth movements, LOC, changes in HR/BP/colour, other signs • yawns, sneezes, nasal stuffiness, excessive sucking, regurgitation/projectile vomiting, loose/watery stools • medications (e.g. phenobarbital, phenytoin, sedatives)
Surgical Conditions	➢ Anterior abdominal wall defect ➢ Vomiting or inability to swallow ➢ Abdominal distention ➢ Delayed passage of meconium or imperforate anus	• intactness of skin • presence of wounds, incisions, petechiae, rashes, scars • tissue turgor, anterior fontanel, mucous membranes, weight loss/gain • measurement of abdominal girth • treatments • fluid balance sheet	• presence/type of defect • open lesion, location, size, colour, peritoneal sac • abdominal distention, soft, tense, visible bowel loops, colour • bowel sounds in all 4 quadrants • abdominal girth • aspirates, volume, color • bloody stools • vomiting, projectile, • excessive salivation, copious secretions • choking, coughing, inability to swallow • dry mucous membranes, sunken anterior fontanel • jaundice, pale • location/type of dressing, bowel bag • NGT/OGT, Replogle tube, open barrel/low intermittent suction

Sequence	Alerting sign	Areas to assess	Descriptive terms
Fluid & Glucose Management	➤ Blood glucose < 2.6 mmol/L ➤ At risk for hypoglycemia ➤ Not feeding or should not be fed	• fluids/hydration • weight gain, loss • intake vs output • abdomen • stools/emesis • ability to feed • neurologic status • catheters/collection devices • treatments • phototherapy • medications & effects	• type of solution, volume, route, frequency • total fluids • intake output balance • urine colour (pale/amber/dark) • stools passed (soft/hard/meconium /loose/yellow, brown, green/seedy/bloody) • dry mucosa, sunken fontanel, skin elastic/non-elastic • able to coordinate suck/swallow, gag reflex • not latching, not sucking, incoordinated, not interested, not waking
Thermoregulation	➤ T < 36.3 or > 37.2°C axillary* ➤ Increased risk for temp instability	• type of thermal management • room temperature • compare body to limb temperature by touch • axillary temperature trend	• radiant warmer/incubator, cot/crib • above/below/within recommended thermal environment • nested • skin warm/hot/cold to touch • pale, mottled, flushed
Infection	➤ Risk factors for infection ➤ ACoRN alerting sign with * ➤ Clinical deterioration	• respiratory • cardiovascular • neurology • abdominal distention • axillary temperature trend • venous/arterial sites • diagnostic tests • medications & effects	• presence of thermal instability, apnea, bradycardia, lethargy, feeding intolerance • pallor, mottling, cyanotic, petechiae • reddened, pinpoint rash • respiratory distress, apnea, tachycardia • lethargic, irritable, poor feeding • skin broken, excoriated, reddened, swollen • CBC results, cultures • medications (e.g. antibiotics, antiviral, antifungal)
Support	➤ Baby ➤ Family ➤ Health care team	• response to handling • sleep/wake patterns • environmental • presence of pain • medications, effects • involvement in baby's care • visiting patterns • ability to express feelings & concerns • support systems • knowledge needs • cultural beliefs	• tolerates handling • able to self-console • startles to noise, irritable with handling • unable to achieve quiet sleep • grimacing, crying • sleeps between feeds, settles easily • effect of sedation (e.g. morphine)

Appendix B
Resuscitation Skills

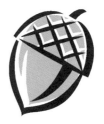

The resuscitation skills discussed in this Appendix are:
1. Free flow oxygen administration
2. Bag-and-mask ventilation
3. Endotracheal intubation
4. End-tidal CO_2 detector
5. Laryngeal mask airway
6. Chest compressions
7. Emergency vascular access – Umbilical vein catheterization
8. Emergency vascular access – Intraosseous vascular access
9. Epinephrine
10. Volume expander
11. Sodium bicarbonate

ACoRN considers the AAP/AHA Neonatal Resuscitation Program (NRP)[1] as a pre-requisite. This is because

- the skills taught in NRP may be needed for resuscitation of babies who become sick after birth
- in some cases, neonatal resuscitation may immediately precede the ACoRN process.

©AAP/AHA

In this textbook, the NRP logo indicates resuscitation skills[2] that are taught by the AAP/AHA Neonatal Resuscitation Program. These skills are included in this Appendix with an ACoRN perspective for the sole purpose of providing a review for professionals with current training in NRP. Review or completion of this Appendix does not constitute an NRP activity.

The ACoRN logo indicates a review of resuscitation skills that are not taught in the AAP/AHA Neonatal Resuscitation Program.

---

[1] Kattwinkel J, ed. Textbook of Neonatal Resuscitation. Dallas: American Academy of Pediatrics and American Heart Association, 2000.

[2] All NRP diagrams reproduced in ACoRN have been kindly provided by the American Academy of Pediatrics (AAP) / American Heart Association (AHA).

©AAP/AHA

Free-flow oxygen administration during resuscitation

Indication   Central cyanosis in a spontaneously breathing baby

Goal   To increase the concentration of inspired oxygen

Equipment
- source of 100% oxygen, oxygen/air blender and flowmeter
- flow-inflating bag or an oxygen mask or oxygen tubing, in order of preference
  - a flow inflating bag can also be used for administration of CPAP or ventilation
- pulse oximeter

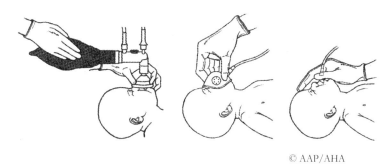

© AAP/AHA

Oxygen administration during resuscitation:

| Flow inflating bag | Oxygen mask | Oxygen tubing |

Procedure
1. Set oxygen flow rate to 5 L/minute.
2. Administer 100% oxygen. Once the baby's colour becomes pink, the supplemental oxygen should be gradually withdrawn to the lowest concentration at which the baby remains pink.
3. Use in conjunction with pulse oximeter monitoring if oxygen administered for more than 3 to 5 minutes, aiming for SpO_2 between 88 to 95%.
4. An oxygen air blender facilitates adjusting the concentration of inspired oxygen to values under 100% once the baby is pink and the target SpO_2 between 88 to 95% is achieved.

Potential complications
- Prolonged flow of non-humidified, non-warmed oxygen may dry the respiratory mucosa and cool the baby.

©AAP/AHA

Bag-and-mask ventilation

Indications   Absent or inadequate respiratory effort: apnea or gasping respirations
HR < 100 bpm

Goal   To provide positive pressure ventilation

Equipment
- source of 100% oxygen, oxygen/air blender and flowmeter
- flow-inflating bag (with manometer) or self-inflating bag (with pressure-release valve) with an oxygen reservoir attached
- appropriate-sized face mask
- orogastric tube
- pulse oximeter

Procedure
1. Select bag capable of delivering 90% to 100% oxygen with an appropriate sized face mask; connect to an oxygen source (preferably via a blender).
2. Set the flowmeter to 5 to 10 L/minute.
3. Test bag for leaks, function of pressure-release valve, and the integrity of the valve assembly and pressure manometer (if any).
4. Position the bag-and-mask onto the baby's face.
5. Ventilate at a rate of 40 to 60 breaths/minute, with sufficient pressure (15 to 20 cmH$_2$O for normal lungs; 20 to 40 cmH$_2$O for "stiff" lungs) to cause the chest to rise.

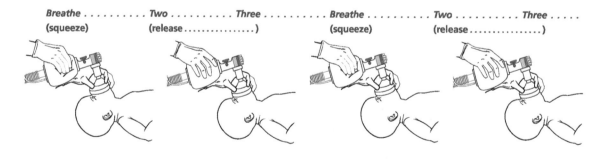

© AAP/AHA

6. Auscultate the chest for presence of bilateral breath sounds. Observe the baby's color and measure the heart rate.
7. If the chest does not rise, check for inadequate seal, reposition the head, suction if appropriate, open the mouth slightly, then reapply the facemask.
8. If the chest still does not rise, consider increasing inspiratory pressure.
9. Adjust the concentration of inspired oxygen to achieve a target SpO$_2$ between 88 to 95%.
10. If bag-and-mask ventilation is required for more than several minutes, insert an orogastric tube to decompress the stomach and aspirate contents.

Potential complications

- Hyperventilation, leading to hypocarbia (decreases respiratory drive and brain blood flow).
- High airway inflation pressure (increases lung injury and risk for air leaks, such as pneumothorax).
- Gastric distention (leads to decreased diaphragmatic excursion, difficulty inflating the lungs, and possibly aspiration of stomach contents).

©AAP/AHA

Endotracheal intubation

Indications

Ineffective ventilation with bag-and-mask technique
Inability to maintain a patent airway
Need or anticipation of need for prolonged ventilation
Need for endotracheal suctioning
Route for instillation of certain medications (e.g. epinephrine, surfactant)
To avoid gastric distension in babies with congenital diaphragmatic hernia or anterior abdominal wall defects

Goal

To establish direct access to the trachea

Equipment

- source of 100% oxygen, oxygen/air blender and flowmeter
- bag and mask system
- suction apparatus and catheters (6, 8, 10, 12 Fr)
- laryngoscope handle
- straight laryngoscope blades (size 00, 0, 1)
- selection of endotracheal tubes and stylets
- end-tidal CO_2 detector
- scissors, tape, and stethoscope
- pulse oximeter

Tube size (mm ID)	Weight (g)	Gestational age (weeks)
2.5	< 1,000	< 28
3.0	1,000 to 2,000	28 to 34
3.5	2,000 to 3,000	34 to 38
3.5 to 4.0	> 3,000	> 38

Procedure

1. Position the baby's head in a midline position with neck slightly extended.
2. Turn laryngoscope light on.
3. Hold the laryngoscope in the left hand, between the thumb and first two or three fingers, with the blade pointing to the baby. Keep one or two fingers free to rest on the baby's face to provide stability.
4. Stabilize the baby's head with the right hand.
5. Slide the laryngoscope blade over the tongue, along the midline, and advance the blade until the tip lies in the vallecula, just beyond the base of the tongue.
6. Lift the entire blade slightly upwards in the direction the handle is pointing, thus lifting the tongue out of the way to expose the pharyngeal area.
7. Look for landmarks. Suctioning secretions may improve visualization.
8. Insert the endotracheal tube from the right side of the baby's mouth (to prevent the tube from blocking the view of the glottis until the vocal cord guide is at the level of the cords (wait for the cords to open if they are together).
9. Note the centimeter mark at the level of the lips.
10. Stabilize the position of the tube, and remove the stylette and the laryngoscope.
11. Initiate bag ventilation.
12. Secure the endotracheal tube in place.

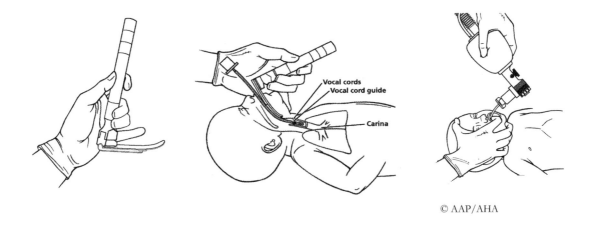

© AAP/AHA

13. Confirm endotracheal tube placement:
    • tube is seen passing through the vocal cords
    • end-tidal CO_2 detector changes colour from purple to yellow
    • mist is seen within the tube during expiration
    • breath sounds are equal bilaterally
    • chest rises with ventilation
    • heart rate, colour, and oxygen saturation improve
14. Chest radiograph demonstrates mid-tracheal position with the tip of the tube 1 cm proximal to the carina.

15. Adjust the concentration of inspired oxygen to achieve a target SpO_2 between 88 to 95%.

Potential complications
- Inadvertent placement in the esophagus.
- Trauma to the lips, gums, tongue, larynx/trachea.
- Right main stem bronchus intubation.
- Vagal response at the time of intubaton leading to bradycardia.
- Pain and discomfort.

Notes
- Intubation requires 2 people: one to perform the procedure and the other to assist
- Consider premedication prior to elective or semi-urgent intubation

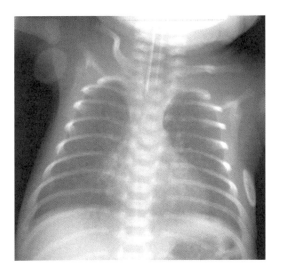 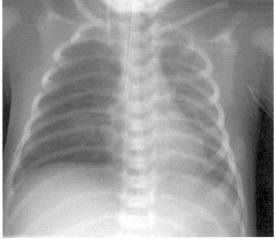

- ○ Correct placement.
- ○ Tube in the trachea, above the carina.

- ○ Incorrect placement.
- ○ Right main stem bronchus intubation (also shows right internal jugular line).

 ### *End-tidal CO_2 detector*

Indications   Adjunct for endotracheal intubation

Goal   To confirm, rapidly and reliably, correct placement of the endotracheal tube.

Principles   Carbon dioxide (CO_2), produced in the body during cellular metabolism, is carried back through the venous system to the lungs. In the lungs, CO_2 diffuses from the pulmonary capillaries into the alveoli where it is exhaled.

Exhaled (end-tidal) CO_2 detection has been found to be the most rapid and reliable method for confirming endotracheal tube (ETT) position.

The end-tidal CO_2 detector is positioned between the ETT connector and the manual bagging device.
- The end-tidal CO_2 detector changes color from purple to yellow when it comes into contact with exhaled CO_2.
- Color ranges marked on a reference chart indicates the approximate CO_2 concentrations in the baby's exhaled tidal volume.

The reagent used by CO_2 detectors is metacresol purple, a non-toxic pH-sensitive substance.

Application

Once the baby is intubated and the end-tidal CO_2 detector is in place, the detector is read as follows:
- Purple < 4 mm Hg CO_2 = Correct tube placement is unlikely (little CO_2 present)
- Tan < 15 mm Hg CO_2 = Tube may not be in correct place
- Yellow 15 to 38 mm Hg CO_2 = Confirmatory of correct ETT placement

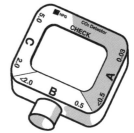

Equipment

End-tidal CO_2 detector

Procedure

1. Visualize the ETT going through the vocal cords.
2. Initiate ventilation, ensuring that there are breath sounds in both lungs, and no sounds over the stomach
3. Observe for chest movement.
4. Place the end-tidal CO_2 detector between the bagging system and endotracheal tube.
5. Reinitiate ventilation observing the end-tidal CO_2 detector for color change, from purple to yellow within 4 to 6 breaths.
6. Document the presence or absence of color change for each intubation attempt.

Notes

There may be a false negative in the presence of,
- poor cardiac output
- decreased pulmonary blood flow
- , very low exhaled CO_2 (for example, extremely low birth weight baby with severe lung disease)

Bibliography

Bhende MS. End-tidal carbon dioxide monitoring in pediatrics - clinical applications. Jouranl Postgrad Med. 2001 Jul-Sep; 47(3): 215-8.

DeBoer S & Seaver M. End-tidal CO2 verification of endotracheal tube placement in neonates. Neonatal Network. 2004 May-Jun; 23(3): 29-38.

Kattwinkel J, ed. Textbook of Neonatal Resuscitation. Dallas: American Academy of Pediatrics and American Heart Association, 2000.

Laryngeal mask airway

Indications   When bag and mask technique is ineffective in providing ventilation and endotracheal intubation is not possible

Goal   To provide an airway for assisted ventilation

Principles   Laryngeal mask airways (LMA) have an inflatable silicone mask at the end of a rubber shaft connecting tube. The silicone mask is designed to fit over the larynx and block entry of air into the esophagus. Once the mask is properly placed and inflated, it provides a seal over the larynx so that air/oxygen can be delivered to the lungs.

Equipment
- LMA mask size '1'
- 5 mL syringe for cuff inflation
- bag and mask system attached to oxygen source
- water soluble lubricant
- stethoscope
- tape to secure LMA

Procedure
1. Suction pharynx and empty stomach.
2. Inspect the LMA for tears and leaks by inflating the cuff with a maximum of 4 mL of air.
3. Deflate the cuff and mask prior to insertion.
4. Lubricate the back of the mask and tube; avoid getting lubrication on the anterior surface of the cuff and bowl of the mask.
5. Position baby for intubation (head extended and midline).
6. Hold the LMA by the shaft, like a pen, as near as possible to the mask to prevent the mask from turning over.
7. Place the anterior cuff and bowl end of the LMA against the palate.
8. Using index finger, follow the palate groove while advancing the mask into the pharynx, ensuring that the mask remains flat.
9. Press mask into posterior pharyngeal wall using index finger.
10. Grasp the LMA shaft with other hand and gradually withdraw index finger.
11. Press the LMA gently against the larynx to ensure mask is fully inserted.
12. Inflate mask with 3 to 4 mL of air; the shaft may rise up as the mask is inflated.
13. Connect LMA to bagging system and initiate ventilation.
14. Confirm placement by listening for breath sounds, and observing chest expansion.

Potential Complications	• Inhalation of lubricant. • Leak around the cuff specially if high pressure is required. • Trauma to upper airway. • Aspiration. • Dryness of throat/mucosa.
Notes	• Not to be used for endotracheal suctioning or instillation of medication.
Bibliography	Pennant JH, White PF. The Laryngeal Mask Airway. It's Uses in Anesthesiology. Anesthesiology 79: 144, 1993. Brimacombe JR, Brain AIJ. The Laryngeal Mask Airway: A Review and Practical Guide. WB Saunders, 1997.

©AAP/AHA

Chest compressions

Indications	Heart rate < 60 bpm after 30 seconds of effective ventilation with 100% oxygen.
Goal	To improve cardiac output until effective ventilation improves oxygenation and cardiac contractility.

Procedure	1. Continue ventilation.
	2. Apply two-fingers or two–thumbs over the lower third of the sternum, just below the nipple line.
	   • the two-thumb technique is considered more effective than the finger technique, but it limits access to the umbilical cord.
	3. Compress to a depth of one-third of the anterio-posterior diameter of the chest.
	4. Perform 3 chest compressions and 1 ventilation every two seconds,
	   • there should be 120 events per minute, 90 compressions and 30 ventilations
	   • the person doing the compressions should count aloud: "one-and-two-and-three-and-breathe-and" while the person ventilating squeezes during "breathe-and" and releases during "one-and"
	5. Pause after 30 seconds of ventilation and compressions to determine the heart rate by auscultation,

- reinitiate ventilation and compressions if the heart rate is ≤ 60 bpm
- stop compressions but continue ventilation if heart rate > 60 bpm.

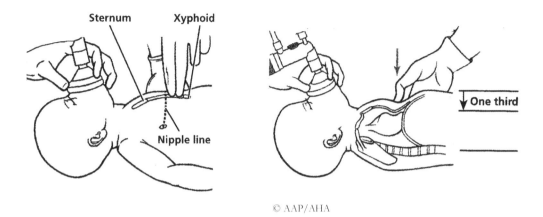

© AAP/AHA

Potential complications
- Trauma to the chest and/or intra-abdominal organs (for example, the liver).
- Impediment to ventilation if compressions and ventilations are not coordinated.

Notes
- Chest compression is a 2-person procedure.
- Hypoxemia is the cause of persistent bradycardia and low cardiac output in most cases requiring resuscitation. Cardiac output improves as effective ventilation is established. If bradycardia persists, suspect poor ventilation technique, mechanical obstruction of the airway, or pneumothorax.

©AAP/AHA

Emergency vascular access – Umbilical vein catheterization

Indications
Actual or anticipated need for volume expansion
Intravascular drug administration
Blood sampling during resuscitation

Goal
To access the intravascular space on an emergency basis

Equipment

- antiseptic solution
- mask, sterile gloves
- sterile procedure tray with forceps, umbilical tape, and gauze
- umbilical catheters size 3.5 F (< 1500 grams) and 5.0 F (≥ 1500 grams)
- feeding tube size 5.0 F can be utilized for very short term if no venous catheter is available in an emergency
  - more clots are formed around feeding tubes
- stopcock, 10 mL syringe, and sterile 0.9% NaCl
- #10 scalpel blade

Procedure

1. Wash hands.
2. Mask and glove.
3. Assistant opens equipment onto sterile field.
4. Connect umbilical catheter, stopcock and syringe. Flush with 0.9% NaCl. Close the stopcock to the catheter to prevent fluid loss and air entry.
5. Cleanse the cord stump and the skin immediately surrounding the stump area.
6. Using sterile technique, tie umbilical tape loosely around the cord stump.
7. Grasp cord stump with forceps, cut off the umbilical clamp with the scalpel blade leaving about 1 to 2 cm of cord stump. If necessary, control bleeding by gently tightening the umbilical tape.
8. Insert the fluid-filled catheter into the umbilical vein. Continue inserting the catheter to just below the skin surface (2 to 4 cm) until blood return occurs when gently drawing back on the syringe. Using a catheter positioned at this level to infuse fluids and medications for emergency use is considered safe. Inserting the catheter beyond 4 cm below the skin surface is associated with the risk of infusing vasoactive or hypertonic fluids into the liver and causing tissue damage.
9. Secure the line by holding it firmly in place and suturing it to the cord stump as soon as possible.
10. Ensure the stopcock is closed toward the baby when the catheter is not in use.
11. Make sure no air is injected into the vein.

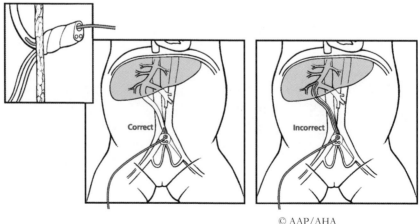

© AAP/AHA

Potential complications
- Perforation of the vessel.
- Insertion into the portal venous system resulting in infusion of fluid and/or drugs into the liver.
- Blood loss with catheter dislodgement.
- Air embolism.
- Infection.

Note

This route is only available for the first few days of life.

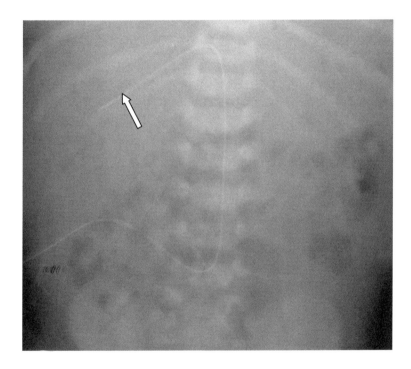

○ Incorrect placement.
○ An umbilical venous catheter incorrectly placed in the portal venous system.

 Emergency vascular access - Intraosseous vascular access

Indications

When attempts at venous cannulation fail in term babies with life-threatening situations.

Goal

To access the intravascular space on an emergency basis.

Principles

The marrow cavity is in continuity with the venous circulation.

- Blood can be withdrawn for analysis (hemoglobin, pH, PCO_2, crossmatch, electrolyte determination, and culture).
- Crystalloid, blood products, and medications may be syringed or infused by pump into the marrow cavity.

The intraosseous (IO) route is one of the quickest and most effective ways to establish vascular access in an emergency.

IO vascular access must be achieved aseptically to reduce the risk of osteomyelitis.

IO infusions should be considered a short-term solution (i.e. a few hours) only until venous access is established.

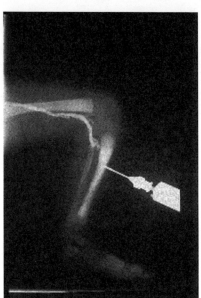

Equipment

- antiseptic solution
- mask, sterile gloves
- sterile procedure tray with forceps, umbilical tape, and gauze
- needles, in order of preference:
  - intraosseous or bone marrow needle (16 or 18 g)
  - short spinal needle with stylet (18 or 20 g)
  - short hypodermic needle (18 or 20 g)
  - consider using the bone injection gun (BIG). Note: there is less possibility of leakage or breaking a bone with the BIG.

The photograph illustrates how quickly and directly the injected material enters the major circulation after intraosseous injection.
(courtesy Dr. Dan Waisman, Haifa, Israel)

- 1% lidocaine without epinephrine in a syringe with a 25 or 30 g needle attached for skin infiltration
- 5 mL syringe filled with preservative-free 0.9% saline solution, attached to a 3-way stopcock
- 50 mL syringe with IV solution or IV solution bag with an IV infusion pump
- protective cover
- restraints - to protect established IO infusion

Procedure

1. Palpate the tibial tuberosity. Cannulation site is 1 to 2 cm below the tuberosity on the flat, antero-medial surface of the tibia.
2. Apply sterile gloves then drape the site.
3. Clean the skin.
4. Inject lidocaine without epinephrine into the skin, subcutaneous tissue, and onto the periosteum.

5. Stabilize the limb with counter-pressure directly opposite the proposed site of penetration to avoid bone fracture (sand bag or towel roll can be used).

6. Advance the needle at a near-90-degree angle with the tip directed 10 to 15° away from the epiphyseal (growth) plate. Use a twisting or boring motion until the cortex is penetrated. Penetration is signaled by a sudden decrease in resistance, often described as a "give" or "pop". Stop inserting further. Penetration depth is rarely more than 1 cm in a baby.

7. Remove the stylet from the needle. Attach saline-filled syringe and stopcock. Aspirate marrow to confirm position. Aspiration is not always successful with smaller gauge needles.

8. Flush needle with 2 to 3 mL saline while palpating the tissue adjacent to the insert site to detect extravasation. There should be only mild resistance to fluid infusion. If marrow cannot be aspirated or significant resistance to infusion is met:
   • the hollow needle may be obstructed by bone plugs
   • the bevel of the needle may not have penetrated the cortex
   • the bevel of the needle may be lodged against the opposite cortex.
   Advance or withdraw the needle slightly and try to flush again.

9. When needle position is confirmed, secure the needle in place with sterile gauze and strapping. Secure the limb. Apply a protective covering to maintain a clean infusion site while the needle is in place.

10. Attach IV tubing and begin infusion of fluid or drugs via IV pump or syringe pump.

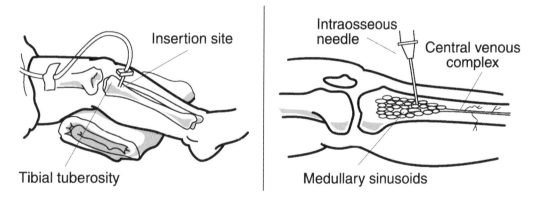

Insertion site	Intraosseous needle
Tibial tuberosity	Central venous complex
	Medullary sinusoids

Potential complications
- Bone fracture.
- Extravasation of fluid from the puncture site.
- Osteomyelitis, cellulitis, subcutaneous abscess, or sepsis.
- Damage to the epiphyseal plate.
- Compartment syndrome.

Note:
- Intraosseous infusion cannot be established on a bone punctured by a previous IO attempt.
- The intraosseous route should be replaced as soon as a normal vein can be cannulated and within a few hours. The longer the period of use, the greater the risk of complications.

Bibliography

Claudet I, Fries F, Bloom MC, Lelong-Tissier MC. Etude retrospective de 32 cas de perfusion intraosseus. Archives of Paediatrics 1999; 6: 566-9.

MacDonald MG, Ramasethu J, eds. Atlas of Procedures in Neonatology. Philadelphia: Lippincott, Williams & Wilkins, 2002.

McGillvary D. Vascular access in under 90 seconds: Intraosseous infusion. Paediatric Child Health 1997; 2(1): 27-8.

Shulman HM. Intraosseous infusions: the impossible line. Can J CME 1995: 28-32.

©AAP/AHA

Epinephrine

Indications

Persistent heart rate < 60 bpm after 30 seconds of chest compressions with effective ventilation using 100% oxygen.

Goal

To increase the rate and strength of cardiac contractions

Supplied

Epinephrine 1:10,000 (0.1 mg/mL)
- draw solution into a 1 mL syringe

Administration

IV, UV, IO or ETT.
- Absorption is more reliable with intravascular administration, but it takes time to establish intravenous access.
- Give as a rapid bolus, followed by 0.5 to 1.0 mL of 0.9% NaCl.

Dose

0.1 to 0.3 mL/kg (based on estimate of weight)
- dose may be repeated every 3 to 5 minutes

Incompatibility
- phenobarbital
- sodium bicarbonate

Adverse effects / precautions
- Cardiac arrhythmias.
- Tissue necrosis if extravasated.
- Severe hypertension with possible intracranial/intraventricular hemorrhage.
- Renal vascular ischemia.

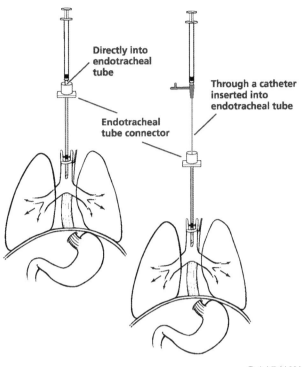

Endotracheal administration of epinephrine

Volume expander

Indications   Known or suspected intravascular volume depletion

Goal   To increase circulating intravascular volume

Supplied   0.9% NaCl (normal saline), Ringer's lactate, or O negative blood
- draw the prescribed volume into a 30 or 50 mL syringe

Administration   IV, UV, or IO
- infuse over 5 to 10 minutes

Dose   10 mL/kg (based on an estimate of weight)
- dose may be repeated

Adverse effects / precautions
- Volume overload leading to heart failure.
- Intraventricular hemorrhage with rapid volume expansion.

©AAP/AHA

Sodium bicarbonate

Indications
Confirmed or presumed metabolic acidosis occurring with prolonged resuscitation

Goal
To improve myocardial function and increase myocardial response to epinephrine during prolonged resuscitation.

Supplied
4.2% (0.5 mEq/mL)
- draw the prescribed dose into a 10 mL syringe

Administration
IV, UV or IO
- infuse slowly (no faster than 0.5 to 1 mEq/kg/minute)

Dose
1 to 2 mEq/kg (2 to 4 mL/kg)

Incompatibility
- epinephrine
- calcium gluconate

Adverse effects / precautions
- Rapid infusion of hyperosmolar solution is linked to intraventricular hemorrhage.
- Tissue necrosis if solution extravasates.
- If ventilation is inadequate, CO_2 accumulates, leading to respiratory acidosis.

Monitoring
Follow acid/base status by checking blood gases.

Notes
- Use of sodium bicarbonate is discouraged during brief CPR.
- Do not give sodium bicarbonate unless the lungs are adequately ventilated.

Appendix C
Procedures

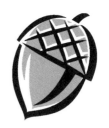

The procedures discussed in this Appendix are:
1. Blood pressure measurement
2. Blood sampling, capillary
3. Bowel bag application
4. Cardiorespiratory monitoring
5. Continuous positive airway pressure (CPAP)
6. Mechanical ventilation
7. Pneumothorax – Chest transillumination
8. Pneumothorax – Chest tube insertion
9. Pneumothorax – Needle aspiration
10. Pulse oximetry

ACoRN

Blood pressure measurement

Indications
Arterial blood pressure is a critical measurement of cardiovascular function and should be evaluated in every at-risk or unwell baby.

Goals
- To detect the alterations in blood pressure which result from cardiovascular instability.
- To evaluate the effect of therapeutic interventions for shock and other causes of cardiovascular instability.
- To monitor a baby's cardiovascular stability during procedures.

Principles
Arterial blood pressure indirectly reflects the
- force of cardiac contraction
- volume of cardiac output
- circulating blood volume, and
- vascular tone.

Blood pressure is measured in mmHg. The mean arterial blood pressure (MAP) is the most reproducible and frequently quoted value in newborns.

The arterial blood pressure can be measured non-invasively using oscillometry. This technique uses an inflatable blood pressure cuff that encircles a limb. The cuff is automatically inflated above systolic pressure and then electronically deflated. A computerized blood pressure monitor senses the amplitude (size) of the arterial pulsation transmitted to the air within the cuff. The monitor analyzes the pulsations, thereby estimating systolic, mean and diastolic blood pressure, as well as heart rate.

On the first day of life for the purpose of stabilization, the lower limit of mean arterial blood pressure approximates to the gestational age in weeks. This value rises by 2 to 3 mmHg in the following few days. As an example, only 10% of newly born 34 week gestation babies would be expected to have a mean arterial blood pressure less than 34 mm Hg in the first day of life, rising to 37 to 38 mm Hg in the first week.

Other measurements of cardiovascular function such as heart rate, perfusion and color are essential when interpreting an "abnormal" blood pressure.

Application
Blood pressure monitors should be maintained and used according to the manufacturers' specifications. Computerized oscillometric blood pressure monitors may require configuration for neonatal/pediatric use to avoid excessive cuff pressure and possible injury during cuff inflation.

The choice of blood pressure cuff depends on the size of the baby. The ideal size is the largest cuff that will encircle the upper arm or leg without the bladder overlapping.

A symbol (usually an arrow) indicates the position of the cuff with reference to the underlying artery.

The cuff should connect to the monitor via an airtight tubing ensuring there is no leak or open port.

The blood pressure of a baby who is agitated or upset does not reflect his/her baseline condition.

Equipment

- non-invasive oscillometric blood pressure monitor
- neonatal/pediatric cuffs (sizes # 1 to 5)

Procedure

1. Turn on the monitor and enable the start-up procedure.
2. Select the largest cuff that will encircle the upper arm or leg without the bladder overlapping. A cuff that is too small will give a false high value. The opposite is true for cuffs with bladders too large or too loose for the baby.
3. Encircle the upper limb with the cuff, securing it firmly using the cuff's adhesive/fabric tab(s). Applying the cuff too tightly will restrict blood flow and thus give a false low value.
4. Ensure the centre of the bladder is aligned with the arterial pulse.
5. Connect the cuff tubing to the monitor ensuring an airtight seal.
6. Hold the baby's arm or leg straight.
7. Initiate inflation of the cuff.
8. Observe the baby while the cuff inflates and deflates, providing comfort if agitation occurs.
9. Document systolic, diastolic and mean pressure as well as heart rate and time.
10. Set the monitor to cycle at regular intervals as needed. Repeat measurements after interventions.

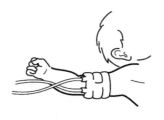 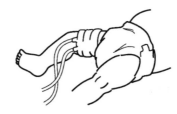 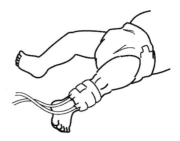

Potential complications

- Agitation and movement of the baby's limb can result in artifact and incorrect results.
- Oscillometry may be unreliable in very low birth weight babies or if cuff size is inappropriate.
- Adult default settings on the machine or repeated/excessive cycling may result in injury to the limb: attention should be paid to the area encircled by

the cuff and the distal limb.
- Obtaining a blood pressure measurement from the thigh is painful in children and adults. It is not known if neonates perceive it as painful.
- Check all abnormal results or alarms clinically to confirm the baby has not deteriorated.

Bibliography

DINAMAP™ Adult/Pediatric and Neonatal Vital Signs Monitor Operation Manual. Tampa, Florida: Critikon Inc, 1983.

Fletcher MA, MacDonald MG. Atlas of procedures in neonatology. Philadelphia: J.B. Lippincott Company, 1993.

Kattwinkel J, Cook LJ, Hurt H, Nowacek GA, Short JG. Neonatal Care: Book II - Perinatal Continuing Education Program. Charlottesville: University of Virginia, 2002.

 Blood sampling, capillary

Indications

To obtain a small blood sample for point of care or small-volume laboratory testing.

Equipment

- warm compress (not > 40° C) for foot
- gloves
- sterile micro lancet, tip not longer than 2.5 mm
- alcohol swabs
- sterile 2 x 2 gauze
- adhesive bandage
- blood collection device(s) appropriate for the blood tests ordered

Procedure

1. Assemble equipment and supplies.
2. Establish increased regional circulation by wrapping the foot with a warm, moist compress for 5 to 10 minutes. The heel should be warm at the time of puncture.
3. Wash hands and apply gloves.
4. Hold the baby's foot by the heel.
5. Select the puncture site in the soft lateral or medial area of the plantar surface of the heel.

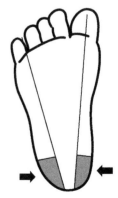

6. Cleanse the sampling site with alcohol swabs, allowing the alcohol to dry.
7. Using aseptic technique and standard precautions, puncture the heel with a depth restricted sterile micro lancet so the puncture will be no more than 3 mm deep.
8. Wipe off the first drop of blood; this sample may be inaccurate as alcohol used to cleanse the site may alter results.
9. Collect blood into appropriate specimen tubes.
   - When collecting capillary blood gases, rapidly fill heparinized capillary tubes without introducing air. Firmly seat both capillary tube end-caps. Mix blood and anticoagulant by rolling tubes.
10. Dry the heel with sterile gauze, apply pressure until the bleeding stops, and cover site with adhesive bandage.

Potential complications

- Bruising of foot or leg from excessive squeezing.
- Injury to nerves, tendons and cartilage if sampling outside the indicated areas or too deeply.
- Infection.
- Repeated punctures over the weight bearing area of the heel can cause formation of scar tissue resulting in pain, delayed walking and/or abnormal gait.

Notes

- Check your facility's policies and certification process for capillary blood sampling.
- Venipuncture is more appropriate for the collection of larger blood samples and blood cultures.

Bibliography

Kattwinkel J, Cook LJ, Hurt H, Nowacek GA, Short JG. Neonatal Care: Book II - Perinatal Continuing Education Program. University of Virginia, Charlottesville, 2002.

Deacon J, O'Neill P (eds): Core Curriculum for Neonatal Intensive Care Nursing/AWHONN NANN AACN. WB Saunders, Philadelphia, Pennsylvania, 1999.

 Bowel bag application

Goals

To cover and protect an abdominal wall defect.

Principles

Babies born with an abdominal wall defect risk damaging the exposed tissues, and are at higher risk for cold stress and infection due to exposed abdominal contents.

Bowel bags minimize the risk of breakdown, infection, and thermal, fluid and electrolyte losses. Bowel bags also provide clear visualization of the exposed bowel.

Traditionally, sterile, warm saline gauzes were used to cover the exposed bowel and other abdominal contents. These should be avoided as they do not allow direct visualization, are rough on the exposed surfaces, absorb fluid from the lesion, and may leave residual particles.

Equipment

- sterile bowel bag
- non-latex sterile gloves

Procedure

1. Administer vitamin K prior to applying bowel bag.
2. Open bowel bag, maintaining the inside of bag as sterile as possible.
3. Use non-latex sterile gloves when handling the exposed bowel and inside of bag.
4. Contain the exposed bowel and place on top of the abdomen.
5. Have an assistant place the baby into the bag feet first, drawing bag up to the nipple level, or high enough to fully cover the defect.
6. Position the bowel on top of abdomen in as midline a position as possible within the bag. Avoid torsion/twisting of the bowel.
7. Pull tie tapes closed snugly under arms to completely enclose the defect and to secure the bag to baby.
8. Position the baby supine – do not allow bowel to flop to one side or the other. Alternatively, position baby in a side-lying position and support exposed bowel with rolls to prevent torsion or pulling on bowel. If the defect is particularly large and the bowel cannot be stabilized in a midline position, gently wrap rolled gauze around the bowel over the bowel bag.

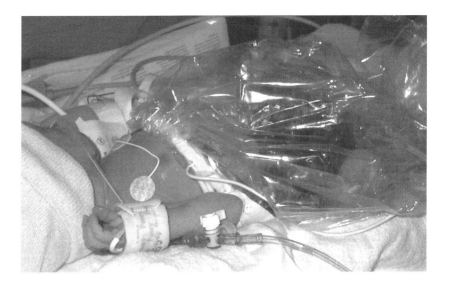

Notes

- If umbilical lines are to be inserted, cut a vertical slit in the bag to allow access to the umbilical cord for insertion. Once lines are in situ and secured, bring lines out through the bag and re-tape the bag closed to maintain moisture.

- Ensure bowel is supported in a midline position at all times prior to surgery. Protecting the integrity and perfusion of the bowel preoperatively assists in better bowel recovery post-operatively.

Bibliography

Howell, K. (1998). Understanding gastroschisis: An abdominal wall defect. Neonatal Network, 17(8), 17-25.

Strodtbeck, F. (1998). Abdominal wall defects. Neonatal Network, 17(8), 51-53.

 Cardiorespiratory monitoring

Indications

All at-risk and unstable babies require continuous monitoring of heart rate and respiratory rate.

Goals

- Detection of acute cardiac conditions such as bradycardia and tachycardia.
- Detection of acute changes in respiratory rate, particularly apnea.
- Trending of cardiorespiratory data over time.
- Monitor baby during procedures.

Principles

Cardiorespiratory monitoring measures both heart rate and rhythm, and respiratory rate.

Cardiac activity is detected electrically using electrodes attached to the baby's skin. The monitor interprets the electrical discharge of the heart with each beat to measure heart rate and displays the heart rhythm on a screen or paper print out.

The electrodes attached to each side of the chest also measure changes in chest size caused by breathing. Expansion of the chest results in a change in the body's ability to conduct electricity that can be detected electronically. Respiratory rate is depicted numerically or as a waveform. Apnea is the absence of respiratory activity for a set time.

Application

Electrodes are normally composed of electrical conducting gel with an adhesive surface. A pre-attached wire and plug connect each electrode to a common plug that connects to the monitor. Plugs are enclosed in plastic sheaths to prevent incorrect connection or disconnection, or inadvertent connection to live electric outlets and subsequent risk of electrocution.

Electrodes, leads, and/or plugs are colour-coded for optimal placement and should be connected to the monitor in the correct sequence:

- Right arm – WHITE
- Left arm – BLACK
- Left leg – RED

Once turned on, the monitor will default to preset alarms for heart and respiratory rate which differ from pediatric and adult cutoffs. Recommended settings for the newborn are:

- heart rate:
  - low: 90 to 100 bpm
  - high: 180 to 200 bpm
- respiratory rate:
  - apnea is defined as no respiratory movements for 20 seconds
  - the default apnea alarm is set to 20 seconds.

Equipment

- cardiorespiratory monitor
- 3 neonatal electrodes with wires and plugs
- socket and cable for electrodes

Procedure

1. Apply electrodes to clean, dry, healthy skin according to color code. Placement can be on the torso or shoulders and thighs depending on the size of the baby. Avoid placing electrodes onto nipples.
2. Connect electrodes to monitor via socket and cable.
3. Turn on monitor and ensure alarm defaults are set as described above.
4. Note that waveforms (if portrayed) should be sharp and clear. Some monitors provide different options for visualizing electrocardiogram waveforms; most use lead II as a default.
5. Document heart rate and respiratory rate displayed on monitor. Confirm the monitor is functioning properly by checking the heart rate using a stethoscope and respiratory rate by visualization.

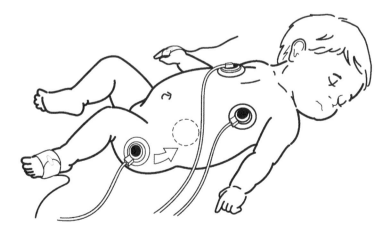

Precautions

- Use neonatal electrodes that are appropriately sized for the baby to avoid skin injury.
- Do not use leads which are damaged or frayed.
- Do not disable alarms.
- Do not reuse disposable electrodes.
- Check all abnormal results or alarms clinically to confirm the baby has not deteriorated.
- Chest electrodes do not detect obstructive apnea until the heart rate decreases or oxygen saturation decreases.

Bibliography

Fletcher MA and MacDonald MG. Atlas of Procedures in Neonatology. Philadelphia: J.B. Lippincott Company, 1993.

Kattwinkel J, Cook LJ, Hurt H, Nowacek GA, Short JG. Neonatal Care: Book II - Perinatal Continuing Education Program. Charlottesville: University of Virginia, 2002.

MacDonald MG, Ramasethu J, eds. Atlas of Procedures in Neonatology. Philadelphia: Lippincott, Williams & Wilkins, 2002.

Continuous positive airway pressure (CPAP)

Indications

Respiratory conditions associated with decreased lung compliance, increased work of breathing and poor oxygenation.

Goals

- Stabilize the lungs to decrease tendency to atelectasis at end-expiration
- Stabilize the airways to decrease tendency to obstructive apnea

Principles

Lungs with decreased compliance are "stiff". The alveoli tend to collapse, reducing overall lung volume. This leads to areas that are poorly ventilated and unable to participate in gas exchange. Babies attempt to compensate by exaggerated use of the accessory muscles of breathing in order to generate sufficient pressure to pull air into the lungs during inspiration.

When inspiratory and expiratory airway pressures are maintained by CPAP at levels above ambient pressure throughout the respiratory cycle,
- lung mechanics is stabilized
- the collapse of distal airways is prevented
- atelectatic alveoli are recruited
- airway resistance is reduced

- the volume of air remaining in the lung at the end of a normal expiration (functional residual capacity, FRC) increases
- the lung becomes more compliant, allowing the delivery of a greater tidal volume for a given pressure
- the work of breathing is decreased
- oxygenation improves because there is a greater surface for gas exchange.

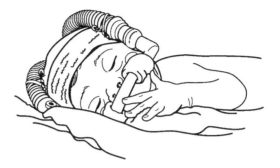

Application

The seal between the nasal prongs and the nares needs to be maintained in order for CPAP to remain constant throughout the respiratory cycle. The amount of positive pressure depends on whether the baby's mouth is open or closed.

For the purpose of stabilization, a gastric tube may be placed to decrease gastric distension. Although nasal CPAP by itself is not a contraindication to feeding, gastric distention may decrease feeding tolerance.

Equipment

- source of continuous positive pressure such as,
  - free flow of gas exiting through an underwater seal (bubble CPAP) or expiratory valve
  - CPAP demand flow system
  - mechanical ventilator on CPAP mode
  - flow inflating bagging system (short term)
- nasal prongs (the size depends on the size of the baby's nares)
- bonnet or hat (the size depends on the size of the baby's head)
- pulse oximeter.

Procedure

1. Position baby prone, lateral, or in a supported supine position.
2. Select the appropriate size nasal prongs and hat.
3. Place the hat on the baby's head and position the ties or Velcro straps as per the manufacturer's instructions. If the bonnet is too large it will slip down over the eyes, if it is too small it will ride upwards pulling the prongs hard against the nose.
4. Insert the nasal prongs into the nares. If there is blanching of the nares, smaller sized prongs are indicated in order to prevent excoriation. Ensure the prongs are kept off the nasal septum to avoid septal erosion.

5. Secure the CPAP tubing to the hat using the ties (Velcro straps).
6. Set the desired CPAP level (usually 5 cmH$_2$O), oxygen concentration, low pressure alarm, and apnea alarm.
7. Monitor respiratory frequency, work of breathing, oxygen requirements (pulse oximetry) and presence/absence of apnea before and after application.

Notes

CPAP can also be administered through an endotracheal tube whose tip is located in the posterior nasal pharynx (NPT – nasopharyngeal tube CPAP).

• NPT are prone to accumulation of secretions and mucous plugs not only in the tube but also around it; these secretions may not clear by just suctioning the NPT.

CPAP cannot be administered endotracheally in newborns as the size of the ETT is too small and the tube resistance too high for spontaneous unassisted breathing.

Bibliography

Hutchinson AA. Advances in nasal continuous positive airway pressure (NCPAP). Validation of an improved design. Neonatal Intensive Care. 1999; 12: 16-18.

Kamper J. Early nasal continuous positive airway pressure and minimal handling in the treatment of very-low-birth-weight infants. Biol Neonate. 1999; 76: S22-S28.

 Mechanical ventilation

Indications

• Apnea
• Existing or anticipated respiratory failure
• Prolonged or ineffective bag-and-mask ventilation
• Diaphragmatic hernia
• When paralysis or heavy sedation is required because of the clinical condition or to facilitate a surgical procedure or radiological examination

Principles

The goal of mechanical ventilation is to assist or take over the work of breathing, improve oxygenation, and restore/improve the respiratory component of the acid base balance system.

A mechanical ventilator is designed to mimic the rhythmic cycling of breathing.

- To achieve inspiration, a quantity of gas is delivered to the lungs (tidal volume $= V_T$) over a period of time (inspiratory time $= t_I$) using sufficient pressure to expand the alveoli (peak inspiratory pressure $=$ PIP).
- To allow expiration to occur, the ventilator provides time (expiratory time $= t_E$) for the chest wall and lung to recoil.
- To prevent the alveoli from collapsing, distending pressure in the airway should remain positive at end expiration (positive end-expiratory pressure $=$ PEEP).
- The number of breathing cycles per minute is known as the respiratory rate or frequency (f).
- Within a breathing cycle, the relative time spent in the process of inspiration versus expiration is known as the inspiration to expiration (I:E) ratio.

Application

Mechanical ventilators are classified on the basis of
1. how they cycle:
   - time cycled ventilators deliver a breath (cycle) on a set schedule
   - patient triggered (synchronized) ventilators deliver a breath when cued by the baby's attempt to inspire
   - combined modes: patient triggered with back up time cycling
2. how they limit the delivery of inspiratory gas:
   - volume-limiting ventilators deliver a set V_T (in mL) while the PIP varies from breath to breath depending on the "stiffness" of the lung
   - pressure-limiting ventilators deliver a set PIP (in cmH_2O) while the V_T varies depending on the "stiffness" of the lung

The degree of ease or difficulty to inflate the lungs is referred to as compliance. The stiffer or less compliant the respiratory system (lung plus chest wall), the greater the PIP required to deliver a V_T.

Compliance is expressed mathematically as: $\quad C \; = \; \dfrac{\text{change in volume}}{\text{change in pressure}}$

Clinical situations that can decrease compliance of the respiratory system include,
- respiratory distress syndrome
- meconium aspiration syndrome
- pneumothorax
- congenital thoracic dystrophies
- diaphragmatic hernia
- other space-occupying lesions in the chest.

Volume-limited ventilators have been less commonly used for newborn ventilation because accurate measurement of the small V_T characteristic of newborns is difficult. New technology has overcome this obstacle, but the resulting ventilators require a high level of training and expertise by the operator.

Equipment
- neonatal ventilator and circuit tubing
- heated humidifier with thermostat control in the circuit and sterile distilled water
- oxygen blender and air and oxygen hoses

Procedure
1. Connect the assembled circuit tubing and humidifier to the ventilator.
2. Connect the air and oxygen hoses to the corresponding wall outlets.
3. Set the initial ventilator parameters (pressure-limited, time-cycled ventilator) guided by the settings being used with the bagging system and information in the table below.

Parameter	Preterm baby or LBW baby with lung disease	Term baby with lung disease	Normal lungs (for example, apnea with no lung disease)
PIP (cmH_2O)	20	25	15
PEEP (cmH_2O)	5	5	3
f (per min)	40 to 60	40 to 60	30
t_I (sec)	0.3	0.4	0.3 to 0.4
t_E (sec)	0.7 to 1.2	0.6 to 1.1	1.6
% oxygen	100	100	30
Flow (L/min)	6 to 8	10 to 15	6 to 10

*The T_I is initially set at 0.25 to 0.30 sec for a patient-triggered ventilator

4. Check the integrity of the patient circuit by occluding the tubing, noting whether the PIP and PEEP settings are reached.
5. Turn on and set all ventilator alarms (low and high pressure, volume, apnea, and oxygen analyzer).
6. Connect the ventilator circuit to the endotracheal tube.
7. Immediately check the baby's response to the initial ventilator settings by assessing:
   - degree of chest expansion
   - quality of spontaneous respiratory efforts
   - quality of breath sounds bilaterally
   - oxygen saturation.
8. Adjust the ventilator settings according to the baby's response, or in discussion with a consultant or referral centre.

Clinical sign	Action
Poor chest expansion or decreased breath sounds	Increase PIP
Chest expansion visible and breath sounds heard	Maintain PIP
Chest appears to be expanding excessively	Decrease PIP
Chest expanding but baby fighting against the ventilator	Increase f Consider sedation

Adjust inspired oxygen concentration to maintain oxygen saturation 88 to 95%

9. After 15 to 30 minutes of mechanical ventilation, obtain arterial (P_{CO_2}, P_{O_2}, and pH) or venous/capillary (P_{CO_2} and pH) blood gas and adjust ventilation based on the results:

Pa_{CO_2} (cmH$_2$0)	Inspired O$_2$ < 50%	Inspired O$_2$ 50 to 60%	Inspired O$_2$ > 60%
> 50	Increase f, if pH < 7.25	Increase f, if pH < 7.25	Increase PIP
40-50	Maintain PIP and f	Maintain PIP and f	Increase PEEP
< 40	Decrease PIP	Decrease f	Increase PEEP

Notes

- The adjustment table above is for reference purposes only; guidance on actual adjustments should be sought from an experienced consultant physician, as required.
- The requirement for high PIPs should signal the need to rule out reversible causes of inadequate chest movement such as: atelectasis, endotracheal tube obstruction by secretions or pneumothorax.
- Optimal PEEP for a particular baby and disease condition increases compliance; however, either too much or too little PEEP can lead to decreased compliance.
- Fighting against the ventilator may indicate the need to adjust f in order to synchronize with the baby's intrinsic respiratory effort.
- Increasing t_I may improve chest expansion in larger babies and babies with stiff lungs. Enough expiratory time should be available to allow for a full expiration and prevent air trapping.
- The initial oxygen concentration may be high for babies with lung disease. Weaning should occur as quickly as possible while maintaining SpO_2 within the desired range.
- For new style patient-triggered ventilators, a flow sensor will need to be set up according to the manufacturer instructions.

Bibliography

American Physiological Society and ACCP-ATS Committee on Pulmonary Nomenclature. Respiratory Care standard abbreviations and symbols. Resp Care 1997; 42: 637-642.

Goldsmith JP, Karotkin EH. Assisted Ventilation of the Neonate. 4th ed. Philadelphia, PA: Saunders; 2003.

Pneumothorax – Chest transillumination

Indication

Acute respiratory deterioration, after ruling out mechanical causes (equipment malfunction, obstructed airway or endotracheal tube, or displaced endotracheal tube).

Goal

To attempt to detect pneumothorax at the bedside in the absence of a chest radiograph.

Principles

Free air in the thorax glows more intensely and over a larger area than air within the lung when a focused beam of high intensity light is applied directly to the chest wall in a darkened environment.

When a pneumothorax is present, a glow or halo is seen through the skin surrounding the light source. The glowing area may extend to the middle of the chest. The presence of a unilateral pneumothorax is more easily detected by the asymmetry of the rim of light between the two sides of the chest.

Transillumination works optimally in premature babies, whose skin is more translucent and chest wall is thinner than term babies.

Equipment

- a fiberoptic transilluminator to deliver focused, high intensity, cold light
- a blanket to shield surrounding ambient light

Procedure

1. Position the baby supine.
2. Darken the room as much as possible.
3. Observe the chest wall as you firmly place the fiberoptic light flat against the baby's chest at the following sites:
   - mid clavicular line above the nipple
   - mid axillary line.
4. Compare both sides of the chest.

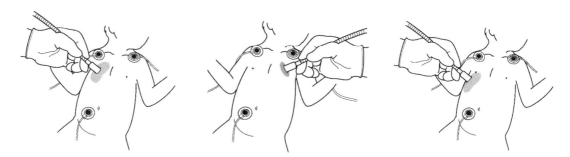

Transillumination at the level of the right mid-clavicular line (left panel) shows a large halo when compared to the identical position on the left mid-clavicular line (middle panel). A similar difference would be seen when comparing the glow effect at the level of the right anterior-axillary line (right panel) and the left anterior axillary line (not shown).

Notes

It is imperative that the two sides of the chest be compared to each other because the pattern of transillumination is affected by the size of the baby, thickness of skin, presence of edema, brightness of the light, and darkness of the room. A significant reproducible discrepancy between the two sides of the chest using a similar technique is consistent with the presence of a pneumothorax.

False negative chest transillumination can occur in the presence of a small unilateral pneumothorax or bilateral pneumothoraces due to a lack of difference in transillumination between the two sides of the chest.

Transillumination during needle aspiration of a pneumothorax is helpful to confirm drainage of air.

Other uses of transillumination include identification of blood vessels for IV insertion and peripheral arterial line.

Bibliography

Rennie JM, Roberton NRC. A Manual of Neonatal Intensive Care. London: Arnold, 2002

 Pneumothorax – Chest tube insertion

Indication

To drain a pneumothorax or pleural effusion

Principles

Gas or fluid within the pleural space constitutes a space occupying lesion, reduces the ability of the lung(s) to expand thereby limiting gas exchange, and impedes venous return to the heart.

A chest tube inserted between the ribs and connected to an underwater seal is an optimal way to drain free air, blood or fluid collected in the pleural cavity.

Application

Generally a chest tube to drain air should aim its tip towards the anterior pleural space, while one placed for drainage should aim its tip posteriorly. This is because air will generally rise to the anterior part of the chest while fluid will settle to the basal region. In a newborn, the point of entry to the chest may be similar in both cases.

Equipment

- sterile gloves and sterile drapes
- cleansing solution
- 1% lidocaine without epinephrine
- 1 mL syringe and 27G needles to infiltrate lidocaine
- sterile hemostats, straight and curved
- scalpel handle and blade
- one rubber tipped curved forceps for each chest tube inserted
- sterile gauze (4x4), transparent occlusive dressing, waterproof tape and scissors
- chest tube with trocar (sizes 8, 10 and 12 Fr)
- suture kit
- thoracic drainage system/underwater seal device

Procedure

1. Prepare the thoracic drainage system: fill the suction control chamber to the 5 to 10 cm mark and the water seal chamber to the 2 cm mark.
2. Connect the drainage system to wall suction.
3. Review chest radiograph to confirm location of the pneumothorax.
4. Ensure that cardiorespiratory monitoring is in place and that all leads and wires are removed from the area of chest tube insertion.
5. Position the baby with the affected side up at a 45 to 60 degree angle and a roll behind the back.
6. Raise the baby's arm on the affected side over his head.
7. Locate the 4th intercostal space in the mid to anterior axillary line (care should be taken to avoid the nipple area).
8. Cleanse the area with the cleansing solution and inject a small amount of 1% lidocaine intradermally and subcutaneously in the area of insertion just below the 4th intercostal space. Do not inject more than 0.3 mL/kg of the lidocaine preparation.
9. Mask, scrub and don sterile gown and gloves.
10. Cleanse the insertion site and surrounding area with cleansing solution; allow the solution to dry and wipe off with sterile water (cleansing solutions can be very irritating to immature skin).
11. Cover the area with sterile drapes.
12. Make a 0.5 cm long, transverse incision along the top of the 5th rib
13. Determine the necessary length of chest tube insertion (approximately the distance from skin incision to the sternum). Note this distance on the black markings of the chest tube.

14. Insert the chest tube using one of two techniques:

   Blunt dissection method:
   - Remove the trocar from the chest tube.
   - Take the small curved hemostat and insert the closed tip into the skin incision.
   - Bluntly dissect the subcutaneous tissue and slide the forceps over the 5th rib into the 4th intercostal space (always dissect just over the top of the rib to avoid hitting the intercostal artery which runs below each rib).
   - With the forceps, punch through into the pleural space. A gush of air may be heard or fluid may be released.
   - Carefully advance the chest tube (without the trocar) to the pre-determined distance, aiming anteriorly toward the baby's opposite shoulder.

   Using a trocar:
   - Take a small piece of gauze and place around chest tube (with trocar in place), securing it with the curved forceps at approximately 2 cm from the tip of the tube.
   - Take the small curved hemostat, insert the closed tip into the skin incision and bluntly dissect the subcutaneous tissue. Insert the chest tube with trocar and forceps guard into the tunnel created. The forceps clamped across the tube will prevent the tube from penetrating too far, with the trocar in place.
   - When the chest tube "pops" into the pleural space, release the clamp and remove the trocar from the tip of the chest tube.
   - Carefully advance the chest tube to the pre-determined distance, aiming anteriorly toward the baby's opposite shoulder. The trocar should be pulled out as the chest tube is advanced. Condensation will be noted within the chest tube as the trocar is removed.

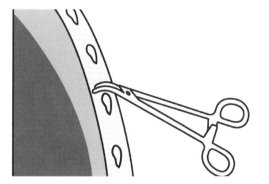 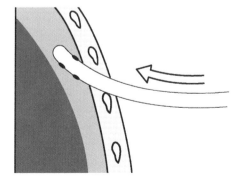

14. Have your assistant attach the chest tube to the drainage system tubing using a universal adapter. Tape the connection with waterproof tape.
15. Secure the chest tube with a suture through the skin and wrapped around the tube. Tape the tube in place ensuring no tension is placed on the chest tube while this is done. Cover the insertion site with a sterile dressing.
16. Turn on the wall suction until slow bubbling occurs in the suction control chamber.
17. Repeat a chest radiograph to ensure proper placement of chest tube and drainage of the pneumothorax or effusion.

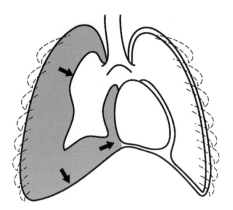 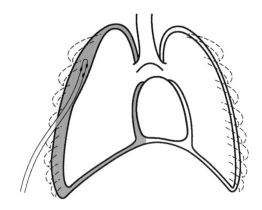

Potential complications

- Puncture of the lung.
- Bronchopleural fistula.
- Hemorrhage.
- Rupture of great vessels or cardiac chambers.
- Incorrect placement of chest tube outside the pleural cavity.

Notes

- Chest tubes should never be left open to the air. A Heimlich valve should be attached to the free end of the chest tube in the event that a closed system is not available or to transport of a baby with a chest tube in place. The valve will allow air and fluid to drain out of the tube and prevent air from being drawn into the pleural space on inspiration.
- Small spontaneous pneumothoraces occur in up to 3% of normal term babies; these often resolve without intervention.

Bibliography

MacDonald MG, Ramasethu J. Atlas of Procedures in Neonatology 3rd ed. Philadelphia, PA: Lippincott Williams & Wilkins; 2002.

Pneumothorax – Needle aspiration

Indication   Tension pneumothorax while preparing to insert a chest tube.

Goal   Needle aspiration of a pneumothorax is an emergency procedure used for the temporary, short-term decompression of a tension pneumothorax.

Principles   A tension pneumothorax occurs when there is a leak or tear in the lung causing a check valve effect, allowing air to enter the pleural space. The air trapped in the pleural space limits the ability of the ipsilateral lung to expand. A pneumothorax under tension will displace the mediastinum and impede the venous return and function of the contralateral lung. The tension pneumothorax must be relieved urgently for normal ventilation to resume.

The insertion of the needle into the affected side will allow for a temporary relief for the baby and clinical improvement. Transillumination may confirm drainage as will a rapid improvement in cardiorespiratory signs.

With the baby in the supine position, free air within the thorax will collect anteriorly. To aspirate air until a chest drain can be placed, place a butterfly needle anteriorly into the second intercostal space at the midclavicular line.

Air is withdrawn using a syringe with a three-way stopcock. The needle is then connected to extension tubing and a bottle of sterile water to maintain an underwater seal after the aspiration of air. Air under tension within the pleural space will continue to bubble out.

Although needle aspiration can be a very useful tool for the immediate relief of a tension pneumothorax, it is not appropriate for longer-term management. Care must be taken to ensure the needle does not travel further into the chest cavity and cause lung or vascular injury. Chest drain insertion should be considered in all babies who require needle aspiration of a pneumothorax.

Equipment
- sterile gloves and cleansing solution
- 1% lidocaine without epinephrine (time allows for local infiltration in most circumstances)
- 21 or 23 gauge butterfly needle or 18, 20 or 22 over needle cannula
- three way stopcock
- large syringe (20 ml)
- IV extension tubing
- small container of sterile water

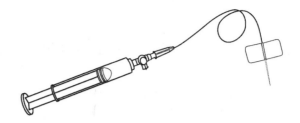

Procedure
1. Connect butterfly needle to a stopcock, and stopcock to syringe.
2. Connect IV extension tubing to the free port of the stopcock.
3. Position the baby supine.
4. Identify the second intercostal space in the midclavicular line on the side of the chest on which the pneumothorax is suspected and swab the area with an alcohol wipe.
5. Insert the butterfly needle perpendicular to the chest, just over the top of the rib.
6. Once the needle is in place, attach the stopcock with a syringe and tubing. Turn the stop cock to ensure the needle is open to the syringe.

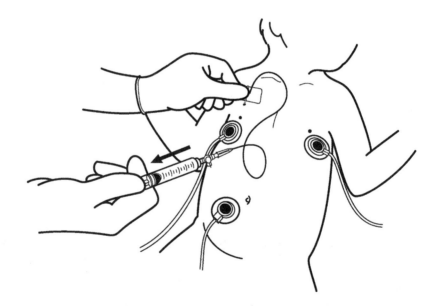

7. Pull back on the syringe to aspirate the air in the chest.
8. When the syringe is full, turn the stopcock off to the butterfly needle and empty the syringe.
9. These steps can be repeated until the baby improves or you are no longer aspirating air.
10. While awaiting chest tube placement, the needle can be held in place and attached to an underwater seal by placing the free end of the IV extension tubing in the water bottle.

Potential complications

- Puncture of inflated lung resulting in development of a pneumothorax.
- Puncture of vascular structure resulting in bleeding.
- Puncture of liver or bowel abnormally placed within the thorax (e.g. congenital diaphragmatic hernia).
- Caution: great care should be taken when expelling air from the syringe to ensure that this air is not being re-injected into the chest cavity.

Bibliography

Bowman ED, Levi SM, Presbury FE, McLean A.. Editors. Stabilization and transport of newborn infants and at-risk pregnancies. In Newborn Emergency Transport Service, 4th Edition, 1998.

MacDonald MG, Ramasethu J. Atlas of Procedures in Neonatology 3rd ed. Philadelphia, PA: Lippincott Williams & Wilkins; 2002.

 Pulse oximetry

Goal

- To determine the need for supplemental oxygen administration
- To evaluate the response to an oxygen enriched environment and adjust the concentration of inspired oxygen

Principles

The term oxygen saturation (SO_2) indicates the proportion of hemoglobin molecules that are carrying oxygen. Pulse oximetry estimates saturation by sensing the differences in the absorption spectra of oxygenated and reduced hemoglobin at the time of maximal arterial pulsation. This allows pulse oximetry to estimate the oxygen saturation of the arterial blood (SaO_2).

An oximeter probe contains two diodes that emit light at specific wavelengths, one in the red band and one in the infrared. The amount of light transmitted through the tissue (finger, toe, foot etc.) is measured with a photodectector. The red/infrared absorption ratio of these pulsatile differences computes the pulse oximeter reading (SpO_2).

The most common extrinsic factors that interfere with pulse oximetry include either too little signal (difficulty to identify the arterial pulsation due to improper probe placement or low perfusion) or too much noise (excessive motion artifact or ambient light). A pulse waveform display and audible pulse beep must coincide with each heartbeat to determine if the pulse oximeter is detecting valid pulses or interfering signals.

Intrinsic interference results from factors that affect the absorbance of light such as high concentration of circulating carboxyhemoglobin or methemoglobin.

Fetal hemoglobin has a greater affinity for oxygen than adult hemoglobin, thus it will become fully saturated at a lower PaO_2.

Equipment

- pulse oximeter with visual display, audible beep and alarm system
- pulse oximetry probe
- a method to secure the probe

Procedure

1. Assemble all the equipment and ensure normal functioning.
2. Pulse oximetry probes are either reusable or single patient use.
3. Attach the probe's sensor to the hand, foot or wrist of the baby.
4. Ensure the sensor is properly aligned with the light placed on one side of the tissue and the receiver (photodiode) on the opposite side. When alignment is poor the photodiode will not detect all the light transmitted through the tissue and the pulse oximeter will not function properly.
5. Secure the sensor in place, firmly but not tightly. Excessive pressure can impede the circulation and affect readings and/or result in tissue injury at the site. The sensor should be moved to a different site every six to eight hours.
6. Set the high and low alarm limits for SpO_2 and heart rate.
7. Ensure the pulse oximeter is detecting an adequate pulse by comparing the heart rate reported with the cardiorespiratory monitor. The heart rate detected should not differ by > 5 beats/minute.
8. Document the SpO_2, respiratory rate, heart rate, and state (for example, crying, sleeping, awake and quiet, feeding, and undergoing a procedure).
9. Ensure the target SpO_2 range is well documented. In general, the SpO_2 is maintained between 88 to 95%. Clinical condition, unit guidelines or physician choice may result in different targets.

Bibliography

Anderson CG, Benitz WE, Madan A. Retinopathy of prematurity and pulse oximetry: a national survey of recent practices. J Perinatol. 2004 Mar; 24(3): 164-8.

Clarke M. Oxygen saturation: what is the appropriate range in neonates? The Perinatal Newsletter 1996; 13(3): 3-4.

Salyer JW Neonatal and pediatric pulse oximetry. Respir Care. 2003 Apr; 48(4): 386-96.

Appendix D
Interpretation of investigations

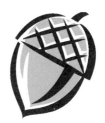

 The three investigations discussed in this Appendix are:
1. Blood gases
2. Complete blood count and differential
3. Chest radiographs

Blood gas interpretation

Goals
To determine the ventilation, oxygenation, and acid-base status to aid in diagnosis and treatment.

Principles
pH estimates the blood total acid load, which mostly reflects dissolved CO_2 but may also include metabolic acids such as lactic acid.

P_{CO_2} indicates how well the lung is removing CO_2 from the blood (ventilation).

Pa_{O_2} (arterial P_{O_2}) indicates how well the lung is transferring oxygen to the blood (oxygenation) in relation to % inspired oxygen.

Base deficit, BD, estimates how much metabolic acid is present in the blood. Base excess (BE), the negative value of BD, and bicarbonate are also used to describe the acid-base status.

The presence of an acidosis with pH ≤ 7.25 and $P_{CO_2} \geq 55$ is an indication of poor ventilation (respiratory acidosis).

Arterial, capillary or venous samples are nearly equally useful for the determination of ventilation, pH and base deficit.

Sp_{O_2} can be used as a continuous estimate of oxygenation.

Application
Arterial, venous or capillary blood samples can be used for blood gas analysis; the choice depends on the ability to obtain a sample as well as the primary purpose of the analysis. Arterial blood gas sampling is necessary when a P_{O_2} value is required. Capillary and venous samples are never appropriate for assessment of P_{O_2}. The use of pulse oximetry to monitor oxygen saturation in babies has decreased the need to determine arterial P_{O_2} in order to assess oxygenation.

If arterial sampling is not possible or desirable, capillary sampling is most commonly used in the newborn. The accuracy of capillary blood gas pH depends on good perfusion at the site of sampling (the heel is used in babies). A sample taken from a poorly perfused area results in a false low pH. Warming the heel to promote vasodilatation and arterial inflow (arterialization) can minimize this effect. In situations where peripheral perfusion is poor, venous gases will give a better estimate of acid base status.

The result for each parameter may be either increased, decreased or within a range of generally accepted normal values:

	Decreased	Normal	Increased
pH	< 7.35 acidosis	7.35 to 7.45	> 7.45 alkalosis
P_{CO_2}	< 35mmHg hypocapnia respiratory alkalosis hyperventilation	35 to 45 mmHg	> 45mmHg hypercapnia respiratory acidosis hypoventilation
Base deficit	< 0 mmol/L metabolic alkalosis too much buffer	0 to 4	> 4 mmol/L metabolic acidosis too little buffer
Pa_{O_2}	< 50mmHg hypoxemia	50 to 80 mmHg	> 80mmHg hyperoxia

Blood gases are considered satisfactory in acute respiratory illness when the pH is 7.25 to 7.40 and the P_{CO_2} 45 to 55 mmHg.

Interpretation

Step One: determine the pH as normal, decreased (acidosis) or increased (alkalosis).

Step Two: determine the primary type of acidosis or alkalosis.

pH	P_{CO_2}	Base deficit	Interpretation
Decreased	Increased	Normal	Respiratory acidosis
Decreased	Normal	Increased	Metabolic acidosis
Increased	Decreased	Normal	Respiratory alkalosis
Increased	Normal	Decreased	Metabolic alkalosis

Step Three: assess arterial oxygenation to classify the P_{O_2} as normal, increased (hyperoxia), or decreased (hypoxemia).

Notes

- Most acid-base problems in babies result from inadequate lung function, leading to respiratory acidosis.
- If there is metabolic acidosis, the goal is to support the system that may be causing it. Most often it is due to circulatory insufficiency.
- Interpretation of abnormal blood gases and decisions regarding corrective measures should be performed by experienced care providers, or in consultation with referral centers.

> o   Although treatment generally aims for the accepted normal range, the desired P_{CO_2} and Pa_{O_2} may be higher or lower depending on the specific clinical situation.

Bibliography

Brouillette RT, Waxman DH. Evaluation of the newborn's blood gas status. Clin Chem 1997;43:215-221.

Shapiro BA, Penuzzi WT, Templin R. Clinical Application of Blood Gases. 5th ed. Toronto, Ont: Mosby; 1994.

 Complete blood count and differential interpretation

Indications

A hemoglobin/hematocrit should be checked in babies who are pale or plethoric or when blood loss is suspected.

A complete blood count (CBC) with white count and differential should be done when infection is suspected.

A platelet count should be done when bleeding, clotting, or infection are being investigated.

Goals

To evaluate hematologic indices in at-risk or unwell babies.

Principles

CBC consists of: red and white blood cells, and platelets.
- Red blood cells contain hemoglobin which carries 97 to 98% of the oxygen contained in the blood. The hemoglobin concentration measures the amount of hemoglobin contained in each volume of blood. The hematocrit measures the relative volume of red cells in a spun sample of whole blood.
- White blood cells are part of the body's immune system.
- Platelets are components that participate in clotting.

Application

Arterial, venous or capillary blood samples can be used for a CBC analysis. The hematocrit is higher in capillary samples than in venous or arterial blood.

Normal ranges for term babies during the first 12 hours of life (capillary samples)

	Mean value ± SD	Range
Hemoglobin (g/L)	193 ± 22	150 to 220
Hematocrit (%)	61.0 ± 7.4	45 to 66
Total white blood cell count (WBC) x 10^9/L	24.0 ± 6.1	16.2 to 31.5
Total neutrophil count x 10^9/L	15.6 ± 4.7	6.0 to 26.0
Immature neutrophil count (bands) x 10^9/L	2.5 ± 1.8	0.7 to 4.3
Immature to total neutrophil (I/T) ratio	0.16 ± 0.10	0.05 to 0.27
Platelets x 10^9/L		150 to 350

Interpretation

Hemoglobin/hematocrit:

These vary with postnatal age and gestational age.
- The hemoglobin and hematocrit normally increase in the first 12 hours due to hemoconcentration and then gradually decline. By four weeks of life, the hemoglobin in a term baby drops to a mean of 110 g/L (as low as 70 g/L in low birth weight babies).
- Preterm babies have lower hemoglobin at birth.
  - The hemoglobin in g/L for babies born at 23 to 31 weeks gestation on the first day of life ranges from 145 ± 16 to 162 ± 17 (mean ± SD).
  - The corresponding hematocrit (%) is 43.5 ± 4.2 to 48.0 ± 5.0.

White blood cell count:

The WBC count also increases over the first 12 hours and then declines. The normal range in the first month of life is 5 to 15 x 10^9/L. During the first few days of life, WBC counts obtained during CBC analysis must be based on manual examination as automated counts are unreliable.

In babies with systemic bacterial infection, the WBC may be increased, decreased, or normal. The neutrophil count may be increased, decreased or show an increased number of immature neutrophils or bands (left shift). A left shift is reflected by an increase in the immature to total (I/T) neutrophil ratio.

Findings suggestive of a bacterial infection include:
- leucopenia (< 5 x 10^9/L)
- neutropenia (< 2 x 10^9/L)
  - neutropenia in newborns is highly significant and may be the first clue to infection.
- I/T ratio > 0.25
- thrombocytopenia (< 100 x 10^9/L) is highly significant.

Platelets:

The bleeding time is prolonged in thrombocytopenic babies, particularly in those with platelet counts below $100 \times 10^9/\text{L}$. Thrombocytopenia can result from many causes, including sepsis, coagulation disorders, and chronic intrauterine TORCH infection.

Warning!

The WBC and differential count is not a reliable predictor of bacterial sepsis.
- The decision to treat sepsis in sick babies is a clinical one.
- Do not delay antibiotic treatment while waiting for the results of a manual WBC, differential count, band count or I/T ratio.

Notes

The interpretation of a CBC should take into account the baby's clinical circumstances. For example,
- stress can cause an increase in the number of immature white cells (left shift)
- a baby born to a mother with HELLP syndrome (hemolysis, elevated liver enzymes, low platelets), or with marked intrauterine growth restriction may have neutropenia and thrombocytopenia for several days.

Bibliography

Alur P, Devapatla SS, Super DM, Danish E, Stern T, Inagandla R, Moore JJ. Impact of race and gestational age on red blood cell indices in very low birth weight infants. Pediatrics 2000; 106: 306-10.

Fanaroff AA, Martin RJ, Eds. Neonatal-perinatal medicine: Diseases of the fetus and infant, 7th Ed. 2002. Mosby Inc.

Manroe BL, Weinberg AG, Rosenfeld CR, Browne R. The neonatal blood count in health and disease: I. Reference values for neutrophilic cells. J Pediatr 1979; 95: 89-98.

Mouzinho A, Rosenfeld CR, Sanchez PJ, Risser R. Revised reference ranges for circulation neutrophils in very-low-birth-weight infants. Pediatr 1994; 94: 76-82.

 Chest radiograph interpretation

Goal

To assist in the diagnosis of respiratory and cardiac conditions.

Principles

Radiographic film, before an image is taken, is transparent and appears white on a view box. When a radiograph is taken, x-rays pass through the intervening tissue to reach the film (photographic plate). The more x-rays that are able to pass through, the darker the area will appear on the film. If an object has little density, such as an aereated lung, most of the X-ray beam will pass to the film and the image will appear black. If an object is dense, such as a bone, less X-rays reach the film and the image will appear white.

Application

Anatomic structures seen on a radiograph can be identified by their characteristic density. There are five radiographic densities in order of increasing brightness: air, fat, fluid, bone, and metal. The lungs appear dark ('air density') because they are filled with air whereas the heart, which is largely composed of water, is brighter than the lungs ('fluid density').

Interpretation

1. Check the labels for the baby's name, date and time taken, and R/L markers.
2. Assess the general quality of the radiograph.
   - if the image is centered (medial ends of the clavicles should be equidistant from the spinous processes of the vertebrae)
   - the penetration or exposure of the entire film (over- or under-exposed)
3. Identify extra objects on the radiograph.
   - ECG leads
   - endotracheal tube: note placement and position of the tip of the tube in relation to the carina
   - UA or UV line: note placement and location of the catheter tip
   - oro- or nasogastric/chest tubes: note placement and location of the catheter tip
4. Identify the anatomic structures beginning from the centre of the radiograph and working toward the edges.
5. Look for abnormalities in each of the following zones:
   - mediastinum
     o trachea, left/right mainstem bronchi
     o aortic arch and descending aorta
     o left/right pulmonary arteries
     o heart shadow size and shape, and the right and left heart borders (the ratio of the heart diameter to thoracic diameter is normally < 0.6)
     o thymus
     o esophagus (not normally seen unless containing a radio-opaque oro- or nasogastric tube)
   - lung fields
     o lung tissue should fully extend to the chest wall
     o most conditions affecting the lung tissue displace the air in the alveoli, resulting in abnormalities often described as streaky, grainy, patchy, bubbly, fluffy, hazy, dotty, white-out
     o horizontal fissure separating the right upper and middle lobes
     o pulmonary vascular pattern
   - chest wall
     o bones, including clavicles and twelve pairs of ribs
     o soft tissues

- diaphragms
  - right hemi-diaphragm is upwardly displaced by the liver
  - on inspiration, both hemi-diaphragms usually located at the level of the 9th rib
  - costophrenic angles, should appear sharply defined
  - check under the diaphragm for free air
- upper abdomen
  - position of the stomach bubble

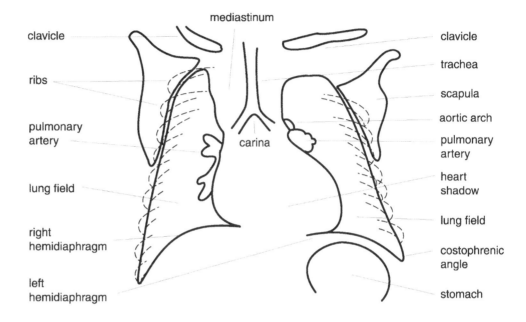

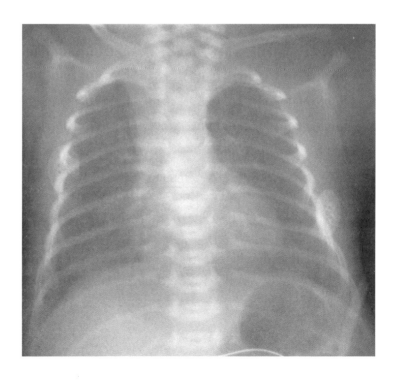

Notes

The 3 most common observations:
1. abnormal lung markings:
   - absent (pneumothorax)
   - reduced (cyanotic congenital heart disease)
   - increased (pulmonary edema)
   - diffuse (RDS)
   - focal (pneumonia)
2. abnormal heart shape or size
   - small (hypovolemia)
   - normal
   - large (cardiac disease)
3. placement of ETT and lines

For examples of radiographs of common respiratory and cardiac conditions, please refer to the Respiratory Chapter (pages 3-12 to 25) and Cardiovascular Chapter (pages 4-12 to 13).

Bibliography

Banerjee A. Radiology made easy. London: Greenwich Medical Media Ltd., 2000.

Ouellette H, Tétreault P. Clinical Radiology made ridiculously simple. Miami: Medmaster Inc., 2002.

Appendix E
Medications

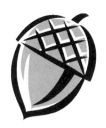

 The medications discussed in this Appendix are:
1. Ampicillin
2. Cefotaxime
3. Cloxacillin
4. Dopamine
5. Fentanyl
6. Gentamicin
7. Morphine
8. Penicillin G
9. Phenobarbital
10. Phenytoin
11. Premedication prior to intubation
12. Prostaglandin E_1
13. Surfactant
14. Vancomycin

Explanatory notes

- Renal function and clearance of antibiotics are influenced both by the gestational age (GA) and the postnatal age. Therefore, in infants more than 7 days old, it might be useful to consider the postconceptional age (PCA) in the dosing schedule.

- In babies whose PCA is not readily known, the dosing schedule can be based on the body weight categories, which approximate the PCA.

Bibliography

Bradley JS, Nelson JD, eds. Nelson's Pocket Book of Pediatric Antimicrobial Therapy. 15th Ed. Lippincott, Williams and Wilkins, 2002-2003.

Smyth J, McDougal A, Vanderpas E, eds. Neonatal Drug Dosage Guidelines. Vancouver, BC: Children's and Women's Health Centre of British Columbia, 2004.

Young TE, Mangum B. Neofax 2004. 1 7th Ed. Raleigh NC: Acorn Publishing Inc, 2004.

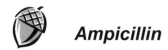 ***Ampicillin***

A semisynthetic penicillin with broad spectrum bactericidal action

Indication Treatment of infection with group B *streptococcus*, *Listeria monocytogenes*, and susceptible *E. coli* species.

Supplied Powder for injection in 250 mg and 500 mg vials – reconstitute using sterile water for injection.

Recommended concentration for IV infusion is 50 mg/mL. Maximum concentration for IV infusion is 100 mg/mL.

Administration IV administration: slow IV push over 5 minutes not to exceed a rate of 100 mg/minute.

IV administration preferred but may be given IM.

Dose 50 mg/kg/dose
100 mg/kg/dose for meningitis

PCA (weeks)	Use body weight (g) if PCA not known	Postnatal (days)	Interval (hours)
≤29	< 1200	0 to 28 > 28	q12h q6h
30 to 36	1200 to 2000	0 to 7 8 to 28 > 28	q12h q8h q6h
≥ 37	> 2000	0 to 7 > 7	q8h q6h

Y-site injection compatibility D2/3 and 1/3NS, D5%W, D10%W, 0.9%NS, 0.45%NS, calcium gluconate, heparin, hydrocortisone, magnesium sulfate, morphine, potassium chloride.

Y-site injection incompatibility Amikacin, dopamine, epinephrine, gentamicin, midazolam, parenteral nutrition solutions, sodium bicarbonate, tobramycin.

Flush IV line or allow time for IV line to clear between medication administrations.

Adverse effects / precautions
- Hypersensitivity reactions are rare in neonates.
- Very large doses may result in seizures.

Monitoring   With prolonged therapy, monitor renal, hepatic, and hematologic function.

Notes
- Clearance is primarily by the renal route and increases with postnatal age.
- Increase dosing interval in severe renal failure.
- Do not mix ampicillin and aminoglycosides (amikacin, gentamicin and tobramycin) in the same line or administer concurrently. Flush line between medications or separate administration times by a least 1 hour.

 ### *Cefotaxime*

A preferred third generation cephalosporin in neonates

Indication   Treatment of neonatal sepsis and meningitis caused by susceptible gram negative organisms.

Supplied   Powder for injection in 500 mg vials - reconstitute using sterile water for injection.

Recommended concentration for IV infusion is 100 mg/mL.

Administration   IV infusion over 20 minutes

Dose   50 mg/kg/dose

PCA (weeks)	Use body weight (g) if PCA not known	Postnatal (days)	Interval (hours)
≤29	< 1200	0 to 28 > 28	q12h q8h
30 to 36	1200 to 2000	0 to 7 > 7	q12h q8h
≥ 37	> 2000	0 to 7 > 7	q12h q8h

Y-site injection compatibility   D2/3 and 1/3NS, D5%W, D10%W, 0.9% NS, 0.45% NS, acyclovir, heparin, magnesium sulfate, metronidazole, morphine, parenteral nutrition solutions.

Y-site injection incompatibility

Sodium bicarbonate, vancomycin.

Flush IV line or allow time for IV line to clear between medication administrations.

Adverse effects / precautions

- Rare
- Resistance may develop during treatment for some gram negative infections (e.g. those caused by Enterbacter species)

Monitoring

With prolonged therapy, monitor renal, hepatic, and hematologic function.

Notes

- Increase dosing interval in severe renal impairment.
- Cefotaxime may be substituted for an aminoglycoside (e.g. gentamicin) for broad spectrum coverage in the first week of life, when renal function/urine output is a concern or the inability to monitor drug levels.
- Do not mix cefotaxime and vancomycin in the same line or administer concurrently. Flush line between medications or separate administration times by a least 1 hour.

 Cloxacillin

A penicillinase-resistant penicillin

Indication

Treatment of neonatal infections caused by penicillinase producing staphylocooci (e.g. staphylococcus aureus).

Supplied

Powder for injection in 500 mg vial – reconstitute using sterile water for injection.

Reccomended concentration for IV infusion is 100 mg/mL.

Administration

IV infusion over 20 minutes or IM.

Dose

25 mg/kg
50 mg/kg/dose for meningitis

PCA (weeks)	Use body weight (g) if PCA not known	Postnatal (days)	Interval (hours)
≤29	< 1200	0 to 28 > 28	q12h q6h
30 to 36	1200 to 2000	0 to 7 8 to 28 > 28	q12h q8h q6h
≥ 37	> 2000	0 to 7 > 7	q8h q6h

Y-site Injection compatibility

D2/3 and 1/3NS, D5%W, D10%W, 0.9%NS, 0.45%NS, calcium gluconate, heparin, midazolam, morphine, parenteral nutrition solutions, potassium chloride.

Y-site injection incompatibility

Amikacin, gentamicin, tobramcyin, sodium bicarbonate.

Flush IV line or allow time for IV line to clear between medication administrations.

Adverse effects / precautions

- Phlebitis
- Tissue irritation (IM route not recommended)
- Interstitial nephritis
- Hypersensitivity rash

Monitoring

Periodic CBC, platelet count, urinalysis, urea, serum creatinine and liver enzymes.

Notes

- Increase dosing interval in severe renal impairment.
- Do not mix cloxacillin and aminoglycosides (amikacin, gentamicin and tobramycin) in the same line or administer concurrently. Flush line between medications or separate administration times by a least 1 hour.

 Dopamine

A sympathomimetic medication

Dose-dependent pharmacological action:

- renal vasodilation   2 to 4 mcg/kg/minute
- beta-1 inotropic effect   5 to10 mcg/kg/minute
- alpha vasoconstrictive effect   > 10 mcg/kg/minute

In neonates, dopamine is primarily used to increase blood pressure by increasing systemic vascular resistance through peripheral vasoconstriction.[1]

Indication

Treatment of hypotension.

If the cause of hypotension is due to hypovolemia, volume expansion should be given to correct the hypovolemia first before starting dopamine therapy.

Supplied

200 mg in 5 mL = 40 mg/mL vials for injection.

Dopamine must be diluted prior to use. Maximum concentration should not exceed 3.2 mg/mL. Concentrations as high as 6 mg/mL have been used safely via central lines.

Administration

Continuous IV infusion by syringe pump.

Central line prefered as it provides a secure line and avoids the complications associated with peripheral line extravasation.

Dose

Initial dose: 2 to 5 mcg/kg/minute

Maintenance infusion: Titrate gradually up to a maximum of 20 mcg/kg/minute, balancing desired cardiac/vascular effects (blood pressure and heart rate) with adverse effects.

Quick calculation for dopamine infusion where 1 mL/hr = 10 mcg/kg/minute

15 x weight (kg) = # mg dopamine to be added to IV fluid to make total volume of 25 mL

30 x weight (kg) = # mg dopamine to be added to IV fluid to make total volume of 50 mL

60 x weight (kg) = # mg dopamine to be added to IV fluid to make total volume of 100 mL

Example: for a 3 kg baby who is to receive 10 mcg/kg/minute dopamine add 45 mg (15 x 3 kg) to IV fluid to make a total volume of 25 ml.

Y-site injection compatibility

D2/3 and 1/3NS, D5%W, D10%W, 0.9%NS, 0.45%NS, alprostadil (PGE₁), calcium chloride, calcium gluconate, dobutamine, epinephrine, fat emulsion 20%, fentanyl, heparin, isoproterenol, magnesium sulfate, midazolam, milrinone, morphine, pancuronium, parenteral nutrition solutions (amino acid/dextrose), potassium chloride, ranitidine.

---

[1] Zhang J, Penny DJ, Kim NS, Yu VYH, and Smolich, JJ. Mechanisms of blood pressure increase induced by dopamine in hypotensive preterm neonates. Arch. Dis. Child. Fetal Neonatal Ed. 1999; 81: F99-F104.

Y-site injection incompatibility

Amphotericin B, sodium bicarbonate, THAM (tromethamine).

Flush IV line or allow time for IV line to clear between medication administrations.

Adverse effects / precautions

- Tachycardia and arrhythmias
- Increased pulmonary artery pressure
- Tissue sloughing following extravasation
- Peripheral circulatory impairment

Monitoring

- Heart rate and rhythm
- Clinical assessment of circulation (skin color, capillary refill time, temperature of extremities, pulses, and blood pressure, preferably via an arterial line)
- Check IV site for signs of extravasation to prevent tissue sloughing

Notes

- Admixtures exhibiting color change should not be used.
- Use high doses with caution in persistent pulmonary hypertension of the newborn.
- If infused peripherally, white tracking (due to peripheral vasoconstriction) may appear along the course of the vein.
- The commercial preparation of dopamine contains sodium bisulfite, which has been reported to cause anaphylaxis.
- Some infusion pumps, when run at rates < 0.5 mL/hr, deliver an undesirable pulsatile flow instead of a steady flow of fluid. This is a function of syringe size (larger syringe has more variability due to stiction) and drug concentration. Avoid the use of syringes > 30 mL and high drug concentrations.

 Fentanyl

A narcotic analgesic.

Indications

Pain management
Premedication for noxious procedures

Supplied

50 mcg/mL

Route

IV

Dose

- Sedation: 1 to 2 mcg/kg/dose slow IV push (~ 3 minute) q2 to 4 hour prn
- Analgesia: 3 to 5 mcg/kg/dose slow IV push (~ 3 to 5 minute) q2 to 4 hour prn
- Continuous infusion: 1 to 4 mcg/kg/hour (usually 2 mcg/kg/hour) preceded by a loading dose of 3 to 5 mcg/kg slow IV push

Y-site injection compatibility

D2/3 and 1/3NS, D5%W, D10%W, 0.9%NS, 0.45%NS, amikacin, atropine, caffeine citrate, calcium chloride, calcium gluconate, cefazolin, cefotaxime, cefoxitin, ceftazidime, cefuroxime, chloramphenicol, cloxacillin, clindamycin, dexamethasone, digoxin, dobutamine, dopamine, epinephrine, erythropoietin, erythromycin, esmolol, fluconazole, furosemide, ganciclovir, gentamicin, heparin, hydrocortisone, indomethacin, insulin, isoproterenol, linezolid, magnesium sulfate, metronidazole, midazolam, milrinone, morphine sulfate, naloxone, pancuronium, penicillin G,phenobarbital, piperacillin, potassium chloride, pyridoxine, rantitidine, sodium bicarbonate, THAM (tromethamine), tobramcyin, vancomcyin.

Y-site injection incompatibility

Amphotericin B, ampicillin, hydralazine, phenytoin.

Flush IV line or allow time for IV line to clear between medication administrations.

Adverse effects / precautions

- Respiratory depression, apnea
- Chest wall rigidity, especially with rapid administration and large dose, reversible with naloxone
- Bradycardia with rapid IV injection
- Decreased GI motility (delayed gastric emptying, constipation, ileus)
- Urinary retention

Resuscitation equipment including a suction apparatus, mask, self-inflating bag and source of oxygen must be immediately available.

The narcotic antagonist naloxone (Narcan®) can be used to reverse respiratory depression associated with fentanyl use, but it should **never** be given to babies with neonatal abstinence syndrome or babies born to mothers with long-term history of narcotic use. Naloxone dose is 0.1 mg/kg IV push, IM or ET. May repeat in 3 to 5 minutes if no response.

Monitoring

- Monitor respiratory and cardiovascular status, urine output, and level of sedation/pain relief.
- Observe for abdominal distention and auscultate for bowel sounds.

Notes
- Fentanyl is more potent than morphine (by as much as 50 to 100 times). Clinically a ratio of 10: 1 (morphine: fentanyl) is generally used for dose conversion (i.e. 10 mcg morphine = 1 mcg fentanyl).
- Fentanyl is the preferred opioid analgesic for babies with compromised cardiovascular function or at risk of persistent pulmonary hypertension of the newborn.

 Gentamicin

An aminoglycoside antibiotic.

Indication   Treatment of infection with aerobic gram-negative bacilli, including *Pseudomonas*, *Klebsiella*, *E. coli*, *Proteus*, and *Serratia*..

Supplied   Injectable solution. Pediatric solution available as 10 mg/mL (recommended)

Administration   IV infusion over 30 minutes
May be given IM

Dose   2.5 mg/kg/dose

PCA (weeks)	Postnatal age (days)	Interval (hours)
< 28	ALL	q24h
28 to 34	ALL	q18h
≥ 35	0 to 7 > 7	q12h q8h

Extended interval dosing   Alternatively, some centers use dose extended interval dosing. There is limited information available for the neonatal population. One reference suggests the following guidelines.[2]

[2] Young TE, Mangum B. Neofax 2004. 1 7th Ed. Raleigh NC: Acorn Publishing Inc, 2004.

PCA (weeks)	Postnatal age (days)	Dose (mg/kg/dose)	Interval (hours)
≤29	0 to 7	5	q48h
	8 to 28	4	q36h
	≥ 29	4	q24
30 to 34	0 to 7	4.5	q36h
	≥ 8	4	q24h
≥ 35	ALL	4	q24h

Y-site injection compatiblity

D2/3 and 1/3NS, D5%W, D10%W, 0.9%NS, 0.45%NS, alprostadil (PGE₁), calcium gluconate, heparin (low concentrations 0.5 to 1 unit/ml), fat emulsion 20%, magnesium sulfate, morphine, pancuronium, parenteral nutrition solutions (amino acid/dextrose), ranitidine.

Y-site injection incompatibility

Ampicillin, amphotericin B, cloxacillin, furosemide, penicillin G, piperacillin. Flush IV line or allow time for IV line to clear between medication administrations.

Adverse effects / precautions

- Renal toxicity
  - dosage must be adjusted in renal insufficiency
  - contraindicated in renal failure
- Vestibular and/or ototoxicity
- Prolonged muscle paralysis when used in conjunction with neuromuscular blocking agents
- Neuromuscular weakness when given to patients with elevated magnesium or pre-existing conditions that depress neuromuscular transmission

Monitoring

Follow serum levels at steady state (usually on day 3 of therapy) in babies without clinical evidence of renal disease. In babies with asphyxia, severe oliguria or increased creatinine, serum concentration measurements should be obtained early and the dosage interval adjusted empirically until serum drug concentration results are available.

Therapeutic serum concentration:
- peak 5 to 10 mcg/mL: draw sample 30 minutes after end of infusion or one hour after IM injection
- trough 0.5 to 1 mcg/mL: draw sample 60 minutes before dose due

If the extended interval dosing is used, peak level may be measured after the first dose, and trough level before the second dose.

Blood samples should be spun and refrigerated or frozen as soon as possible after collection.

Assess renal function.

Notes
- IM injection associated with variable absorption, especially in the very small babies.
- Serum half-life is prolonged in premature and asphyxiated newborns. Clearance is also decreased in babies with a PDA treated with indomethacin.
- Do not mix ampicillin and gentamicin in the same line or administer concurrently. Flush line between medications or separate administration times by a least 1 hour.

 Morphine

A narcotic analgesic.

Indications
- Pain management
- Premedication for noxious procedures
- Treatment of opioid withdrawal and abstinence

Supplied
Injectable solution - 2 mg/mL, 10 mg/mL, 15 mg/ml
Oral solution - 1 mg/mL

Administration
IV, IM, SC, or PO

Dose
Pain management:
- 0.05 to 0.2 mg/kg/dose IV over at least 5 minutes q3 to 4 hours prn
- Same dose may be given IM or SC
- Continuous IV infusion 0.01 to 0.02 mg/kg/hour

Neonatal narcotic abstinence treatment:
- Dosage and weaning schedules vary. Starting dose: 0.03 mg/kg PO q3h. Round dose to the nearest 0.01 mL of oral solution.
- Review dose daily and recalculate based on daily weight, ongoing symptoms, and a weaning schedule.

Y-site injection compatibility
D2/3 and 1/3NS, D5%W, D10%W, 0.9%NS, 0.45%NS, alprostadil (PGE$_1$), amikacin, atropine, caffeine citrate, calcium chloride, calcium gluconate,

cefazolin, cefotaxime, cefoxitin, ceftazidime, cefuroxime, chloramphenicol, clindamcyin, cloxacillin, dexamethasone, digoxin, dobutamine, dopamine, epinephrine, erythropoietin, erythromycin, esmolol, fat emulsion 20%, fentanyl, fluconazole, furosemide, gentamicin, heparin, hydrocortisone, insulin, isoproterenol, magnesium sulfate, midazolam, naloxone, pancuronium, parenteral nutrition solutions (amino acid/dextrose), penicillin G, piperacillin, potassium chloride, pyridoxine, ranitidine, sodium bicarbonate, THAM (tromethamine), tobramcyin, vancomycin.

Y-Site Injection incompatibility

Amphotericin B, ampicillin, ganciclovir, hydralazine, indomethacin, pentobarbital, phenytoin.

Flush IV line or allow time for IV line to clear between medication administrations.

Adverse effects / precautions

- Respiratory depression, apnea
- Hypotension secondary to histamine release
- Decreased GI motility (delayed gastric emptying, constipation, ileus)
- Urinary retention

Resuscitation equipment including a suction apparatus, mask, self-inflating bag and source of oxygen must be immediately available.

The narcotic antagonist naloxone (Narcan®) can be used to reverse respiratory depression associated with morphine use, but it should **never** be given to babies with abstinence syndrome or babies born to mothers with long-term history of narcotic use. Naloxone dose is 0.1 mg/kg IV push, IM or ET. May repeat in 3 to 5 minutes if no response.

Monitoring

- Monitor respiratory and cardiovascular status, urine output, and level of sedation/pain relief.
- Observe for abdominal distention and auscultate for bowel sounds.

Notes

The injectable formulation of morphine contains sodium metabisulfite, which has been reported to cause anaphylaxis. Preservative-free formulations are available, but they are for epidural use and are more expensive.

Bibliography

British Columbia Reproductive Care Program: Substance Use Guideline 4b: Perinatal opioid exposure, care of the newborn. Vancouver, Children's and Women's Health Centre of British Columbia, 1999.

Neonatal drug withdrawal. American Academy of Pediatrics Committee on Drugs. Pediatrics 1998 Jun; 101(6): 1079-88.

Penicillin G

A bactericidal antibiotic.

Indication   Treatment of Group B streptococcal infections, congenital syphilis

Supplied   Use only aqueous crystalline penicillin G for IV administration.

Powder for injection as Pencillin G sodium 1 million unit vial – reconstitute using sterile water for injection.

Recommended concentration for IV infusion is 100,000 IU/mL.

Administration   IV infusion over 20 minutes or IM

Dose   25,000 to 50,000 IU/kg/dose
50,000 IU/kg/dose for meningitis

PCA (weeks)	Use body weight (g) if PCA not known	Postnatal age (days)	Interval (hours)
≤29	< 1200	0 to 28 > 28	q12h q6h
30 to 36	1200 to 2000	0 to 7 8 to 28 > 28	q12h q8h q6h
≥ 37	> 2000	0 to 7 > 7	q8h q6h

Y-site injection compatibility   D2/3 and 1/3NS, D5%W, D10%W, 0.9%NS, 0.45%NS, alprostadil (PGE$_1$), calcium chloride, calcium gluconate, fluconazole, furosemide, heparin, magnesium sulfate, morphine, parenteral nutrition solutions (amino acid/dextrose), potassium chloride, ranitidine.

Y-site injection incompatibility   Aminoglycoside antibiotics, amphotericin B, caffeine citrate.

Flush IV line or allow time for IV to clear between medication administrations.

Adverse effects / precautions   Hypersensitivity has not been seen in neonates.

Notes
- Increase dosing interval in severe renal impairment.
- Do not mix Penicillin G and aminoglycosides (amikacin, gentamicin and tobramycin) in the same line or administer concurrently. Flush line between medications or separate administration times by a least 1 hour.

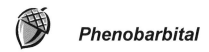 *Phenobarbital*

A barbiturate anticonvulsant

Indication
Neonatal seizures
Sedation for neonatal abstinence syndrome

Supplied
Injectable: Solution 30 mg/mL. Use within 30 minutes of opening the vial.
Oral: Elixir 5 mg/mL

Administration
IV route preferred.
Can be given PR or IM in an emergency.

Dose
- Loading dose (IV): 10 to 20 mg/kg (usual dose is 20 mg/kg) slowly over 10 to 15 minutes (maximum rate for IV infusion is 2 mg/kg/minute)
  - May be repeated up to a maximum of 40 mg/kg
- IV maintenance dose 24 to 48 hours after loading dose: 1.5 to 2.5 mg/kg/dose q12h or 3 to 5 mg/kg/q24h over 10 to 15 minutes
- Oral maintenance dose 24 to 48 hours after loading dose: 1.5 to 2.5 mg/kg/dose q12h or 3 to 5 mg/kg/q24h

Compatibility
D5%W, D10%W, NS

Adverse effects / precautions
- Lethargy and sedation
- Serum half-life varies from 40 to 200 hours in neonates
- Serum levels can increase with concomitant use of phenytoin and valproic acid
- Very hyperosmolar – can cause phlebitis
- Rapid administration and high doses may lead to respiratory depression

Monitoring
- Observe for continuation or suppression of seizures.
- Monitor trough serum concentrations closely. Serum levels are recommended 4 days after starting maintenance dose or changing the maintenance dose.
- Recommended therapeutic range is 70 to 170 mmol/L.
- Check IV site for signs of extravasation and phlebitis

Notes
- Phenobarbital is 50 to 70% metabolized by the liver.

Phenytoin

Indication

For treatment of seizures which are refractory to treatment with phenobarbital.

Supplied

50 mg/mL intravenous preparation.

When the dosage volume is < 0.2 mL, dilute to 5 mg/mL by adding 1 mL of phenytoin 50 mg/mL to 9 mL of sodium chloride 0.9% to produce final concentration of 50 mg/10 mL (5 mg/mL). The lower the concentration the greater is the risk of crystallization. The 5 mg/ml solution in NS is found not to crystallize for up to 4 hours after preparation.

6 mg/mL suspension for oral use (keep at room temperature; shake well prior to each use).

Administration

IV, PO.
DO NOT give IM

Dose

- Loading dose (IV): 10 to 20 mg/kg IV infusion administered slowly.
  - Maximum rate of infusion = 0.5 mg/kg/minute.
- IV maintenance dose: 2 to 4 mg/kg IV infusion q12h.
- Oral maintenance dose: 2 to 4 mg/kg PO q12h
  - Higher dose may be necessary due to variable absorption of drug. Adjust dose according to serum levels.

Compatibility

- Phenytoin is highly unstable in any IV solution. Administer with normal saline only. Flush IV line with saline before and after administration.
- The 5 mg/mL dilution in NS must be used within 4 hour after preparation.
- A 0.22 micron in-line filter is required only for diluted solutions due to the potential of drug precipitation.

Adverse effects / precautions

- Acute following IV administration: hypotension, bradycardia, ventricular fibrillation, vasodilation; venous irritation; pain, thrombophlebitis, skin rash. Observe IV site carefully. Extravasation may cause tissue inflammation and necrosis.
- Chronic use: toxic hepatitis, gingival hyperplasia, hyperglycemia and osteoporosis.

Monitoring

- Monitor respiratory and cardiovascular status, particularly with IV infusion.
- Monitor trough serum concentrations closely. Serum levels are recommended 4 days after starting maintenance dose or changing the

recommended 4 days after starting maintenance dose or changing the maintenance dose.
- Recommended trough serum level: 40 to 80 micromol/L (10 to 20 micrograms/mL).
- <u>DRUG INTERACTION</u> with phenobarbital - levels of phenytoin may increase or decrease (usually decrease); therefore monitor phenytoin levels closely.

Notes
- Observe ECG tracings for cardiac arrhythmias, (eg. ventricular fibrillation) while administering phenytoin.
- Likely to interact with other medications which are metabolized in the liver (e.g. may decrease serum concentrations of theophylline).

Premedication prior to intubation

Premedication prior to laryngoscopy and intubation involves sedation and muscle paralysis. This combination of medication can:
- attenuate or abolish the physiological stress response to the noxious stimulus
- facilitate visualization of the vocal cords, potentially shortening the procedure and resulting in an easier intubation

Indication
Elective and semi-urgent laryngoscopy and intubation.

Administration
Premedication involves a combination of three drugs - an analgesic, an anticholinergic, and a neuromuscular blocking agent.

Morphine 0.1 to 0.2 mg/kg or fentanyl 3 to 5 mcg/kg can be used for analgesia.
- Morphine: There is extensive experience with its use in newborn babies, but its onset of action is slower than the onset of action of both atropine and succinylcholine.
- Fentanyl: The onset of action is fast, but it has potential side effects of chest wall rigidity and laryngospasm.

A neuromuscular blocking agent should only be administered by personnel familiar with its use and skilled in neonatal intubation. When this is not posssible, fentanyl is not recommended due to potential chest wall rigidity. In such situations, morphine and atropine should be used alone.

The drugs are given in the following order: morphine (or fentanyl), followed immediately by atropine, followed 30 to 60 seconds later by succinylcholine.

The baby is pre-oxygenated with 100% oxygen via bag-mask technique while awaiting the onset of action of the premedication (approximately 45 to 60 seconds after the succinylcholine).

Dose

Class	Agent	Dose	Action
Analgesic	Morphine or	0.1 to 0.2 mg/kg IV	Pain relief
	Fentanyl	3 to 5 mcg/kg IV	
Anticholinergic	Atropine	0.01 to 0.02 mg/kg IV	Prevent reflex bradycardia
Neuromuscular blocking agent	Succinylcholine	1 to 2 mg/kg IV	Abolish physical resistance, facilitate visualization

Adverse effects / precautions

- Paralysis leading to apnea
- Bradycardia secondary to the vagal stimulus of laryngoscopy, not counteracted by the atropine

In addition to the equipment used for intubation, resuscitation equipment including a suction apparatus, mask, self-inflating bag and source of oxygen must be immediately available. Ventilation must be supported until the effect of succinylcholine has dissipated.

Monitoring

- Heart rate and pulse oximetry
- Presence of end tidal CO_2 and bilateral breath sounds on auscultation to confirm successful intubation

Notes

- The administration of premedication should not delay urgent intubation where the risk of waiting outweighs the need for pain management.
- When the baby's anatomy is unusual or there is concern that the airway cannot be managed by bag-and-mask ventilation in a paralyzed baby, modification of the premedication regimen should be made. In this circumstance, morphine and atropine are given but succinylcholine is omitted.

Bibliography

Barrington KJ, Byrne PJ. Premedication for neonatal intubation. Am J Perinatol 1998;15:213-216.

Oei J, Hari R, Butha T, Lui K. Facilitation of neonatal nasotracheal intubation with premedication: a randomized controlled trial. J Paediatr Child Health 2002;38:146-50.

Prostaglandin E₁ (PGE₁)

A prostaglandin

Indications

To maintain a patent ductus arteriosus in "duct-dependant" congenital heart disease, including:

- obstruction to pulmonary blood flow with right to left shunts (for example, tricuspid or pulmonary atresia)
- obstruction to systemic blood flow (for example, hypoplastic left ventricle or aortic stenosis)
- mixing of pulmonary and systemic circulations (for example, transposition of the great vessels)

Supplied

500 mcg/mL ampule.

Dilute before administration to a concentration less than or equal to 20 mcg/mL.

Ampules must be refrigerated.

Prepare fresh infusion solutions q24h

Administration

Continuous IV infusion via syringe pump
Peripheral or central venous line

Dose

- Initial infusion rate: 0.05 to 0.1 mcg/kg/minute.
    - Higher initial doses are usually no more effective and are associated with a high incidence of adverse effects
- Maintenance rate: titrate to response, 0.01 to 0.1 mcg/kg/minute (balancing oxygenation and adverse effects).
    - The infusion should be continued at the lowest rate that effectively maintains oxygenation.

Y-site injection compatibility

D2/3 and 1/3NS, D5%W, D10%W, 0.9%NS, 0.45% NS, calcium chloride, calcium gluconate, dobutamine, dopamine, epinephrine, heparin, isoproterenol, midazolam, morphine sulfate, potassium chloride.

Y-site injection incompatibility

No information available.

Quick calculation for preparing an initial PGE₁ infusion

The following is a strategy, applicable for all babies, for quickly mixing and initiating a PGE₁ infusion.

Preparation: Add 1 ampule (500 mcg/mL) to 80 mL D5%W

Infusion rate: Use the baby's birth weight in kg to equal mL,
then PGE₁ infusion rate in mL/h = 0.1 mcg/kg/minute

Examples: For a 3 kg baby, give a PGE₁ infusion of 3 mL/h = 0.1 mcg/kg/minute
For a 4.2 kg baby, give a PGE₁ infusion of 4.2 mL/h = 0.1 mcg/kg/minute

---

Quick calculation for preparing PGE₁ infusion where 1 mL/hr = 0.05 mcg/kg/minute

The following equations provide some alternative PGE₁ dilutions for larger babies in whom volume of IV intake is an issue.

$0.075 \times$ weight (kg) = # mg PGE₁ to be added to IV fluid to make a total volume of 25 mL

$0.15 \times$ weight (kg) = # mg PGE₁ to be added to IV fluid to make a total volume of 50 mL

$0.3 \times$ weight (kg) = # mg PGE₁ to be added to IV fluid to make a total volume of 100 mL

Adverse effects / precautions
- Apnea
- Arteriolar vasodilation leading to hypotension and cutaneous flushing
- Bradycardia or tachycardia
- Fever
- Diarrhea
- Inhibition of platelet aggregation
- Seizure-like activity

Monitoring
- Closely monitor respiration, oxygen saturation, heart rate and rhythm, blood pressure, and temperature.
- The SpO_2 and PaO_2 will rise and colour will improve if the baby is responding to therapy.

Notes
- Expect maximum effect 15 to 30 minutes after infusion begins in cyanotic congenital heart disease and 1.5 to 3 hours (range 15 minutes to 11 hours) in acyanotic congenital heart disease. If PGE₁ is not beneficial within this time frame, the drug should be discontinued and the diagnosis reconsidered.
- Ductus arteriosus begins to close within 1 to 2 hours after drug is stopped.

Surfactant

Surfactant is a lipid/protein material manufactured and secreted by pulmonary alveolar type II cells under the influence of steroids and other hormones during intrauterine life. After birth, surfactant phospholipids form a monolayer at the alveolar-air-liquid interface, reducing the surface tension and decreasing the tendency of the alveoli to collapse. As a result alveoli inflate, and remain inflated, more easily.

There is a primary deficiency of surfactant in respiratory distress syndrome. A secondary deficiency of surfactant may occur when surfactant is inactivated by infection, meconium aspiration or pulmonary hemorrhage.

Indication
- Treatment of moderate to severe respiratory distress syndrome (RDS). Surfactant should be given as early as possible in babies with RDS with a goal of reducing the mortality and morbidity associated with this condition.
- Prophylaxis in preterm babies at high risk of RDS
- Treatment of other pulmonary conditions, such as meconium aspiration syndrome and pnuemonia.

Supplied
Natural surfactants available for use: BLES[R], Survanta[R], Infasurf[R], Curosurf[R]

Route
Surfactant is given directly into the trachea and bronchial tree through the endotracheal tube.

Dose
4 to 5 ml/kg based on manufacturer's instructions (delivering approximately 100mg/kg phospholipid)

Preparation
Stored as per manufacturer's instructions (refrigerated or frozen)

Warm to room temperature by gently rolling the vial between palms - do not use heating devices

Do not shake

Equipment
- Syringe and 18-gauge needle
- 5 French feeding tube OR endotracheal tube connector with side port
- Bagging system or mechanical ventilator

Procedure
1. Prior to surfactant instillation:
   - Establish cardiorespiratory and oxygen saturation monitoring.
   - Ensure that ETT is in proper position
   - Suction the baby's airway
   - Position the baby supine and ensure the head is in the midline position
2. Warm the surfactant to room temperature by gently rolling the vial between your palms. Do not shake the vial, as this will create bubbles in the solution.
3. Draw correct dose of surfactant into syringe.
4. **ETT with Side Port Adapter** – attach syringe to port and administer an aliquot of surfactant with each mechanical inspiration. Total dose is administered as quickly as baby tolerates it.
   ETT without Side Port Adapter - insert the feeding tube attached to the syringe of surfactant into the endotracheal tube and administer the surfactant as fast as tolerated by the baby. Ventilate using a bagging system after each aliquot of surfactant.
5. If reflux of surfactant into the ETT occurs during administration, halt administration and ventilate the infant until the ETT is clear of visible surfactant, then slowly resume administration.
6. Adjust inspired oxygen concentration as required during administration to maintain SpO_2 88 to 95% between delivering aliquots of surfactant. The hypoxemia is very short lived. Stabilize the baby and administer surfactant more slowly.
7. Do not suction the infant for 2 hours post administration unless the need for suctioning is absolutely indicated.

Special considerations

During surfactant administration, many babies desaturate and become transiently bradycardic due to the brief obstruction of the airway. This resolves with hand bagging the baby after the aliquots of surfactant are given. After the surfactant has been administered a dramatic increase in lung compliance can occur. Ventilator changes in peak pressure (PIP) and rate (f) should be anticipated and performed quickly, as required. It is very common for oxygen saturation to improve dramatically, allowing the inspired oxygen concentration to be decreased.

Potential Complications

- Plugging of the ETT. The ETT may need to be suctioned and/or replaced.
- Transient hypoxemia and bradycardia requiring supplemental oxygen.
- Pneumothorax due to rapid changes in pulmonary compliance and failure to adjust the ventilator parameters to compensate.
- Pulmonary hemorrhage (late complication).

Notes   Health care providers administering surfactant must be:
- skilled in neonatal intubation
- prepared to deal with the rapid changes in lung compliance and oxygenation during and after surfactant administration
- able to manage potential complications.

Community hospitals must take into account the skill and experience of their health care providers and distance from referral centers/transport teams when deciding to stock and administer surfactant.

Prophylactic use of surfactant for babies judged to be 'at risk' of developing RDS (intubated babies less than 30 to 32 weeks gestation) has been demonstrated to improve clinical outcome. Babies have less pneumothoraces, less pulmonary interstitial emphysema and a lower mortality.

Bibliography
American Academy of Pediatrics Committee on Fetus and Newborn: Surfactant replacement therapy for respiratory distress syndrome. Pediatrics. 1991 Jun; 87(6): 946-7.

Jobe AH. Drug therapy: Pulmonary Surfactant Therapy. NEJM 1993; 328: 861-868.

Yost CC, Soll RF. Early versus delayed selective surfactant treatment for neonatal respiratory distress syndrome. Cochrane Database of Systematic Reviews 1, 2003.

Soll RF, Dargaville P. Surfactant for meconium aspiration syndrome in full term infants. Cochrane Database of Systematic Reviews. 1, 2003.

 Vancomycin

A bactericidal glycopeptide antibiotic

Indication   Sepsis and meningitis due to methacillin-resistant staphylococci (e.g. staph aureus and staph epidermidis)

Supplied   Powder for injection 500 mg vial – reconstitute using sterile water for injection.

Recommended concentration for IV infusion is 5 mg/mL.

Route   IV infusion by syringe pump over 60 minutes

Dose   15 mg/kg/dose for both sepsis and meningitis, adjusting levels to upper end of therapeutic range for both peak and trough when treating meningitis.

PCA (weeks)	Postnatal age (days)	Interval (hours)
< 27	< 28	q24h
27 to 30	< 28	q18h
31 to 36	< 28	q12h
≥ 37	0 to 7	q12h
	> 7	q8h
ALL	> 28	q8h

Y-site injection compatibility

D2/3 and 1/3NS, D5%W, D10%W, 0.9%NS, 0.45%NS, calcium gluconate, fat emulsion 20%, heparin (concentrations ≤ 1 unit/mL), insulin, magnesium sulfate, midazolam, morphine, parenteral nutrition solutions (amino acid/dextrose), potassium chloride, ranitidine.

Y-site injection incompatibility

Cefotaxime, dexamethasone, heparin (concentrations > 1 unit/mL) pentobarbital, phenobarbital.

Flush IV line or allow time for IV line to clear between medication administrations.

Adverse effects / precautions

- Nephrotoxicity
- Ototoxicity
- Rapid infusion can result in a diffuse red rash and hypotension (red man syndrome).

Monitoring

Monitoring serum levels recommended: peak and trough levels after the second dose in neonates without clinical evidence of renal disease and if planned duration of treatment will be greater than 3 days

Optimal serum concentration: peak (sample taken 60 minutes after end of infusion) 25 to 35 mg/L ; trough (sample taken within 30 minutes prior to next dose) 5 to 10 mg/L

Notes

Do not mix vancomycin and cefotaxime in the same line or administer concurrently. Flush line between medications or separate administration times by a least 1 hour.

Index

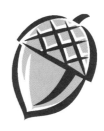